A PRACTICAL GUIDE TO DERMOSCOPY

A PRACTICAL GUIDE TO DERMOSCOPY

Orit Markowitz, MD, FAAD
Director of Pigmented Lesions and Skin Cancer
Associate Professor of Dermatology
Mount Sinai Medical Center
New York, New York

Director of Pigmented Lesions Clinic
Brooklyn VA
Brooklyn, New York

Adjunct Professor, Dermatology
SUNY Downstate Medical Center
Brooklyn, New York

Chief of Dermatology
Queens General Hospital
Jamaica, New York

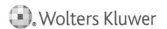
Wolters Kluwer

Philadelphia • Baltimore • New York • London
Buenos Aires • Hong Kong • Sydney • Tokyo

Executive Editor: Rebecca Gaertner
Senior Development Editor: Kristina Oberle
Senior Production Project Manager: Alicia Jackson
Design Coordinator: Teresa Mallon
Senior Manufacturing Coordinator: Beth Welsh
Prepress Vendor: SPi Global

Copyright © 2017 by Wolters Kluwer

11

Printed in the United States of America

Library of Congress Cataloging-in-Publication Data
Names: Markowitz, Orit, author.
Title: A practical guide to dermoscopy / Orit Markowitz.
Description: Philadelphia : Wolters Kluwer, [2017] | Includes bibliographical references.
Identifiers: LCCN 2017003523 | ISBN 9781451192636
Subjects: | MESH: Dermoscopy | Skin Neoplasms—diagnosis | Melanoma—diagnosis | Nevus—diagnosis | Pigmentation Disorders—pathology | Skin Pigmentation
Classification: LCC RC280.S5 | NLM WR 141 | DDC 616.99/477075—dc23 LC record available at https://lccn.loc.gov/2017003523

This book is for my father, Michael Markowitz.
As an electronic engineer and inventor, his passion for science
and discovery was truly infectious. His loss fueled my own passion for
research and innovation at an early age and continues
to drive me all of these years later.
Thank you Dad.

Contributor

Sarah Utz, BA
MD Candidate 2017
Icahn School of Medicine at Mount Sinai
New York, New York

Preface

Dermoscopy has changed the landscape of how we manage pigmented lesions. While the technology is not new, it continues to evolve, and the ways in which residents and physicians learn how to best use this modality is likewise evolving. Well-established methods for learning dermoscopy have focused primarily on pattern recognition, and while this method is a crucial piece toward mastering dermoscopy, this method alone may not work for everyone or for every lesion. During my own training, I was struck by how identifying the pattern algorithm of certain lesions was not possible, specifically for early lesions and particularly for early amelanotic melanomas. I was intrigued by how to diagnose these more effectively, especially given that amelanotic melanoma, while being the most rare, is the most deadly when picked up. As my career evolved and I began teaching students, residents, and fellows, I was pushed to strengthen and actualize the connection between the clinical and dermoscopic exams. I found the most apparent link to be color. Over time, I began to recognize that different colors and color combinations clinically, and then dermoscopically, would correlate with my diagnoses, in some instances bypassing pattern altogether. So I set out to develop my own method of color recognition to complement and streamline the traditional pattern recognition method. At first, I simply began using the Color Wheel in my own practice, but quickly incorporated it into my teaching roles. Now as the Director of Pigmented Lesions of the Department of Dermatology at the Icahn School of Medicine at Mount Sinai and Director of the Pigmented Lesions Clinic at the Brooklyn Veterans Hospital of Downstate University Medical Center, I teach it to the students, residents, and fellows, in addition to directing the Greater New York Dermoscopy course annually for residents in New York. Further, I have lectured nationally and internationally on the Color Wheel's utility in the diagnosis of early malignancies.

This book is truly a labor of love many years in the making. It is my immense pleasure to present my method in a user-friendly manual that can be used by newcomers and experts in the field alike. The majority of pictures and examples are ones that I have collected over the years from my own patients. The figures have been developed in collaboration with a phenomenal graphic designer, Rene Moreno, in order to visually lead us through the book. We begin by presenting and reviewing the traditional methods of dermoscopy, as well as briefly introducing the concepts behind dermoscopy for our newcomers. For our seasoned veterans of dermoscopy, we hope that this guide will be a welcome complement to your already vast knowledge and that you may pick up some new pearls along the way.

I owe a great deal of debt to my mentors of dermoscopy, Dr. Alfred Kopf, Dr. Harold S. Rabinowitz, and Margaret Oliviero, FNP, BC, for their continual support and guidance. And to my mentors of dermatology, Dr. Daniel Siegel and Dr. Mark Lebwohl, who support my research and are fierce advocates for the noninvasive imaging work I do, which all begins with dermoscopy.

Many thanks are due to Sarah Utz, my wonderful medical student at the Icahn School of Medicine, for helping to make this book a reality. She started on this journey with me 3 years ago as a newly minted medical student and is now a budding dermatologist. She was truly instrumental throughout this entire process.

Last, but certainly not least, I would be remiss not to thank my family—my husband Dimitri Vermès and two beautiful children, for without them I would not be where I am today. Their continual love and support has sustained me every step of the way.

Contents

Contributor . . . . *vi*
Preface . . . . *vii*
Introduction . . . . *x*

SECTION I: BASIC OVERVIEW 1

1. Patterns 1
   Intro to Pattern Analysis 1
   Benign Melanocytic Patterns 2
   Malignant Melanocytic Patterns 9
   Malignant Nonmelanocytic Patterns 23
   Nonmelanocytic Patterns 24

2. Equipment 53
   Types of Dermatoscopes 53

3. Color-Wheel Intro 57
   The Basics 58
   The Color Wheel 58
   Flat/Pink-Clear/Red 59
   Elevated/Pink-Clear/Red 62
   Flat/Pink-Clear/Multicolored 64
   Elevated/Pink-Clear/Multicolored 67

SECTION II: CLINICAL PINK-CLEAR 72

4. Flat/Pink-Clear/Red 72
   Benign Lesions 73
   Malignant Lesions 77

5. Elevated/Pink-Clear/Red 85
   Benign Lesions 86
   Malignant Lesions 94

6. Flat/Pink-Clear/Multicolored 104
   Benign Lesions 105
   Malignant Lesions 112

7. Elevated/Pink-Clear/Multicolored 122
   Benign Lesions 123
   Malignant Lesions 137

SECTION III: CLINICAL PALE BROWN 149

8. Flat/Pale Brown/Brown 149
   Benign Lesions 150
   Malignant Lesions 159

9. Flat/Pale Brown/Multicolored 171
   Benign Lesions 172
   Malignant Lesions 184

10. Elevated/Pale Brown/Brown 189

11. Elevated/Pale Brown/Multicolored 196

SECTION IV: CLINICAL **BROWN-BLACK** 202

12. Flat/Brown-Black/Brown 202
     Benign Lesions. 203
     Malignant Lesions 212

13. Elevated/Brown-Black/Brown 215

14. Flat/Brown-Black/Multicolored 225
     Benign Lesions. 226
     Malignant Lesions 234

15. Elevated/Brown-Black/Multicolored 246
     Benign Lesions. 247
     Malignant Lesions 256

SECTION V: CLINICAL OTHER COLORS—YELLOW, **PURPLE, RED** 260

16. Flat/Elevated/Red/Red. 260

17. Flat/Elevated/Purple/Multicolored. 263

18. Elevated/Pink-Clear/Yellow 267

SECTION VI: WHEN DO YOU NOT USE DERMOSCOPY? 272

19. When Do You Not Use Dermoscopy? 272

Index *275*

Introduction

Welcome to the The Color Wheel! Whether this is your first time with dermoscopy or you're a veteran user, we're happy you're here! The Color Wheel has been developed as a new method to simplify the steps needed to best utilize dermoscopy while ensuring that important malignancies are not missed.

The dermatoscope is often thought of as solely a dermatologist's tool. However, its usage is diverse and should be added to many other clinicians' toolboxes, including primary care physicians and subspecialty physicians, such as plastic surgeons and otolaryngologists. Primary care physicians, in particular, have a unique opportunity to enhance their diagnostic acumen by incorporating dermoscopy into their examination routine. They are often the main source of medical referrals for suspicious dermatologic lesions. However, many of these referrals are unnecessary, and their number could be reduced. Arenziano et al. found that primary care physicians trained in dermoscopy significantly increased their referral sensitivity without decreasing specificity.[1]

With this in mind, dermoscopy is an appropriate, noninvasive, and easy screening tool that would greatly benefit many physicians. And in doing so, patients would benefit as well by having potentially life-threatening malignancies diagnosed earlier. The purpose of this book is to provide a useful, engaging, and concise training manual that can be used not only by dermatologists but also by a larger spectrum of medical practitioners who may find use for it in their practices.

There are currently a number of different methodologies that are used to appropriately analyze and diagnose pigmented lesions. Pattern analysis, the ABCD(E) rule, the seven-point checklist, and Menzies method are all commonly used. We will be using pattern analysis as a final step to our approach throughout the book and will delve into more detail in **Chapter 1**.

We will be presenting a new combination method that takes into consideration the many colors seen in different lesions. We will demonstrate how differentiating the colors seen with both the naked eye and the dermatoscope, in conjunction with pattern analysis, greatly enhances one's ability to narrow down the differential diagnosis. When analysis of clinical and dermoscopic colors is combined with basic clinical data such as lesion onset, location, and patient skin type, the potential differential diagnosis becomes very limited. At this point, a pattern analysis can be performed to help determine whether a lesion needs to be biopsied.

For example, if we have a clinically pink macule (flat lesion <1 cm in diameter), there are *at least* seven diagnoses in our differential. However, once we use the dermatoscope and see a connection between faint brown and red vessels, our likely diagnosis is narrowed to only two options: either an amelanotic melanoma or a benign lichen planus–like keratosis (LPLK), leading us essentially to an immediate biopsy unless we see features strongly consistent with a lentigo (sun spot) or a seborrheic keratosis (benign growth). Most dermatologists find such amelanotic melanomas to be the most challenging of lesions, but using color and pattern analysis, diagnosis becomes less intimidating and ultimately helps to save lives.[2,3]

The goal of this manual is to provide both a firm foundation and a useful guide to help you wherever you are on your dermoscopy path. Using this manual as a guide, you will have the tools to expedite your decision-making process and to feel more confident doing so.

We have broken down the book into easy-to-use chapters based on lesion colors. If you're using this book as a reference for a specific lesion, just flip to the chapter with the appropriate clinical and dermoscopic color combination, and there you have it!

We hope you enjoy!

References

1. Argenziano G, Puig S, Zalaudek I, et al. Dermoscopy improves accuracy of primary care physicians to triage lesions suggestive of skin cancer. *J Clinical Oncol.* 2006;24(12):1877–1882.

2. Skvara H, Teban L, Fiebiger M, et al. Limitations of dermoscopy in the recognition of melanoma. *Arch Dermatol.* 2005;141(2):155–160.

3. Thomas NE, Kricker A, Waxweiler WT, et al. Comparison of clinicopathologic features and survival of histopathologically amelanotic and pigmented melanomas. *JAMA Dermatol.* 2014;150(12):1306–1311.

Chapter 1 Patterns

Intro to Pattern Analysis

In the 1980s, the "ABCD" clinical criteria for melanoma enabled the clinician to use an algorithm for melanoma diagnosis and therefore helped with earlier detection of melanoma. In 2004, "E" was added to the rule to produce the commonly used **ABCDE** rule for melanoma diagnosis. These criteria for melanoma diagnosis give the lesion in question a score depending on its **A**symmetry, **B**order, **C**olor, **D**ifferentiating structures/**D**iameter >6 mm, and **E**volution, or noticed change, within the last few months. Each of these categories is given a number score depending on how many criteria they meet within each category. For example, if a lesion had three distinguishable colors, it would receive a number 3 for the color category. The scores are then totaled and weighed; if the lesion has a total score over 5.45, it is considered a melanoma. This method can be a useful tool for patients to assess their nevi at home, but also can be used by clinicians using dermoscopy to assess each feature more closely.[1]

Beginning with the handheld dermatoscope, noninvasive technology now enables clinicians to diagnose melanomas and nonmelanoma skin cancers at earlier and earlier stages, as well as prevent biopsies of otherwise benign lesions. Since the advent of this new technology, we are now making the diagnosis of melanoma for lesions that do not yet demonstrate the classic ABCD and even E's of melanoma and have needed to develop new algorithms for identification and diagnosis.

Pattern analysis provides a stepwise analysis using common patterns and criteria to determine whether a lesion is melanocytic or nonmelanocytic. The lesion is then analyzed to determine which subcategory it falls into and ultimately what the lesion is and therefore whether or not the lesion is suspicious. Whether a lesion is melanocytic or nonmelanocytic can be a very difficult distinction to make, especially when lesions present with very similar patterns; for example, certain types of lentigo lesions (which are nonmelanocytic) can appear similar to a junctional nevus (which is melanocytic). In the color wheel algorithm, it is not as critical to make the distinction between melanocytic and nonmelanocytic or even the final diagnosis of the lesion. Rather, we use pattern analysis as the last step in the algorithm *to confirm the need to biopsy* and to further narrow down a significantly shortened list of possibilities.

The 7-point checklist is exactly as it sounds: seven criteria that determine a score that helps to determine whether or not the lesion in question is melanoma or otherwise. The criteria are split into two groups that are weighted differently: major and minor criteria. The major criteria include an atypical pigment network, gray-blue areas, and atypical vascular pattern; each receives a score of 2, if present. The minor criteria include radial streaming or streaks, irregular diffuse pigmentation or blotches, irregular dots and globules, and regression pattern; each of these criteria receives a score of 1, if present. If a lesion has a total score of three or more, the lesion is given the diagnosis of melanoma.[2]

In an effort to streamline and standardize the various methods and algorithms of dermoscopy, a virtual consensus meeting was held in which 40 expert dermoscopists analyzed and reviewed the diagnostic criteria of over 100 lesions. From this meeting, the 2-point checklist was introduced. The first step determines whether the lesion is melanocytic or nonmelanocytic. This is done by first determining if the lesion has any characteristic melanocytic structures in a specific order. If none are found, then any nonmelanocytic features are assessed and determined (dermatofibroma, seborrheic keratosis, angioma, or malignant basal cell and squamous cell carcinoma [SCC]). If still none are identified, then the lesion is analyzed for blood vessel morphology. If still nothing can be identified, the lesion is termed structureless. The second step is *only* used if the lesion is determined to be melanocytic. The second step uses one of the previous explained algorithms (pattern analysis, 7-point checklist, etc.) to determine whether the lesion is benign or malignant.[3]

As one might expect, these methods have their advantages and disadvantages. If you are familiar with them, you are in a good place to start; if you are not familiar with them, have no fear; everything will be explained as we go along. Our approach synthesizes well-established clinical knowledge of the behavior and characteristics of lesions and presents them in an easy-to-follow series of four steps.

To begin our discussion of how dermoscopy can best assist you in your practice, we need to lay the groundwork for confidently identifying benign versus malignant lesions. In this chapter, we will highlight the basic patterns and colors seen in benign lesions and malignant lesions and where the two are often confused.

Keep in mind that the majority of melanomas <1 cm are *not* clinically obvious, which is precisely why dermoscopy is useful in these situations. When a melanoma is clinically obvious, dermoscopy is not needed. We will be presenting some very challenging clinical pictures of early melanomas, so don't get discouraged! We'll provide you with the skills to tackle these tricky presentations.

Benign Melanocytic Patterns

Figure 1.1 shows the three most common benign melanocytic patterns: reticular, globular, and homogenous. If you are considering benign versus malignant nevi, these are the benign patterns that you should be looking for.

Reticular Pattern

- The reticular pattern is characterized by a uniform network that thins at the periphery (Figures 1.2 and 1.3).
- Figure 1.4 demonstrates six examples of junctional nevi (JN), clinically flat lesions with corresponding dermoscopic images (Figure 1.5) that show a clear uniform network with thinning at the periphery—this is characteristic of JN. Note that there is some faint, hypopigmentation (lightening) around the hair follicles. White is not considered a color, and this feature can make a lesion look like it has asymmetry or color variation at times. However, keep in mind that it is the overall symmetry of the lesion that makes it symmetric.
- Takeaway: Perifollicular hypopigmentation can be seen in both benign and malignant lesions. It **does not contribute** to overall lesion asymmetry or lesion color variation.

The most common Benign Patterns:

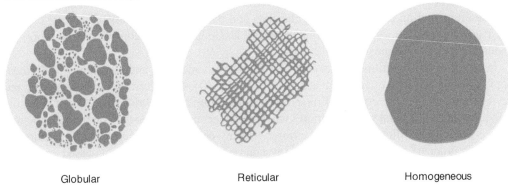

Globular   Reticular   Homogeneous

FIGURE 1.1 An illustration of the most common benign patterns of melanocytic lesions.

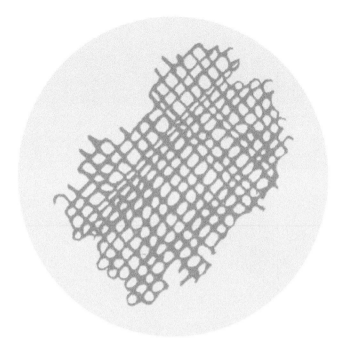

FIGURE 1.2 The reticular pattern is characterized by a uniform network that thins at the periphery.

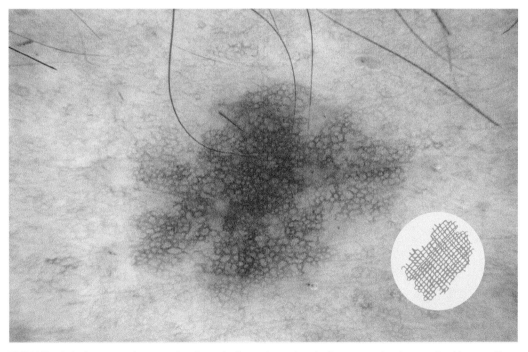

FIGURE 1.3 A dermoscopic example of a reticular pattern. A reticular pattern is characterized by a uniform network that thins at the periphery.

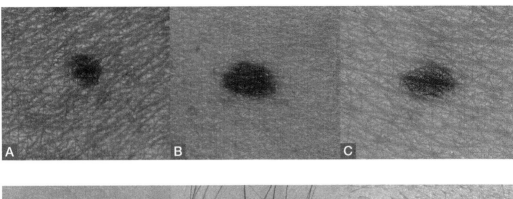

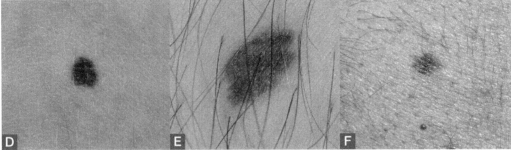

FIGURE 1.4 Six flat clinical lesions characteristic of a junctional nevi (JN).

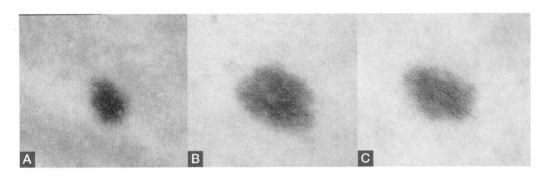

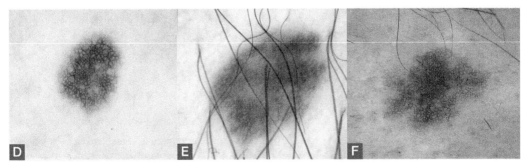

FIGURE 1.5 The corresponding dermoscopic images for the six lesions in Figure 1.4, demonstrating a uniform network thinning at the periphery. Note that there is some hypopigmentation (lightening) around the hair follicles.

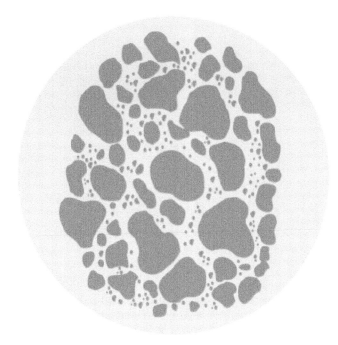

FIGURE 1.6 A dot globular pattern is characterized by diffuse globules throughout the lesion.

Globular Pattern

- The globular pattern is characterized by diffuse globular dots throughout the lesion (Figures 1.6 and 1.7).
- Figure 1.8 demonstrates three examples of congenital nevi (CN), clinically elevated lesions with corresponding dermoscopic images (Figure 1.9) showing a diffuse globular pattern.

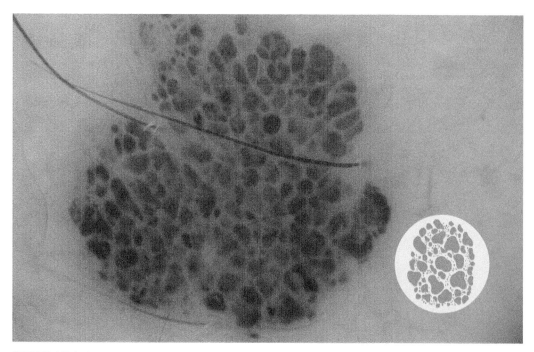

FIGURE 1.7 A dermoscopic example of a globular pattern. A globular pattern is characterized by diffuse dots and globules throughout the lesion.

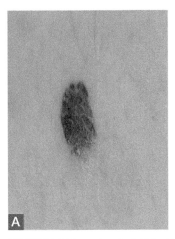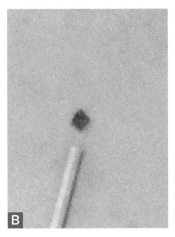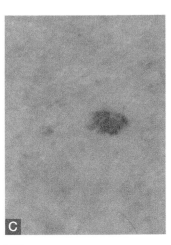

FIGURE 1.8 Three elevated clinical lesions characteristic of congenital nevi (CN).

- Note that there is a **cobblestone** pattern in lesions A and C, as well as some darker dots in lesion B. Asymmetric, dark dots at the periphery of a lesion are often an indication of a malignant feature, but two-tone dark dots **evenly** distributed throughout a lesion, or centrally located, are benign.

Homogenous Pattern

- The homogenous pattern is characterized by a diffuse structureless/nonspecific area. There is neither a reticular network nor globules (Figures 1.10 and 1.11).
- The "Tyndall effect" can also be observed in Figures 1.12 to 1.14. This is a remarkable blue tint that can be seen with lesions that are deep and dense such as intradermal nevi, CN, blue nevi, and, sometimes, seborrheic keratosis in darker-skinned patients.

Pearl

- The Tyndall effect can be confused with the blue white veil is only seen in nodular-type melanoma! Remember your clinical history and evaluation! Intradermal, congenital, and blue nevi will have a long-standing history without change, whereas a melanoma will have appeared recently and developed quickly. Additionally, the blue-white veil is *only* seen in *nodular-type* or *elevated* melanomas, which will often have other malignant signs in addition to the blue-white veil (Figure 1.14).

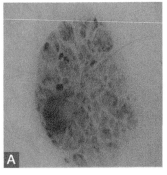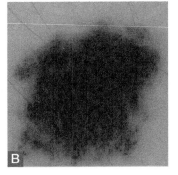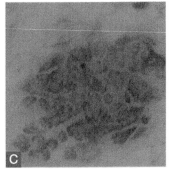

FIGURE 1.9 The corresponding dermoscopic images for the three lesions in Figure 1.8, demonstrating a diffuse dot/globular pattern. Note that there is a cobblestone pattern in lesions **(A)** and **(C)** and some dark dots in lesion **(B)**.

FIGURE 1.10 A homogenous pattern is characterized by a diffuse structure-less area. There is neither a network nor globules.

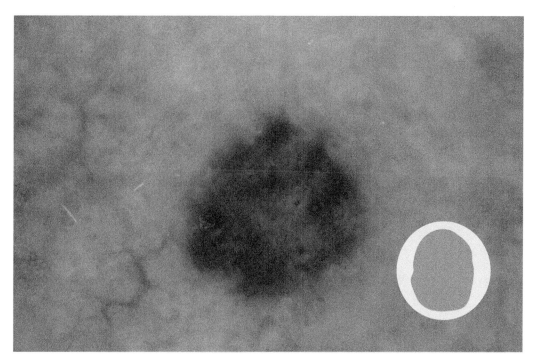

FIGURE 1.11 A dermoscopic example of a homogenous pattern in a blue nevus. A homogenous pattern is characterized by a diffuse structureless area. There is neither a network nor globules. This can be confused with the blue-white veil malignant feature of a nodular melanoma.

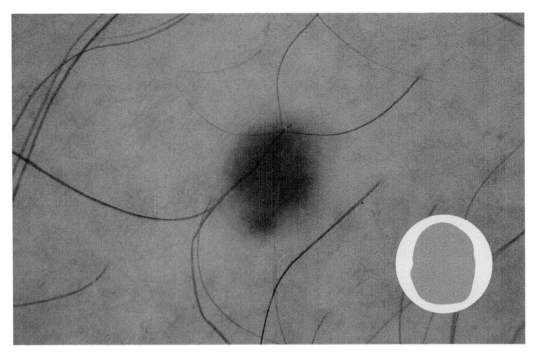

FIGURE 1.12 A dermoscopic example of a homogenous pattern in an intradermal nevus (IN). A homogenous pattern is characterized by a diffuse structureless area. There is neither a network nor globules.

- Figure 1.13 shows a clinical example of an intradermal nevus (IN). This lesion has a well-defined border and resembles other lesions in the neighborhood, which is a good sign of a benign lesion. This clinical picture helps us to not confuse the dermoscopic picture as malignancy.
- Figure 1.15 shows the clinical picture of Figure 1.14, a benign IN. The lesion is *not* elevated and has a well-defined border.

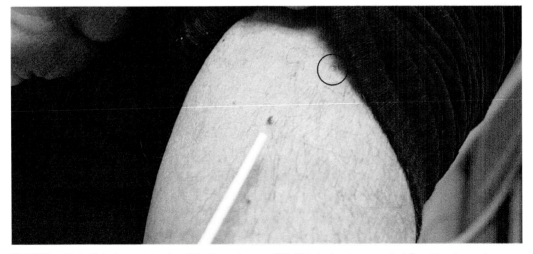

FIGURE 1.13 A clinical example of an intradermal nevus (IN). This lesion has a well-defined border and resembles other lesions, which is often the case with benign lesions.

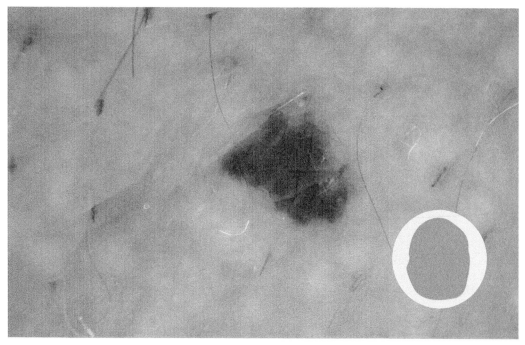

FIGURE 1.14 A dermoscopic example of a homogenous pattern in an intradermal nevus (IN). A homogenous pattern is characterized by a diffuse structureless area. There is neither a network nor globules.

Malignant Melanocytic Patterns

Now that we have a foundation for benign melanocytic patterns, we can introduce the characteristic malignant melanocytic patterns that, if seen in a lesion, raise the suspicion of melanoma (Figure 1.16). Essentially, the malignant patterns are the same as benign, but are no longer diffuse throughout the nevus, but rather disorganized. Then, there are four malignant features that are characteristic of malignant melanomas: blue-gray granularity/dots in superficial lesions,

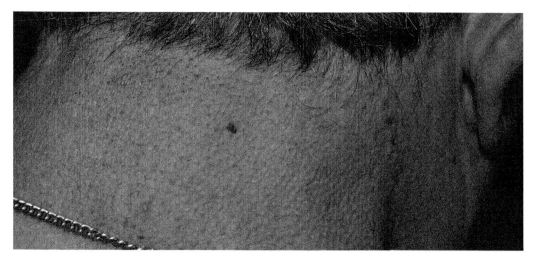

FIGURE 1.15 A clinical example of an intradermal nevus (IN). This lesion has a well-defined border and is not elevated. A blue-white veil is only seen with nodular-type melanoma, and this lesion is not nodular-appearing (not elevated).

In addition to the typically benign patterns that are now disorganized (reticular, globular, homogeneous)

Blue-gray granularity/dots

Blue-white veil

Focal pseudopods/radial streaming

Polymorphous and dotted vessels

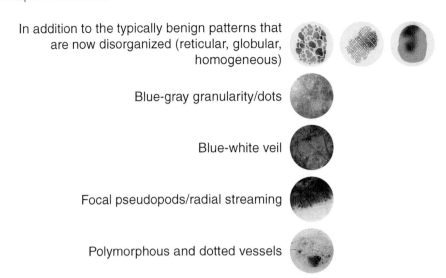

FIGURE 1.16 Malignant features of melanoma. Note that blue-gray granularity is seen in superficial spreading melanoma and also blue-white veil is usually seen in deeper lesions such as nodular melanoma.

blue-white veil in nodular lesions, focal pseudopods/radial stream, and polymorphous or dotted vessels that are clustered together asymmetrically (as opposed to the symmetric defined pigment network of dots and globules). These features, if seen, are an indication to biopsy the lesion. We'll go into each in detail, so don't get overwhelmed!

Also keep in mind that the delineation of benign versus malignant is not so black and white. Benign nevi and malignant melanoma can overlap—these are known as atypical or dysplastic nevi or intraepidermal melanocytic proliferations (Figure 1.17).

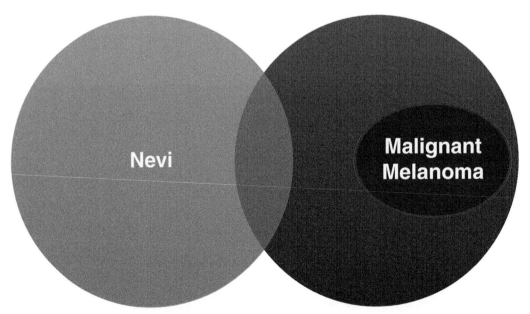

FIGURE 1.17 Benign nevi and malignant melanoma can have overlap. These lesions are known as atypical or dysplastic nevi or intraepidermal melanocytic proliferations.

The most common Malignant Patterns:

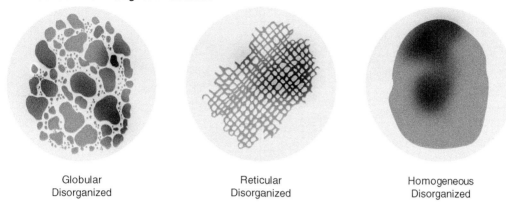

| Globular | Reticular | Homogeneous |
| Disorganized | Disorganized | Disorganized |

FIGURE 1.18 Illustrations of the most common malignant patterns of melanocytic lesions (melanoma).

In Figure 1.18, we see our normal patterns that have become disorganized and are now indicative of melanoma: reticular disorganized, globular disorganized, and homogenous disorganized.

Reticular Disorganized Pattern

- The reticular disorganized pattern is characterized by a nonuniform network that is darkened and thick at the periphery. Figures 1.19 and 1.20 illustrate the schematic and a dermoscopic example.
- Figures 1.21 and 1.22 depict three melanomas that have the characteristic reticular disorganized pattern: nonuniform network with a darkened and thick periphery.

The network is nonuniform and is darkened and thick at the periphery.

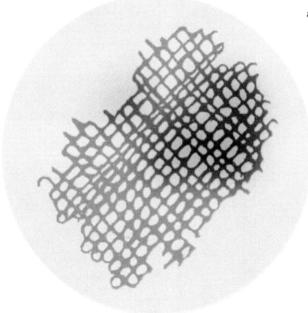

FIGURE 1.19 A reticular disorganized pattern is characterized by a nonuniform network that thickens and darkens at the periphery.

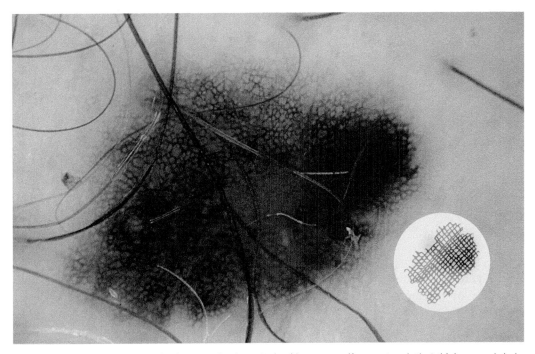

FIGURE 1.20 Reticular disorganized pattern is characterized by a nonuniform network that thickens and darkens at the periphery.

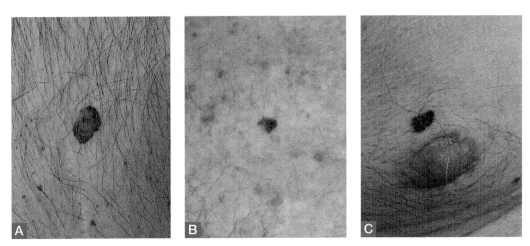

FIGURE 1.21 Three melanomas.

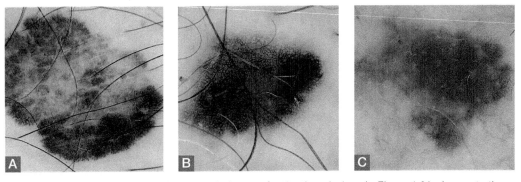

FIGURE 1.22 The corresponding dermoscopic images for the three lesions in Figure 1.21, demonstrating a reticular disorganized pattern. The network is nonuniform and is darkened and thick at the periphery.

Globules different sizes + shapes asymmetrically distributed.

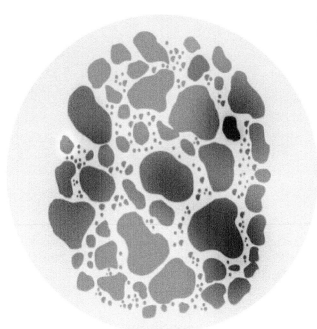

FIGURE 1.23 Dot globular disorganized pattern is characterized by globules of different sizes and asymmetrically distributed shapes.

Globular Disorganized Pattern

- The globular disorganized pattern is easily identified by globules of different sizes and shapes that are asymmetrically distributed. Figures 1.23 and 1.24 illustrate a schematic and a dermoscopic example.

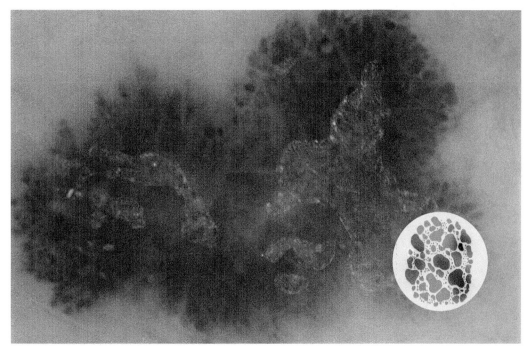

FIGURE 1.24 A dermoscopic example of a disorganized dot globular pattern. Globular disorganized pattern is characterized by globules of different sizes and asymmetrically distributed shapes.

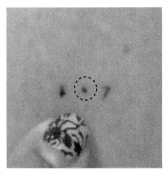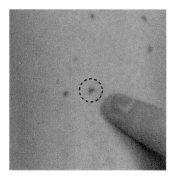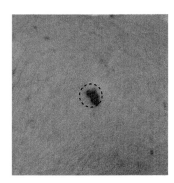

FIGURE 1.25 Three melanomas.

- Figures 1.25 and 1.26 show three examples of corresponding clinical and dermoscopic images of malignant melanomas that clearly demonstrate this globular disorganized pattern. Dots of different colors, sizes, and shapes are scattered asymmetrically throughout each lesion.

Homogenous Disorganized Pattern

- The homogenous disorganized pattern characteristically has neither network or globules nor one defined color, but has many colors, as well as a diffuse homogenous area (Figure 1.27).
- Figure 1.28 is a dermoscopic example of this pattern; there are no definitive networks or globules, but there are clearly different colors of red, pink, and brown spread asymmetrically throughout the lesion.

These malignant patterns can even be seen together in an individual lesion (Figure 1.29). Figures 1.30 and 1.31 show examples of how this may present under the dermatoscope. Oftentimes, people think that melanomas have to be darkly pigmented, but these two examples show how the darkness of the pigment is not a requirement for malignancy; rather, the three malignant patterns can be clearly seen with and without heavy pigment.

As mentioned before with the benign homogenous pattern, oftentimes, we immediately associate the color blue with melanoma. However, this is not always true! There are two instances when blue *does* indicate malignancy: blue-gray granularity in flat/superficial lesions and blue-white veil in nodular/elevated lesions. If you see blue elsewhere, it is just the Tyndall effect discussed earlier in this chapter.

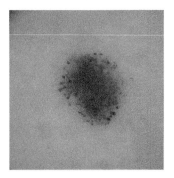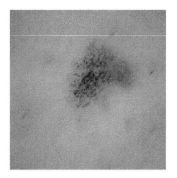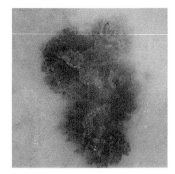

FIGURE 1.26 The corresponding dermoscopic images for the three lesions in Figure 1.25, demonstrating a globular disorganized pattern. Globular disorganized pattern is characterized by globules of different sizes and asymmetrically distributed shapes.

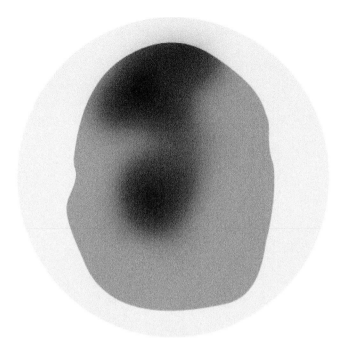

FIGURE 1.27 A homogenous disorganized pattern has no network, no globules, and many colors.

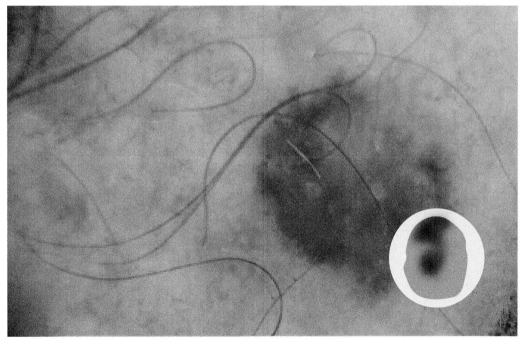

FIGURE 1.28 A dermoscopic example of a disorganized homogenous pattern. A homogenous pattern has no network, no globules, and many colors.

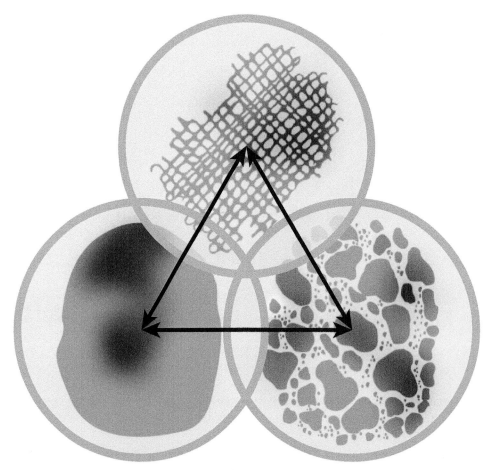

FIGURE 1.29 These disorganized patterns can all be present in a malignant lesion.

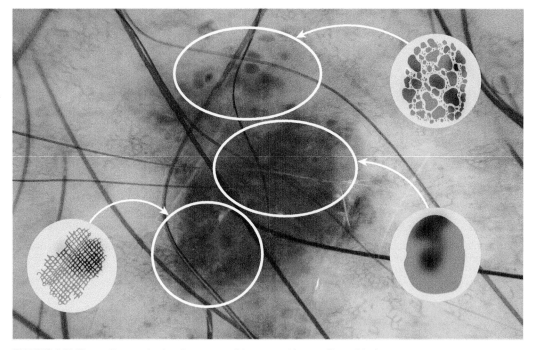

FIGURE 1.30 These disorganized patterns can all be present in a malignant lesion.

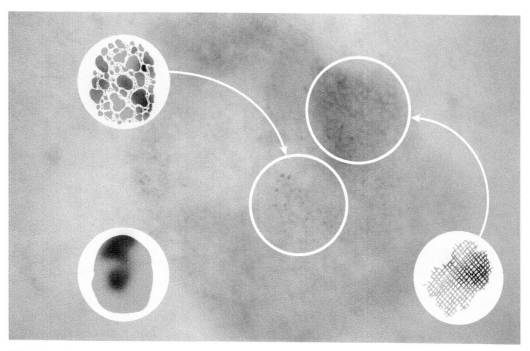

FIGURE 1.31 These disorganized patterns can all be present in a malignant lesion.

Blue-Gray Granularity in Flat Lesions

- Figure 1.32 shows an example of a superficial lesion. In the center, you can see blue-gray granular forms. This is an example of a melanoma in situ.
- What other malignant pattern is appreciable? That's right! Reticular disorganized: you can see the nonuniform network that thickens at the periphery.

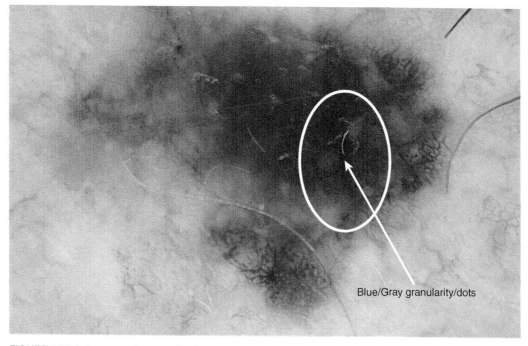

Blue/Gray granularity/dots

FIGURE 1.32 A dermoscopic example of a melanoma in situ, with a disorganized reticular pattern and the malignant feature of blue-gray granularity.

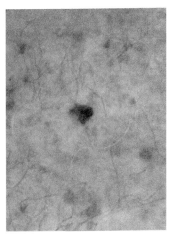 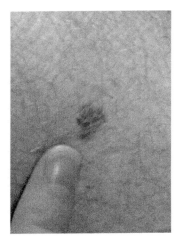 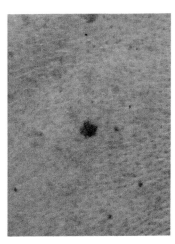

FIGURE 1.33 Three melanomas.

- Figures 1.33 and 1.34 show three clinical examples and their dermoscopic correlates. Figure 1.34 has faint blue-gray granularity in a few places in the center of the lesion. This can be difficult to appreciate, but again, you see the asymmetric, disorganized reticular pattern to lead you to your classification of a malignant lesion.
- These superficial/in situ melanomas are both particularly difficult to diagnose and very harmful—don't get discouraged! ***But when in doubt, take it out!***

Blue-White Veil in Nodular Lesions
- Figure 1.35 shows a dermoscopic example of the blue-white veil seen in nodular melanomas. These lesions are fast-growing, which should be evident by the clinical history.
- In Figures 1.36 and 1.37, we have a brown elevated lesion of 1 month's duration that measured 0.37 mm thick. Dermoscopically, we see an almost hazy, blue-white veil spread over the surface of the nodular lesion. This is very characteristic of a nodular melanoma.

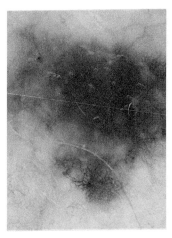 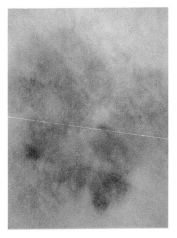 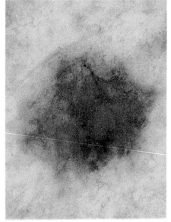

FIGURE 1.34 The corresponding dermoscopic images for the three lesions in Figure 1.33, demonstrating the malignant feature of blue-gray granularity seen in superficial spreading types of melanoma.

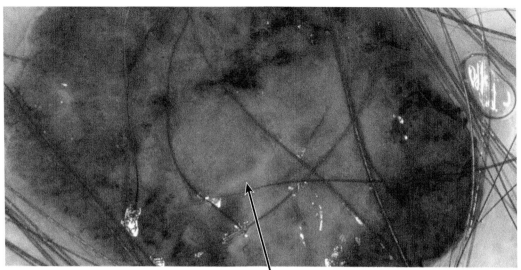

Blue-white veil

FIGURE 1.35 A dermoscopic image demonstrating the malignant feature of blue-white veil seen in fast-growing nodular melanoma.

Focal Pseudopods and Radial Streaming

- The terms focal pseudopods and radial streaming refer to the appearance of peripheral projections that appear to stream out from the border of the lesion. Pseudopods are thick projections and look almost like little feet kicking out of the lesion, while radial streams are thinner and straighter projections.
- Figure 1.38 depicts a clinically flat lesion of unknown duration that on plain sight has some of the ABCDE characteristics of melanoma that were discussed briefly at the beginning of the chapter. The lesion appears **A**symmetric and measures over 6 mm in **D**iameter.
- The corresponding dermoscopic image (Figure 1.39) demonstrates both radial streaming and focal pseudopods, demonstrating the difference between the two.
- Can you see any other malignant features in Figure 1.39? That's right! We can see some blue-gray granularity, as well as a reticular disorganized pattern.

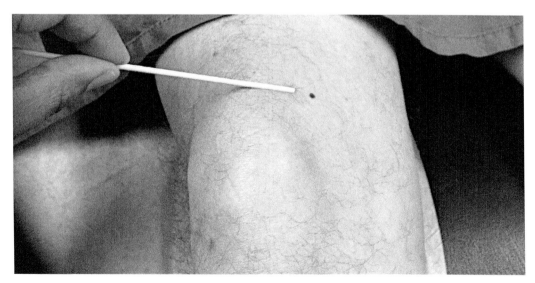

FIGURE 1.36 A brown elevated papule of 1 month duration.

Basic Overview

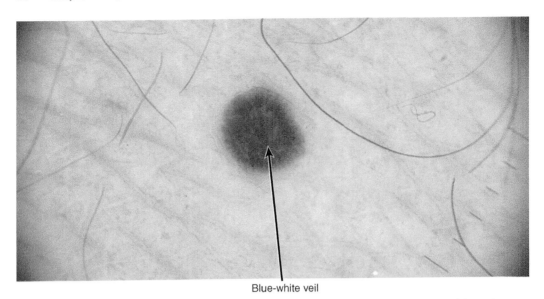

Blue-white veil

FIGURE 1.37 This dermoscopic image demonstrates a blue-white veil, seen in this 0.37-mm nodular melanoma.

Polymorphous and Dotted Vessels

- Vessel morphology seems to be a particularly difficult area for practicing dermoscopy. It can become more complex when we discuss nonmelanocytic patterns (i.e., basal cell carcinoma [BCC] morphology); however, in regard to melanoma criteria, there are only two types of vessels to consider: polymorphous and dotted.

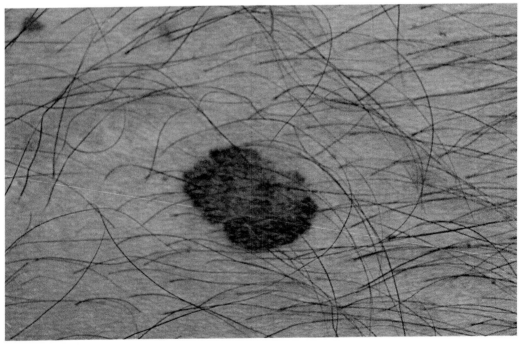

FIGURE 1.38 A clinically brown flat patch with some features of ABCDE of melanoma: **a**symmetry and **d**iameter >6 mm. The patient was unaware of the lesion's duration.

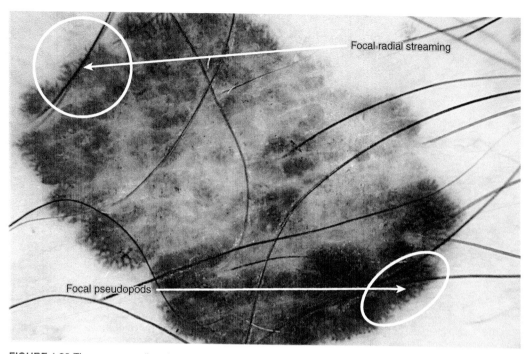

FIGURE 1.39 The corresponding dermoscopic image for the lesion in Figure 1.38, demonstrating the malignant feature of focal radial streaming/focal pseudopods seen in this melanoma in situ superficial spreading type.

- In Figure 1.40, we see an example of a nodular melanotic melanoma with many different shapes of vessels.
- Figures 1.41 and 1.42 show other examples of polymorphous vessels. Some are long and wispy, while others are short and almost dotted. Additionally, we see a negative network,

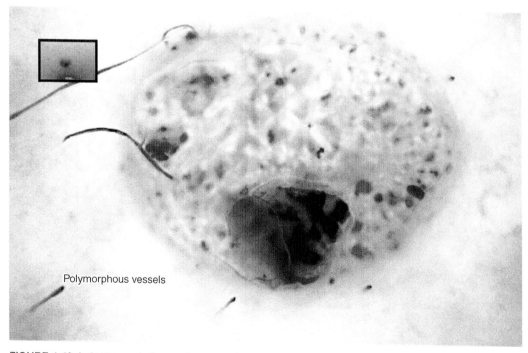

FIGURE 1.40 A dermoscopic image demonstrating the malignant feature of polymorphous seen in malignant melanoma. This example is a nodular melanotic melanoma.

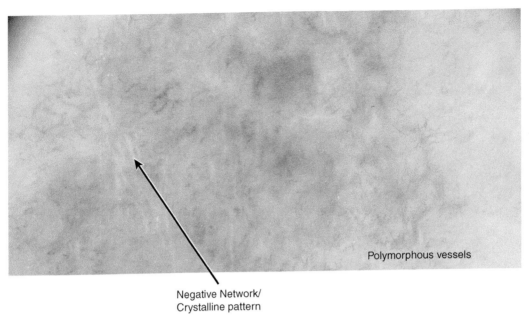

Polymorphous vessels

Negative Network/
Crystalline pattern

FIGURE 1.41 A dermoscopic image demonstrating the malignant feature of polymorphous vessels seen in malignant melanoma. This example is an example of an early amelanotic melanoma, which also has nonspecific pigmentation and a crystalline pattern.

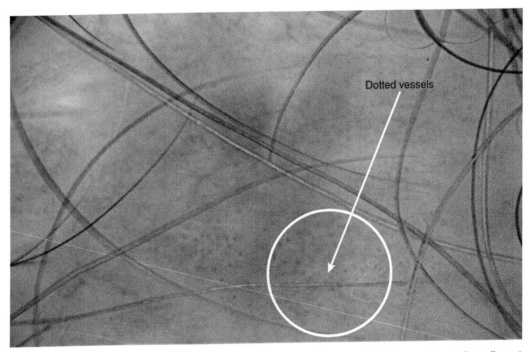

Dotted vessels

FIGURE 1.42 A dermoscopic image demonstrating the malignant feature of dotted vessels seen in malignant melanoma. This example shows an early amelanotic melanoma, which also has nonspecific pigmentation and a crystalline pattern.

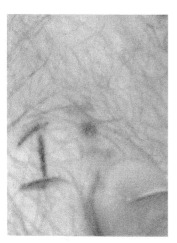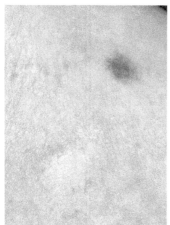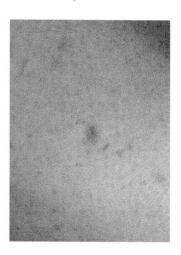

FIGURE 1.43 Three amelanotic melanomas.

called a crystalline pattern, with some nonspecific pigmentation. This is particularly characteristic of an amelanotic melanoma in an early stage. We'll address this again in Chapter 6 Flat/Pink-Clear/Multicolored.

- Figure 1.43 depicts three amelanotic melanomas. These are very difficult lesions to identify, and we specifically chose difficult examples. Figure 1.44 shows the corresponding dermoscopic images, demonstrating the malignant features of dotted vessels and nonspecific faint pigmentation.

Malignant Nonmelanocytic Patterns

Squamous Cell Carcinoma

SCC has certain characteristic patterns that differentiate it from the malignant melanocytic patterns that 've just discussed (Figure 1.45). There are three basic patterns that, if seen, are an indicator of SCC: pink-white shiny areas, a white reflective scaly surface, and ulceration. Additionally, there are three vascular patterns that if seen should also clue you into a diagnosis of SCC. These are dotted vessels, glomeruloid or coiled vessels, and keratinizing vessels.

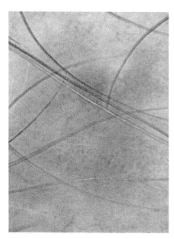

FIGURE 1.44 The corresponding dermoscopic images for the three lesions in Figure 1.43, demonstrating the malignant feature of dotted vessels and nonspecific faint pigmentation.

Patterns of Squamous Cell Skin Cancer

Pink-White
Shiny Area

White Reflective
Scaly Surface

Ulceration

Vascular

Dotted
Vessels

Glomeruloid/
Coiled Vessels

Keratinizing
Vessels

FIGURE 1.45 Illustrations of nonpigmented squamous skin cancer patterns.

Now, some of these vascular patterns are more characteristic in nonpigmented SCCs, whereas some are more characteristic of pigmented SCCs. (We'll address these in each chapter.) Due to the pigmentation, the dotted vessels may appear like brown dots in the pigmented SCCs.

General dermoscopic patterns seen in squamous cell lesions are pink-white shiny areas, white reflective scaly surface, and ulceration. There are three vascular patterns to watch out for, namely, dotted vessels, glomeruloid or coiled vessels, and keratinizing vessels.

Keep in mind that the glomeruloid or dotted vessels can be seen in psoriasis and psoriasiform dermatitis, so don't forget to review the clinical history!

Basal Cell Carcinoma
Figure 1.46 shows the characteristic patterns seen in BCCs. These patterns can also be seen in SCCs, but there are a few that are more indicative of BCC. But remember to NOT LOSE THE FOREST THROUGH THE TREES—these patterns are first and foremost malignant. It is less important to distinguish between BCC and SCC, and more important to ascertain whether or not a biopsy is indicated.

The patterns include ulceration and pink-white to white shiny areas, as seen in SCCs, but additionally include absence of pigmented network, leaf-like structures, large blue-gray ovoid nests or globular structures, spoke wheel areas, crystalline pattern, and a singular vascular pattern—arborizing or tree-like telangiectasias.

Nonmelanocytic Patterns

Seborrheic Keratoses
There is a constellation of patterns that when found together will support a diagnosis of seborrheic keratosis (seb k). These include sharply demarcated borders, milia-like cysts, comedolike openings or crypts, fissures/sulci, ridges/gyri, and looped/hairpin vessels. In addition, you can sometimes see fine vessels surrounded by a halo. Note that many of these features are due to the involvement of keratin associated with these lesions!

Patterns of Basal Cell Skin Cancer

Absence of
Pigmented
Network

Leaf-like
Structures

Large Blue-Gray
Ovoid Nests
or Globular-like
Structures

Arborizing
(tree-like)
Telengectasias
(sharp)

Spoke Wheel
Areas

Ulceration

Pink-White to
White Shiny
Areas

Crystalline
Pattern

FIGURE 1.46 Illustrations of basal cell skin cancer patterns.

Sharply demarcated borders

- Figure 1.47 shows the clear, sharply demarcated border of seborrheic keratosis. Obviously, this feature is not unique to seb k, but it will support your diagnosis.

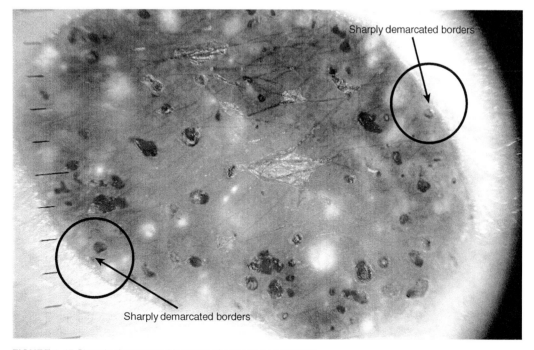

FIGURE 1.47 Sharply demarcated borders of seborrheic keratosis.

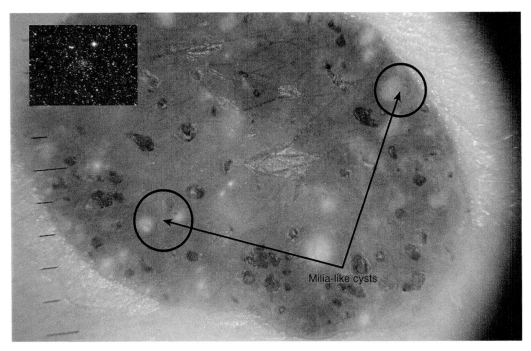

FIGURE 1.48 Milia-like cysts of seborrheic keratosis mimic the stars in the sky.

Milia-like cysts

- Milia-like cysts will appear as round white structures dermoscopically. Figure 1.48 demonstrates what is often described as a "stars in the sky" appearance.
- These correlate with intraepidermal keratin-filled cysts on pathology. See Figure 1.49.
- These also are not unique to seb k, but are a frequent finding. They can also be seen in CN and, occasionally, in BCC.

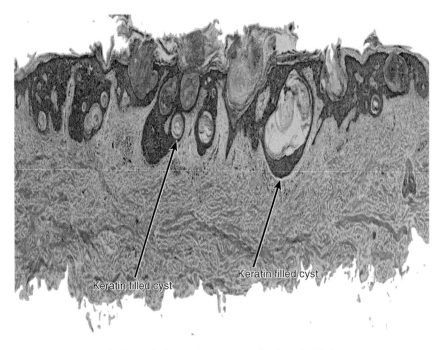

FIGURE 1.49 Milia-like cysts of seborrheic keratosis correspond to keratin-filled cysts.

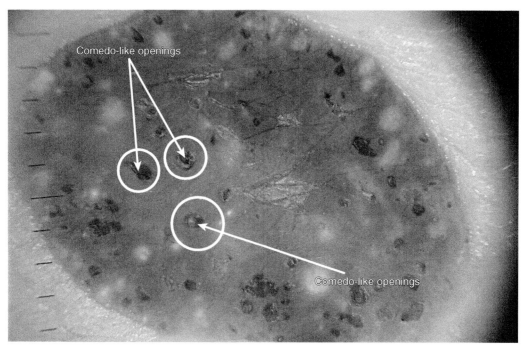

FIGURE 1.50 Comedo-like openings of seborrheic keratosis.

Comedo-like openings (crypts)

- Comedo-like openings are irregularly shaped epidermal craters that, similarly to the milia-like cysts, are filled with keratin. Figure 1.50 shows their irregular shape. Notice that they are not white, like the milia-like cysts.
- Figure 1.51 demonstrates the pathologic correlation of the craters to epidermal plugs of keratin.

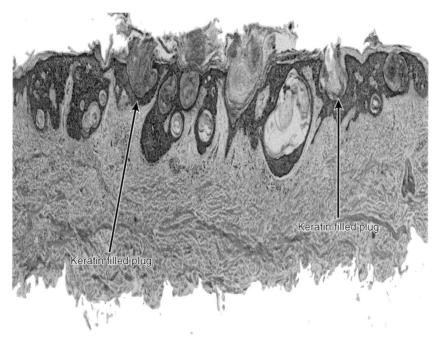

FIGURE 1.51 Comedo-like openings of seborrheic keratosis correspond to keratin-filled plugs.

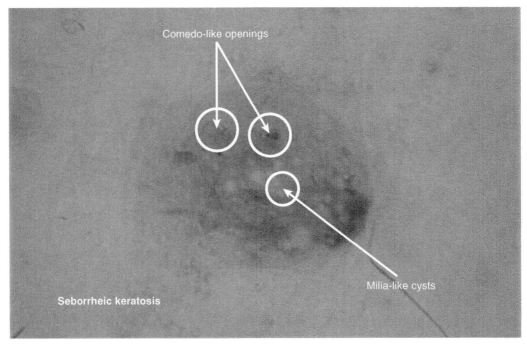

FIGURE 1.52 Comedo-like openings and milia-like cysts of a seborrheic keratosis.

- Figure 1.52 shows both comedo-like crypts and the milia-like cysts side by side. You will notice that the milia-like cysts almost have a glowing appearance to them, whereas the comedo-like openings are darker and more irregular.

Coral pattern: fissures (sulci) and ridges (gyri)

- A coral pattern is often seen in seborrheic keratosis. Figure 1.53 shows the prominent ridges (elevations) and fissures (depressions).
- The ridges are smooth raised portions of the lesion surface; they may have the appearance of finger-like projections (Figures 1.54 and 1.55).

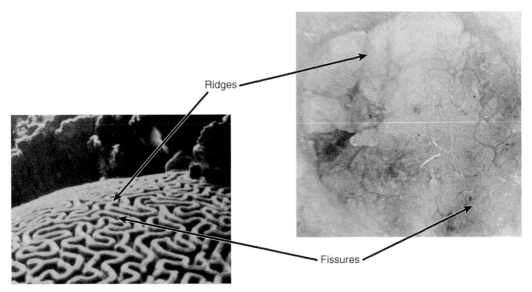

FIGURE 1.53 Coral pattern of seborrhea keratosis demonstrating ridges (elevations) and fissures (depressions). (Coral Image: Jerry Reid, US Fish & Wildlife Service via Wikimedia Commons)

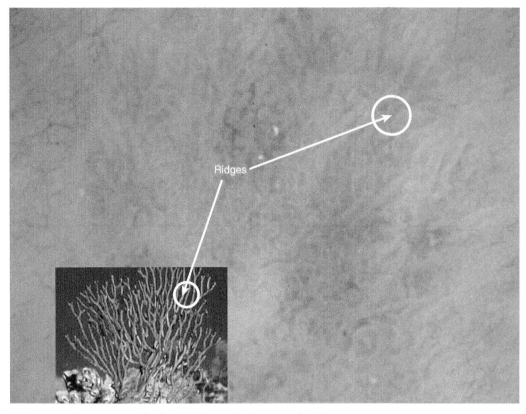

FIGURE 1.54 Coral pattern of seborrheic keratosis demonstrating ridges.

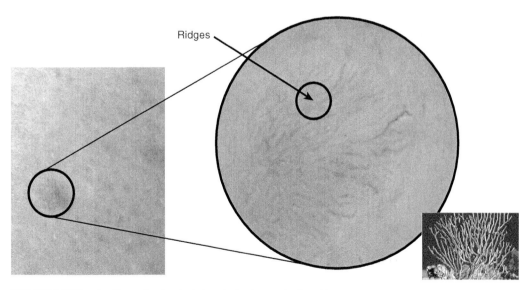

FIGURE 1.55 Coral pattern of seborrheic keratosis demonstrating ridges.

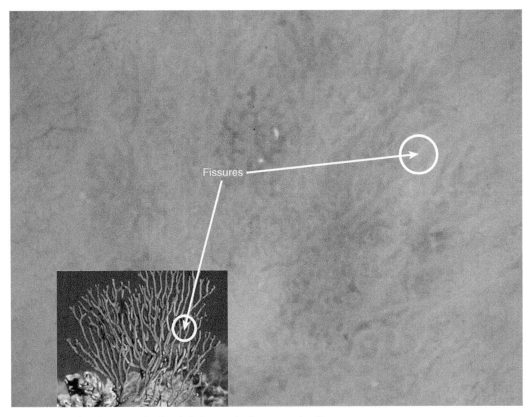

FIGURE 1.56 Coral pattern of seborrheic keratosis demonstrating fissures.

- The fissures are linear epidermal depressions or clefts filled with keratin; they are also termed "sulci" (Figures 1.56 and 1.57).
- Figure 1.58 demonstrates the pathologic correlation to the keratin-filled clefts.

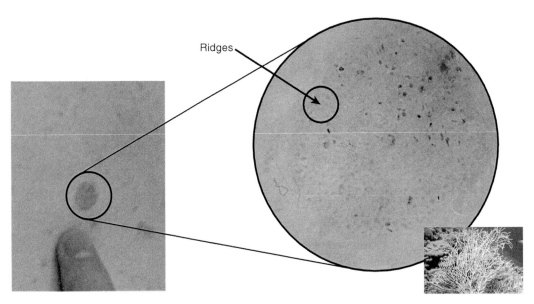

FIGURE 1.57 Coral pattern of seborrheic keratosis demonstrating ridges.

Basic Overview

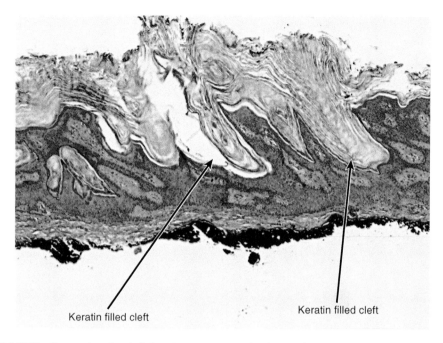

Keratin filled cleft   Keratin filled cleft

FIGURE 1.58 The fissures in seborrheic keratoses correspond to keratin-filled clefts.

Looped (hairpin) vessels and fine vessels surrounded by halo
- Figures 1.59 and 1.60 show the characteristic looped or hairpin vessels that are at the center of a white halo.

Diffuse yellow pigmentation
This is in contrast to a focal yellow pattern that can be seen in SCC.

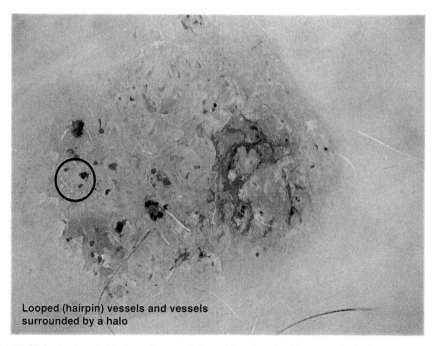

Looped (hairpin) vessels and vessels surrounded by a halo

FIGURE 1.59 Clinically elevated lesions that are pink or skin-colored, with a vascular/red dermoscopic pattern. Irritated seborrheic keratoses have hairpin-like vessels at the center of a white halo.

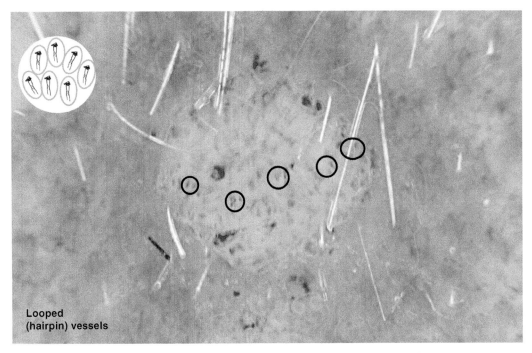

Looped
(hairpin) vessels

FIGURE 1.60 Clinically elevated lesions that are pink or skin-colored with a vascular/red dermoscopic pattern. Irritated seborrheic keratoses have hairpin-like vessels at the center of a white halo.

Test Yourself: Clinical Mimicry!

Figure 1.61 shows two clinically appearing hyperpigmented lesions. Lesion A is flat. Lesion B is raised.

Figure 1.62 illustrates the dermoscopic image of lesion A. Notice the multiple colors and blue-gray dots and granules. Additionally, we see some focal pseudopods and radial streaming, as well as poorly defined borders.

Figure 1.63 shows the dermoscopic image of lesion B, demonstrating sharply defined borders and comedo-like openings. Remember that lesion B is raised!

Lesion A = malignant melanoma in situ (MMIS)

Lesion B = seborrheic keratosis

How did you do?

Comparing these lesions is really like comparing apples and oranges when you consider some basic principles. Both are the same color clinically but one is elevated and the other is flat dark brown/light, the malignant melanoma (MM) is multicolored and flat, whereas the seb k is dermoscopically dark brown/light brown and raised. These characteristics alone put these two lesions into two separate categories. We will discuss this in more depth when we introduce the color wheel, but begin to pay attention to these details.

Solar Lentigo Pearls

Clinically, solar lentigines appear as pale macules and patches on sun-exposed skin. On pathology, they're described as "dirty socks" where the rete ridges have a brown pigment and protrude into the dermis (Figure 1.64).

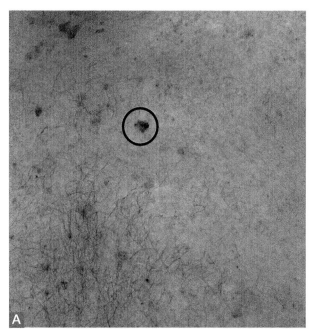

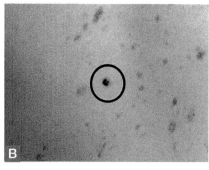

FIGURE 1.61 Clinically similar-appearing hyperpigmented lesions. **(A)** is flat, and **(B)** is elevated.

Characteristic dermoscopic features of solar lentigines include fingerprinting, diffuse light brown structureless area, moth-eaten and/or sharply demarcated borders, and a reticular pattern.

Fingerprinting

- The fingerprinting pattern appears as parallel ridges and short, interrupted lines (Figure 1.65).

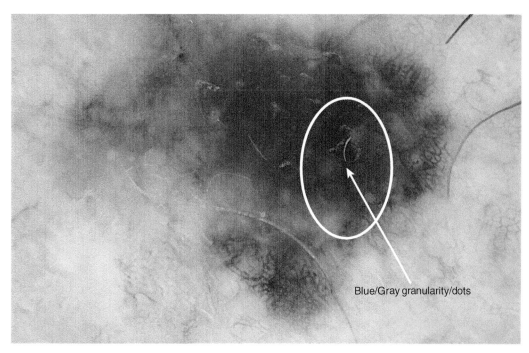

Blue/Gray granularity/dots

FIGURE 1.62 Dermoscopic image of lesion (A) in Figure 1.61 demonstrating blue-gray dots and granules. This is a malignant melanoma in situ (MMIS).

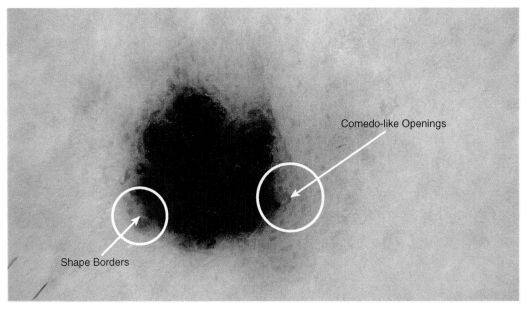

Comedo-like Openings

Shape Borders

FIGURE 1.63 Dermoscopic image of lesion (B) in Figure 1.61 demonstrating comedo-like openings and sharp borders. This is a pigmented benign seborrheic keratosis (seb k).

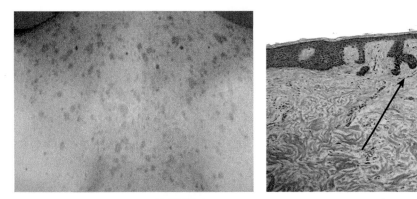

FIGURE 1.64 Solar lentigo appears as pale macules and patches and are related to sun exposure. They are described as "dirty socks" on pathology where rete ridges have brown pigmentation and protrude into the dermis.

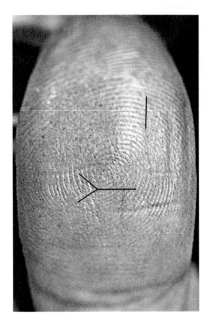

FIGURE 1.65 Solar lentigo has a fingerprint pattern on dermoscopy, with short interrupted lines.

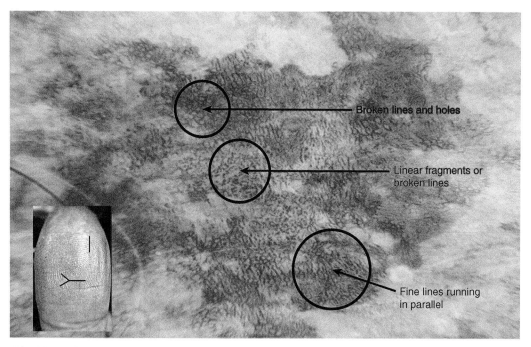

FIGURE 1.66 Solar lentigo has a fingerprint pattern on dermoscopy, with short interrupted lines.

- Figures 1.66 to 1.68 all demonstrate the fingerprinting pattern.

Diffuse light brown structureless area
- Similar to the benign homogenous pattern for melanocytic patterns, solar lentigines can also demonstrate a diffuse, structureless area as shown in Figures 1.69 and 1.70.

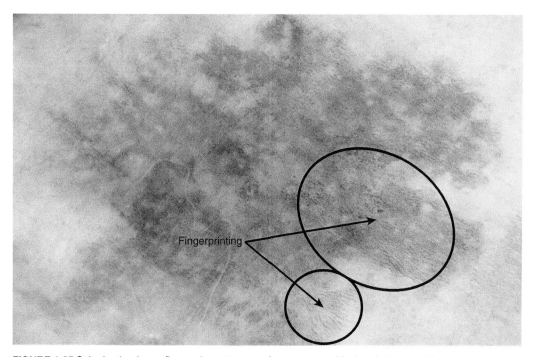

FIGURE 1.67 Solar lentigo has a fingerprint pattern on dermoscopy, with short interrupted lines.

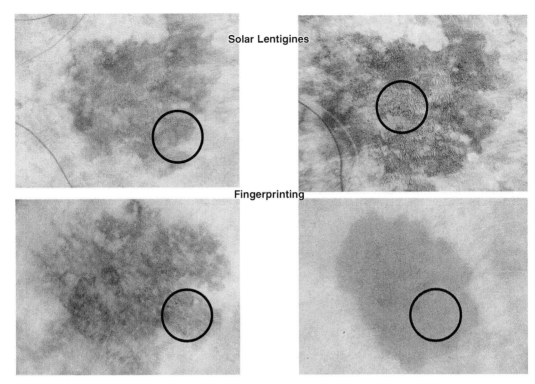

FIGURE 1.68 Solar lentigo has a fingerprint pattern on dermoscopy, with short interrupted lines.

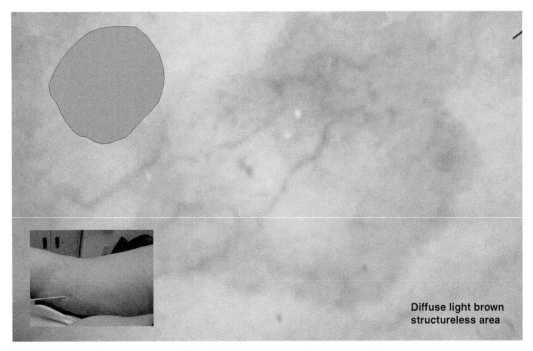

FIGURE 1.69 Solar lentigo can have diffuse light brown structureless areas on dermoscopy.

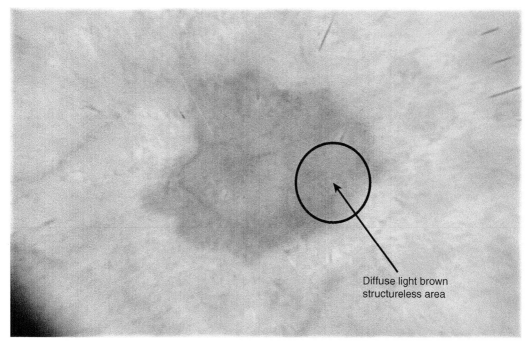

Diffuse light brown
structureless area

FIGURE 1.70 Solar lentigo can have diffuse light brown structureless areas on dermoscopy.

Moth-eaten or sharply demarcated borders

- The moth-eaten borders are characterized by missing pieces around the periphery of the lesion.
- Figures 1.71 to 1.73 illustrate different examples of the moth-eaten boarder pattern.

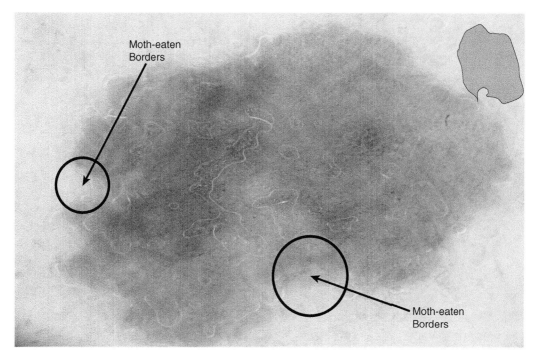

Moth-eaten
Borders

Moth-eaten
Borders

FIGURE 1.71 Solar lentigo has moth-eaten borders.

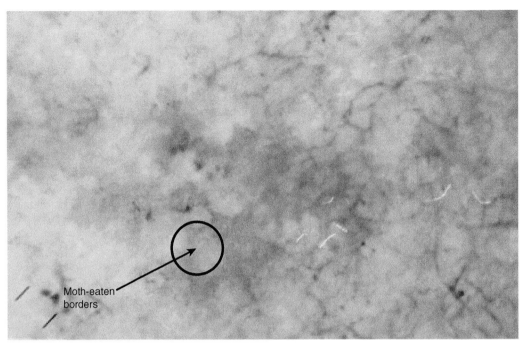

FIGURE 1.72 Solar lentigo has moth-eaten borders.

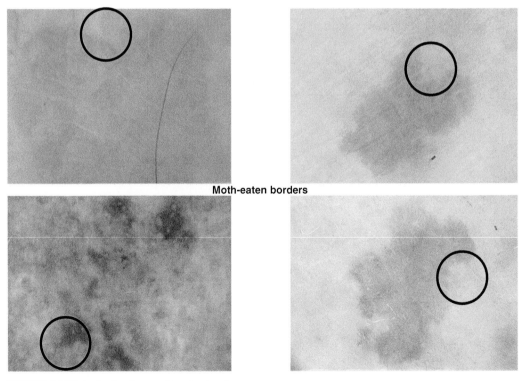

Moth-eaten borders

FIGURE 1.73 Solar lentigo has moth-eaten borders.

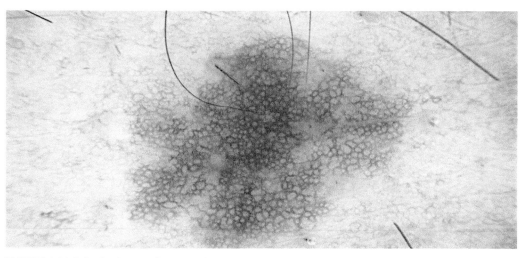

FIGURE 1.74 Solar lentigo can have a reticular pattern similar to the pattern seen in junctional melanocytic nevi.

Reticular pattern

- Another benign melanocytic pattern, solar lentigines, characteristically shows the benign reticular pattern. Often, they can be indistinguishable from a junctional melanocytic nevus (Figure 1.74).
- In solar lentigines, the reticular "holes" correspond to the dermal papillae, and lines correspond to the rete ridges. In junctional melanocytic nevi, there are melanocytes at the rete ridges. Figure 1.75 shows the corresponding pathology.
- Remember that this pattern is seen with JN and lentigines. However, also remember that with the color wheel algorithm, you do not need to know the difference between these two benign lesions, rather a uniform network/reticular pattern is an indication that something is benign. JN are characterized by a reticular network that thins at the periphery (Figures 1.76 to 1.78).

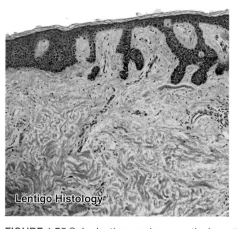
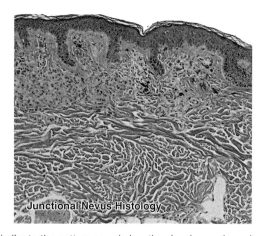

VS

Lentigo Histology

Junctional Nevus Histology

FIGURE 1.75 Solar lentigo can have a reticular pattern similar to the pattern seen in junctional melanocytic nevi (JN). On pathology, holes correspond to dermal papillae, and lines correspond to rete ridges. JNs have melanocytes at the rete ridges.

Basic Overview

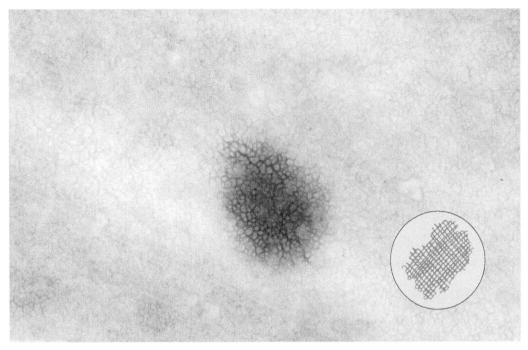

FIGURE 1.76 Solar lentigo can have a reticular pattern similar to the pattern seen in junctional melanocytic nevi (JN).

Pattern pearls

- The dermoscopic feature of evolving seborrheic keratosis can overlap with those of solar lentigines. In both lesions, you can see
  - Fingerprinting
  - Moth-eaten border
  - Focal thickening of network

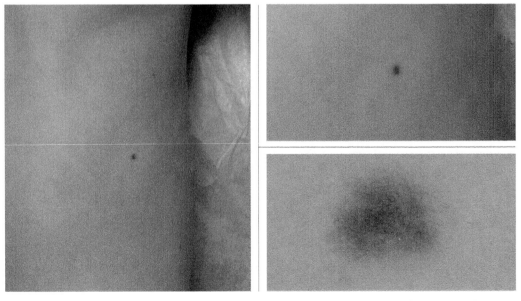

FIGURE 1.77 Solar lentigo can have a reticular pattern similar to the pattern seen in junctional melanocytic nevi (JN).

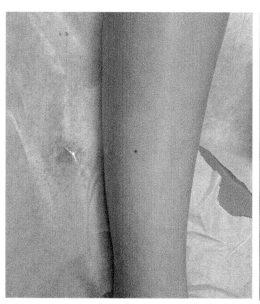
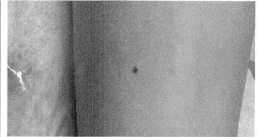
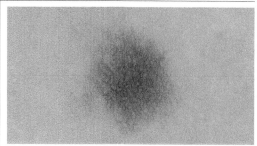

FIGURE 1.78 Solar lentigo can have a reticular pattern similar to the pattern seen in junctional melanocytic nevi (JN).

- Broken interrupted lines
- A few comedo-like openings, ridges, milia-like cysts, and fissures
- Figures 1.79 to 1.83 show examples of early seborrheic keratosis where you see the features of a lentigo, such as a fingerprint pattern and moth-eaten border, and that of a seb k with fat finger projections, sharp borders, milia-like cysts, and comedo-like openings.
  - In Figure 1.79, note the focal thickening ("fat fingers") that starts to occur in the reticular pattern of a lentigo.

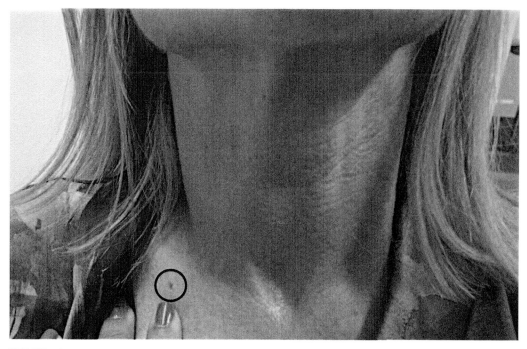

FIGURE 1.79 Clinical image of an early seborrheic keratosis.

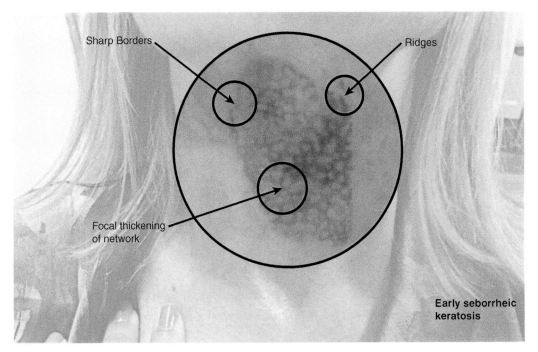

FIGURE 1.80 Dermoscopic image of an early seborrheic keratosis with focal thickening of network, sharp borders, and ridges.

- Figures 1.80 to 1.82 show moth-eaten borders of a lentigo with the formation of ridges seen in a reticulated seb k.
- Figure 1.83 shows the fingerprint pattern of a lentigo along with features of a seb k, such as milia-like cysts, a sharply demarcated border, and ridges.

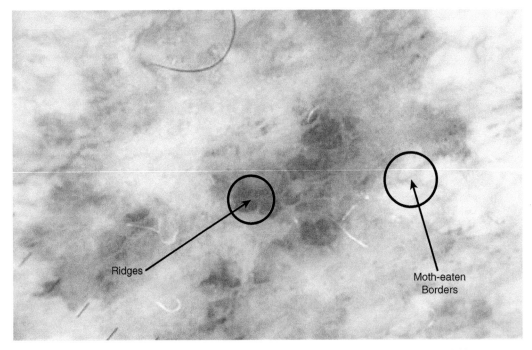

FIGURE 1.81 Dermoscopic image of an early seborrheic keratosis with moth-eaten borders and ridges.

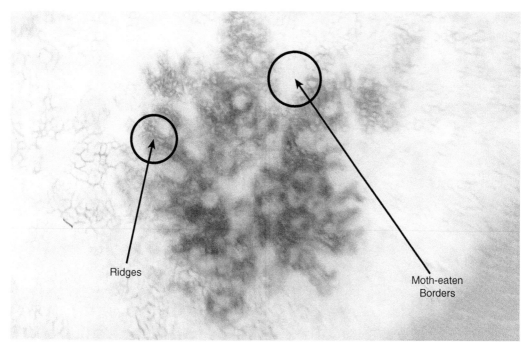

FIGURE 1.82 Dermoscopic image of an early seborrheic keratosis with moth-eaten borders and ridges.

Lichen Planus–like Keratosis/Benign Lichenoid Keratosis

Clinically, a lichen planus–like keratosis (LPLK) is either a solar lentigo undergoing regression or an early seborrheic keratosis undergoing regression. They can be thought of as lentigines or seborrheic keratosis that have become irritated and inflamed. However, don't lose the forest through the trees—focus on benign versus malignant patterns.

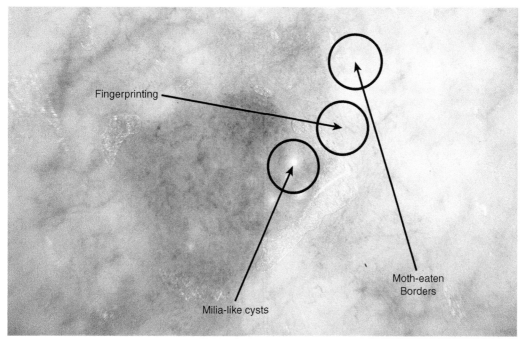

FIGURE 1.83 Dermoscopic image of an early seborrheic keratosis with moth-eaten borders and fingerprinting and milia-like cysts.

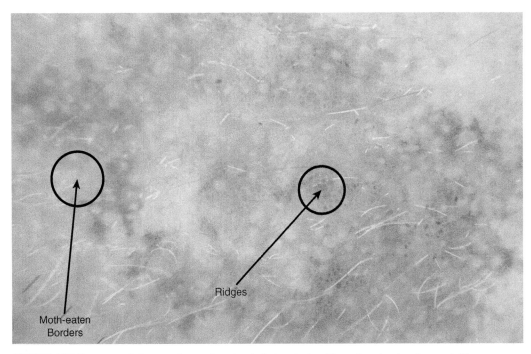

FIGURE 1.84 Dermoscopic image of an early seborrheic keratosis with moth-eaten borders and ridges.

Moth-eaten border

Figures 1.84 and 1.85 show examples of the clinical and dermoscopic picture of an LPLK, a solar lentigo, or a seborrheic keratosis undergoing regression. Notice the diffuse granularity and asymmetry of this lesion; this can look similar to the granularity of malignant melanoma. However, notice the striking moth-eaten border, similar to that seen in solar lentigo.

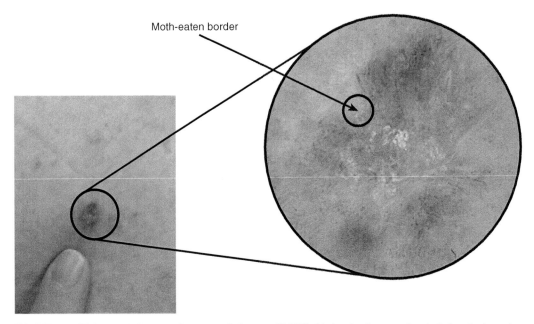

FIGURE 1.85 Clinical and close-up dermoscopic image of LPLK; this is a lentigo or seborrheic keratosis undergoing regression sometimes due to irritation and inflammation. This LPLK has diffuse granularity, which can look similar to the granularity of MM, but this lesion has a moth-eaten border, similar to that seen in lentigo.

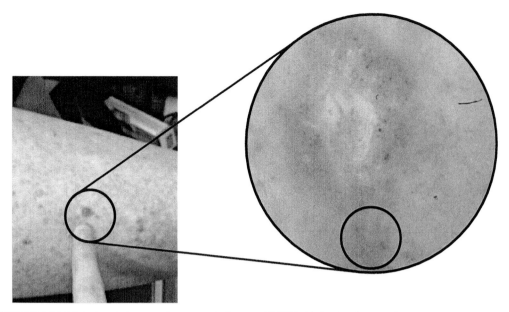

FIGURE 1.86 Clinical and close-up dermoscopic image of LPLK; this is a lentigo or seborrheic keratosis undergoing regression sometimes due to irritation and inflammation. This LPLK has diffuse granularity, which can look similar to the granularity of MM, but this lesion has fingerprint pattern pigmentation.

Fingerprinting

Figure 1.86 shows another clinical and dermoscopic picture of a LPLK, solar lentigo, or seborrheic keratosis. Again, this presentation can be tricky because of the irritation and inflammation often present in these lesions. However, pay attention to the fingerprinting pattern that is evident in the pigmentation of the lesion; this will be different from the pigmentation associated with early amelanotic melanoma.

Figure 1.87 shows a clinical picture of a lesion that is scaly pink, which could be an inflamed seborrheic keratosis or LPLK, but we are suspicious of SCC. Figure 1.88 shows the dermoscopy

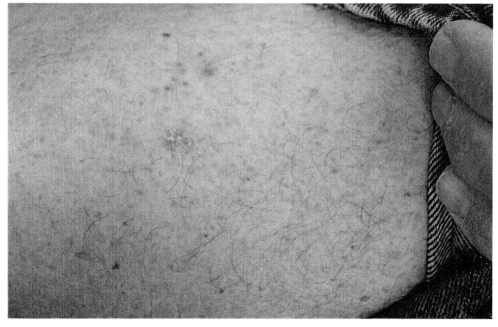

FIGURE 1.87 Clinically pink scaly patch can be an inflamed seb k (LPLK) versus an early squamous cell skin cancer.

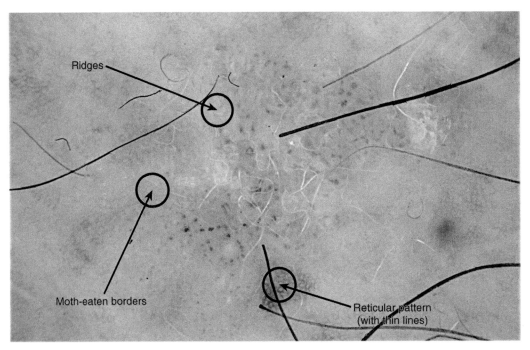

FIGURE 1.88 Dermoscopy of the lesion in Figure 1.87, demonstrating the patterns of a nonpigmented (pink) seborrheic keratosis with ridges, moth-eaten borders, and some reticular pigmentation.

of this lesion, which is more consistent with a nonpigmented seborrheic keratosis or LPLK. The dermoscopic features of ridges, moth-eaten borders, and a reticular pattern with thin lines help to rule out SCC.

Dermatofibroma

Dermatofibromas also have various patterns in their center. Most importantly, a faint pseudo-network-like pattern at the periphery leads to their identification. These central patterns include pigmented network/network-like structures, globules/ring-like globules, central white patch, central vessels and erythema, and a crystalline (scar-like) pattern (Figure 1.89). They can also sometimes appear with diffuse dots and be confused with a flat superficial SCC; however, remember that these will be either elevated or flat, but firmly palpable, and therefore cannot be a superficial SCC.

Faint pseudo-network-like periphery

Figure 1.90 shows a classic dermatofibroma, clinically and dermoscopically. Clinically, the lesion is raised or palpable. Here, we see a central crystalline pattern with the faint pseudo-network-like pattern at the periphery.

Pigmented network

Figure 1.91 shows the dermoscopic and pathologic correlations of the central pigmented network seen in dermatofibromas. As you can see, the pigmented network in the dermoscopic image correlates with the hyperpigmentation of the basal layer of the pathologic image.

Central white patch

Figure 1.92 shows the pathologic correlation of the dermoscopic central white patch seen in dermatofibromas. On pathology, we can see that the white patch is dense collagen bundles.

Central vessels and erythema

Figure 1.93 shows the pathologic correlation of the central vessels and erythema seen in dermatofibromas. On pathology, we see that this is due to increased vascularity.

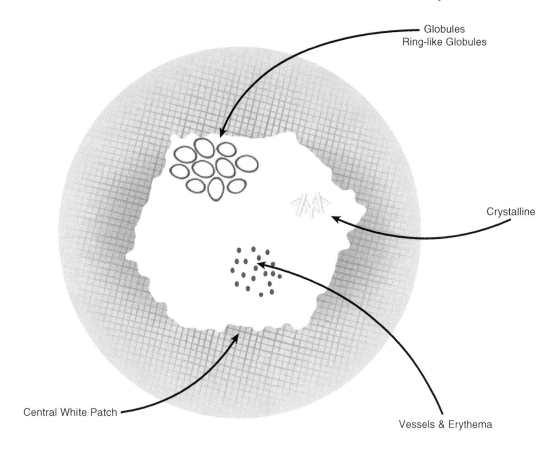

FIGURE 1.89 An illustration of dermatofibromas, which have pigmented network-like structures at the periphery, central white patch, crystalline pattern, ring-like globules, and or vessels and erythema at the center.

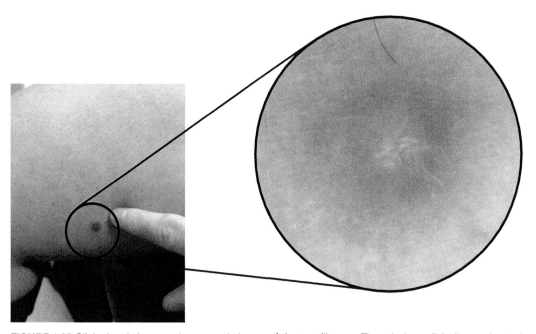

FIGURE 1.90 Clinical and close-up dermoscopic image of dermatofibroma. These lesions clinically are elevated and/or palpable. Dermoscopically, they can have various features at the center; the most important characteristic is a faint pseudo-network-like pattern at the periphery.

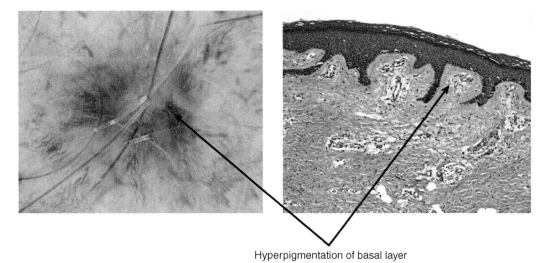

Hyperpigmentation of basal layer

FIGURE 1.91 The pigment network-like structures of dermatofibromas correlate with hyperpigmentation at the basal layer.

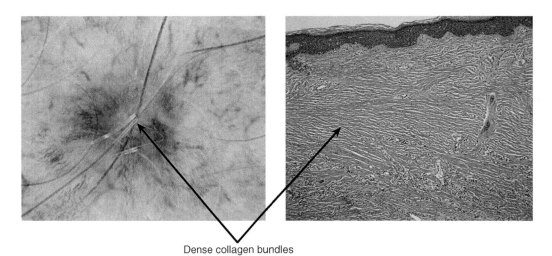

Dense collagen bundles

FIGURE 1.92 The central white patch of dermatofibromas correlates with dense collagen bundles.

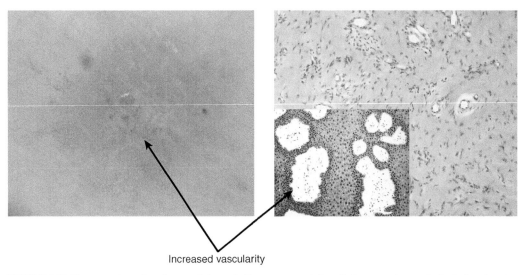

Increased vascularity

FIGURE 1.93 The vessels and erythema of dermatofibromas correlate with increased vascularity in the dermis.

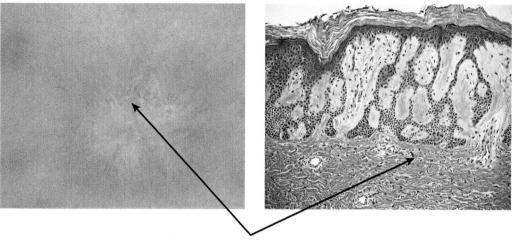

Elongated and broadened rete ridges

FIGURE 1.94 The ring-like globules of dermatofibromas correlate with elongated and broadened rete ridges. The pigmented rete envelopes the papillae, producing the ring-like globules.

Globule-like/ring-like globules

Figure 1.94 shows the pathologic correlation of the globule-like or ring-like globules seen in dermatofibromas. As you can see in the pathologic image, this feature is due to elongation and broadening of the rete ridges. The pigmented rete ridge envelopes the papillae, producing the ring-like globules.

Crystalline structures

Figure 1.95 demonstrates the crystalline structures that can often be seen in the center of dermatofibromas. They are typically shiny, bright white, orthogonal linear streaks seen with polarized dermoscopy. This scar-like pattern correlates with increased collagen in the stroma.

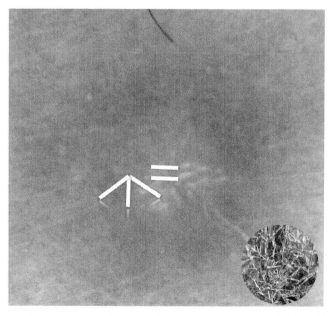

FIGURE 1.95 The crystalline structures of dermatofibromas look like shiny, bright white, orthogonal linear streaks seen with polarized dermoscopy. This scar-like pattern correlates with increased collagen in the stroma.

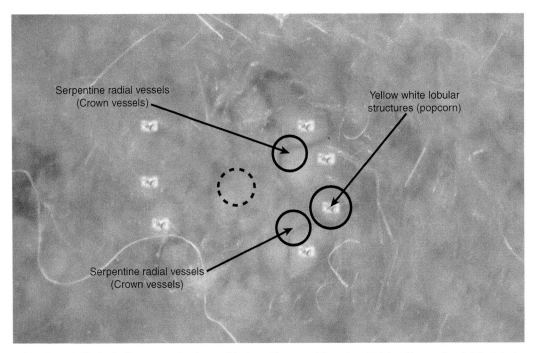

FIGURE 1.96 Clinically flat or mostly elevated lesions that are skin-colored/pink with a yellow/white lobular dermoscopic pattern. This is a dermoscopic example of sebaceous hyperplasia. On dermoscopy, note the white/yellow lobular structures (popcorn) and peripheral serpentine radial vessels (crown vessels), as well as the central indentation (dell).

Sebaceous Hyperplasia

There are three important features to recognize for sebaceous hyperplasia: yellow-white lobular structures resembling popcorn, serpentine radial vessels resembling a crown that do not cross the midline, and central indentation or dell. Figure 1.96 demonstrates these features.

Angioma

The primary feature to recognize in angiomas is the lacunae, but you may also see a whitish veil, erythema, or peripheral erythema (Figure 1.97).

Lacunae

Lacunae are characterized by well-demarcated round or oval structures. They are collections of blood vessels, and depending on the vascularization, they will appear anywhere from bright red to blue-red or dark blue/maroon. When thrombosed, they will appear as homogenous, confluent dark bluish-black pigment (Figure 1.97).

Whitish veil, erythema, peripheral erythema

Figure 1.97 shows the dermoscopic findings of dark lacunae with a whitish veil and peripheral erythema seen in angiokeratoma (4).

Milia/Acne

While seen most often in adolescents and young adults, older populations still experience acne lesions from comedones to large, tender nodules and cysts. Picking can cause irritation and bleeding, making it difficult to differentiate this acne from some presentations of early BCC,

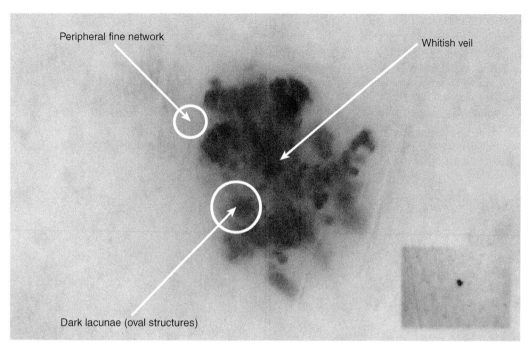

Peripheral fine network

Whitish veil

Dark lacunae (oval structures)

FIGURE 1.97 Clinically flat or mostly elevated lesions that are red/purple with a multicolored lacunae dermoscopic pattern. This is a dermoscopic example of angiokeratoma. On dermoscopy, note the dark oval structures (lacunae) and peripheral erythema and fine network, as well as the whitish veil.

especially in fair-skinned, older adults. Dermoscopic features of acne lesions can include a neutral yellow background and a central punctum.

Neutral yellow background and central punctum

Figure 1.98 is an example of an excoriated acne lesion demonstrating the neutral yellow background and central punctum.

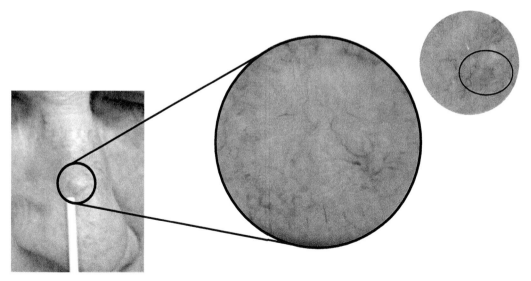

FIGURE 1.98 Clinically flat or mostly elevated lesions that are skin-colored/pink with a yellow/white lobular dermoscopic pattern. These are clinical and dermoscopic findings of excoriated acne vulgaris lesion. **Upper right:** this example illustrates the localized yellow hue that can be seen in an ulcerated BCC.

References

1. Stolz W, Riemann A, Cognetta AB, et al. ABCD rule of dermatoscopy: a new practical method for early recognition of malignant melanoma. *Euro J Dermatol.* 1994;4:521–527.

2. Argenziano G, Fabbrocini G, Carli P, et al. Epiluminescence microscopy for the diagnosis of doubtful melanocytic skin lesions: comparison of the ABCD rule of dermatoscopy and a new 7-point checklist based on pattern analysis. *Arch Dermatol.* 1998;134:1563–1570.

3. Argenziano G, Soyer HP, Chimenti S, et al. Dermoscopy of pigmented skin lesions: results of a consensus meeting via the Internet. *J Am Acad Dermatol.* 2003;48:679–693.

4. Zaballos P, Daufi C, et al. Dermoscopy of solitary angiokeratomas: a morphological study. *Arch Dermatol.* 2007;143:318–325.

Chapter 2 Equipment

Dermoscopy (also called dermatoscopy, epiluminescence microscopy, and surface microscopy) is a method of examining the skin and its underlying structures using handheld magnification. Just as light reflects off the surface of a lake, distorting the view of the rocks and fish, so too does the stratum corneum reflect light off the skin, preventing the structures below from being seen clearly by the naked eye. Dermoscopy uses polarized light or nonpolarized light with a liquid/gel interface to circumvent this problem. The use of nonpolarized light requires applying a liquid/gel medium onto the skin and then placing the lens directly onto the surface of the skin, creating a tight seal, whereas polarized light does not require direct skin contact. Both methods reduce the glare from the stratum corneum and result in an enhanced microscopic (standard 10× magnification) and highly resolute image of the structures just beneath the surface of the skin. With this newly improved vision, the clinician is in a much better position to assess and diagnose various dermatologic lesions, mites, and diseases.

The proper evaluation of the magnified image is an invaluable tool that provides a clinician with greater diagnostic accuracy, sensitivity, and specificity. Vestergaard et al. found a relative diagnostic odds ratio for melanoma to be 9.0 (95% CI 1.5 to 54.6, $p = 0.03$) and a difference in sensitivity of 0.18 (95% CI 0.09 to 0.27, $p = 0.002$) with no significant decrease in specificity.[1] In other words, the odds of diagnosing a melanoma were nine times greater when trained clinicians used dermoscopy, as compared with naked eye examination. Further, they overlooked or missed fewer true positive diagnoses of melanoma (sensitivity), without increasing the number of benign lesions incorrectly diagnosed as melanoma (specificity). One can correctly assume that this advantageous tool allows clinicians to more confidently determine which lesions should be considered for a second opinion or biopsy. Studies have found that, with appropriate use, dermoscopy can decrease the number of unnecessary excisions up to nearly 40%.[2] The benefit of mastering dermoscopy, coupled with its simple and noninvasive nature, unequivocally proves to be an important and useful tool for clinicians. By decreasing unnecessary biopsies and excision of benign skin lesions mimicking malignancies, and increasing accurate diagnosis of a variety of lesions (including malignant melanomas, nonpigmented malignant neoplasms, papulosquamous conditions, and scabies),[3] dermoscopy ultimately provides improvement in patient management and welfare.

Whether you are getting ready to take on dermoscopy for the first time or have been using dermoscopy for some time, it is good to review the differences between different dermatoscopes. While the technologies have improved immensely, the critical differences between contact nonpolarized dermoscopy (CNPD) and contact polarized dermoscopy (CPD) are the same. When thinking about what type of dermatoscope to use, there are a few general and technical considerations to keep in mind.

Types of Dermatoscopes

In general, **nonpolarized dermatoscopes**:
- Will have contact with the skin
- Require a liquid medium
- Are generally a larger size
- Produce nonpolarized images used in atlases and lectures

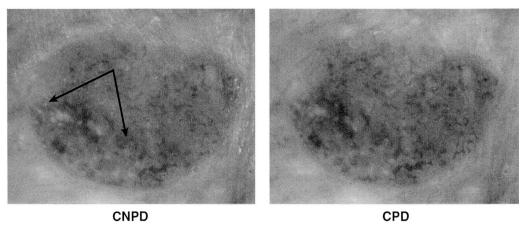

CNPD   **CPD**

FIGURE 2.1 A seborrheic keratosis example. Milia-like cysts and comedo-like openings can be better seen with contact nonpolarized dermoscopy.

In general, **polarized dermatoscopes**:
- Can be used either in contact or without contact of the skin
- Are aided by use of a liquid medium, but it is not necessary
- Are a more convenient, pocket size

The more technical considerations that deal with differences in pattern identification are also important to keep in mind when choosing a dermatoscope.

Dermatoscopic Findings

Examples

We can see in these examples that a nonpolarized dermatoscope is the tool of choice for:
- Epidermal features such as the milia-like cysts, comedo-like openings (Figure 2.1), and ridges (Figure 2.2) that are often seen in seborrheic keratosis
- Regression structures, such as the gray dots and granules seen in a melanoma in situ (Figure 2.3)
- The blue-white veil of a melanoma that is often more prominent with CNPD
  Polarized dermatoscopes are the tools of choice when looking at:
- Vessels and red areas, which are secondary to a vasculature change as seen in this nonpigmented seborrheic keratosis (Figure 2.4) as well as in this dermatofibroma (Figure 2.5)

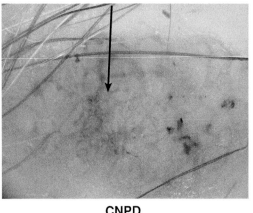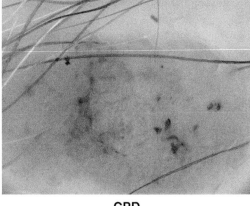

CNPD   **CPD**

FIGURE 2.2 A seborrheic keratosis example. Ridges are more prominent with nonpolarized dermoscopy.

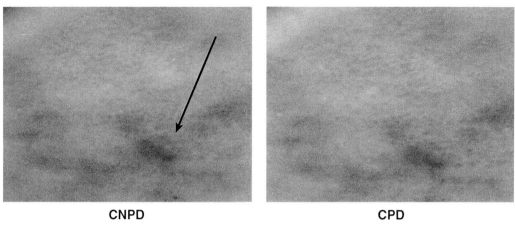

CNPD   CPD

FIGURE 2.3 A melanoma in situ example. Regression structures (*gray dots/granules*) are more prominent with nonpolarized dermoscopy.

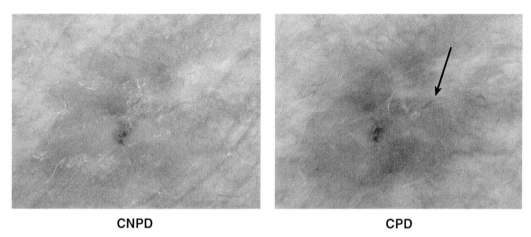

CNPD   CPD

FIGURE 2.4 A nonpigmented seborrheic keratosis example. Vessels and red areas (secondary to vascular changes) are better seen with polarized dermoscopy.

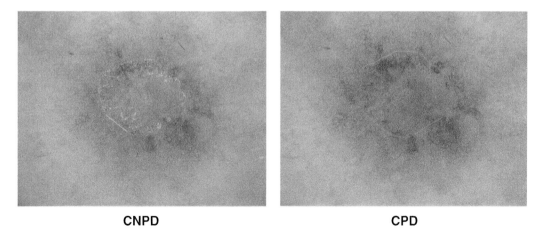

CNPD   CPD

FIGURE 2.5 A dermatofibroma example. *Red* color is more prominent with polarized dermoscopy.

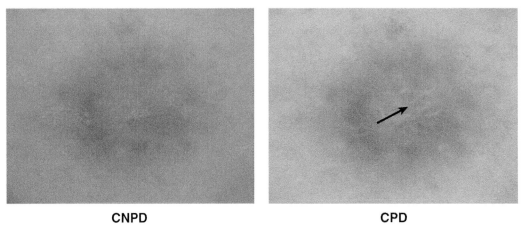

CNPD   CPD

FIGURE 2.6 A dermatofibroma example. The crystalline pattern is more prominent with polarized dermoscopy.

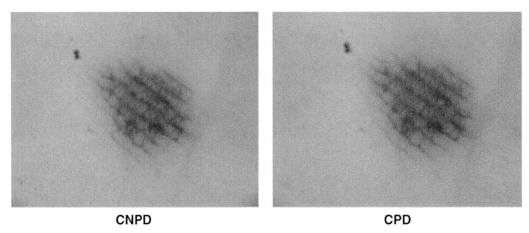

CNPD   CPD

FIGURE 2.7 A junctional nevus example on the sole of the foot. There is no major difference in network morphology between polarized and nonpolarized dermoscopy.

- Altered collagen structures, such as the crystalline pattern seen in this example of a dermatofibroma (Figure 2.6)
- Deeper structures that are often more prominent with CPD

However, there is no major difference between network morphology, when comparing the nonpolarized and polarized dermatoscopes, as seen in this example of a junctional nevus (Figure 2.7). Some dermatoscopes have both contact and noncontact options, as well as both polarized and nonpolarized options all in one scope. However, it is not absolutely necessary to have all capabilities in order to be successful in dermoscopy.

With these considerations in mind, and our discussion of patterns and dermatoscopes tackled, we are ready to introduce you to the color wheel in Chapter 3!

References

1. Vestergaard ME, Macaskill P, Holt PE, et al. Dermoscopy compared with naked eye examination for the diagnosis of primary melanoma: a meta-analysis of studies performed in a clinical setting. *Br J Dermatol.* 2008;159(3):669–676.

2. Argenziano G, Soyer HP, Chimenti S, et al. Impact of dermoscopy on the clinical management of pigmented skin lesions. *Clin Dermatol.* 2002;20(3):200–202.

3. Engasser HC, Warshaw EM. Dermatoscopy use by US dermatologists: a cross-sectional survey. *J Am Acad Dermatol.* 2010;63(3):412–419, 419.e411–412.

Steps: ❶ Flat or Elevated ❷ Color Clinical ❸ Color Dermoscopic ❹ Pattern

Clinical

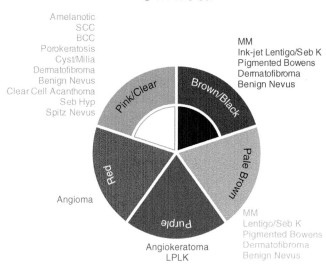

Amelanotic
SCC
BCC
Porokeratosis
Cyst/Milia
Dermatofibroma
Benign Nevus
Clear Cell Acanthoma
Seb Hyp
Spitz Nevus

MM
Ink-jet Lentigo/Seb K
Pigmented Bowens
Dermatofibroma
Benign Nevus

Angioma

MM
Lentigo/Seb K
Pigmented Bowens
Dermatofibroma
Benign Nevus

Angiokeratoma
LPLK

Dermoscopic

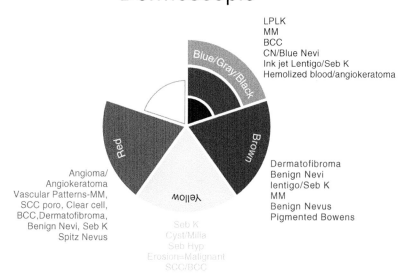

LPLK
MM
BCC
CN/Blue Nevi
Ink jet Lentigo/Seb K
Hemolized blood/angiokeratoma

Angioma/
Angiokeratoma
Vascular Patterns-MM,
SCC poro, Clear cell,
BCC,Dermatofibroma,
Benign Nevi, Seb K
Spitz Nevus

Seb K
Cyst/Milia
Seb Hyp
Erosion=Malignant
SCC/BCC

Dermatofibroma
Benign Nevi
lentigo/Seb K
MM
Benign Nevus
Pigmented Bowens

FIGURE 3.1 The color wheel.

- The Basics
- Flat/Pink-Clear/Red
- Elevated/Pink-Clear/Red
- Flat/Pink-Clear/**Multicolored**
- Elevated/Pink-Clear/**Multicolored**

The Basics

In this chapter, we will go through the steps of the color wheel, using four categories of the wheel as examples. We will also briefly discuss some situations in which it is inappropriate to use the color wheel or dermoscopy.

As discussed in the introduction, the approach that we use in this manual synthesizes these various methods and streamlines the diagnostic algorithm in order to focus on the primary question we are trying to answer with dermoscopy: **Does this lesion need to be biopsied to rule out malignancy?**

The color wheel uses an algorithm for biopsy decision-making that relies first and foremost on our knowledge of clinical history, lesion color, and elevation. Then, only when necessary, dermoscopic pattern recognition is used as the last step.

Even though the color wheel will be a method that streamlines your diagnostic acumen, we must emphasize that your diagnosis should be first and foremost grounded in the clinical history of the patient who is sitting in front of you. There is no replacement for a good clinical history!

The **clinical history** that you want to obtain must include, but is not limited to the following:
- What is your patient's age and sex?
- What is your patient's skin type?
  - Always burn, never tan
  - Always burn, sometimes tan
  - Sometimes burn, but always tan
  - Never burn, always tan
  - Moderately pigmented skin
  - Darkly pigmented skin
- What is their sun exposure history?
- At first glance, how does the lesion look in comparison to other lesions around it? How is it different? Bigger, smaller, asymmetric, symmetric? Where is it located? Head, body, acral? **Remember the lesion that stands out may not necessarily be the darkest or most concerning or "ugliest"-appearing lesion, but rather the "ugly duckling"—the one that does not look like lesions around it.**[1]

After taking note of these considerations, you are ready to look at the lesion more closely. The next important step is to consider the colors in the lesion, and with that, we are going to introduce the color wheel.

The Color Wheel

The color wheel consists of two categories: "Clinical" and "Dermoscopic" colors. The colors you see with your naked eye or "clinical" colors differ from those that you can see with the dermatoscope. We can use these different colors to develop a very focused differential diagnosis and aid in our decision of whether or not to biopsy a lesion.

For each lesion, you'll walk through these steps, with the color wheel at hand to guide you as you're beginning.

Step 1: Is the lesion flat or raised?

Step 2: What color is the lesion on clinical assessment? *(Usually two colors or less)*

Step 3: What is the dermoscopic color/colors?

Step 4: Is further elucidation needed? Is this a malignant or benign pattern?

Simply by taking the first three steps, the differential diagnosis is narrowed down to a short list of possibilities. If the decision to biopsy is still unclear, then dermoscopic pattern recognition is utilized. We previously discussed the necessary patterns in Chapter 1.

Figure 3.1 shows a standard example of the color wheel. The two wheels show the broad differential diagnosis based on each color seen either clinically or dermoscopically. After you determine which colors you are dealing with, you will cross-reference the two lists of differentials to see which diagnosis appears in both lists. This alone will substantially narrow down your differential.

To help you get a feel of how to narrow down your differential using the wheel, we will go into some specific examples.

Flat/Pink-Clear/Red

Figure 3.2 shows an example of how one would evaluate clinically *flat* lesions that are of *pink-clear* color clinically and *red* dermoscopically, with a *vascular dermoscopic pattern.* Let's walk through the steps.

Step 1: Is the lesion flat or raised? **Flat**

Step 2: What color is the lesion on clinical assessment? **Pink-Clear**

Step 3: What is the dermoscopic color? **Red**

Using the color wheel in Figure 3.2, we cross-reference the Clinical and Dermoscopic lists. There are only three malignancies that fit this category: SCC, BCC, +/− porokeratosis.

Keep in mind that we are only considering *Flat* lesions here, so dermatofibroma and intradermal nevi are not considered!

As for the benign lesions, we are considering benign porokeratosis, clear cell acanthoma, or lichen planus–like keratosis/irritated seborrheic keratosis, +/− porokeratosis. Porokeratoses are considered benign, but are often treated similarly to a premalignancy and biopsied or less invasively removed because squamous cell skin cancers can arise within these lesions.

Step 4: Is further elucidation needed to decide whether to biopsy or not? **Yes**

Is this a malignant or benign pattern?

Figures 3.3 to 3.5 show examples of the specific morphologic and vascular patterns seen in the malignancies that we are considering on our differential: BCC and nonpigmented SCC. As you can see, BCC and SCC have very distinct patterns that are distinguishable from the diffuse nonspecific inflammation that one would see with a benign lesion such as lichen planus–like keratosis (Figure 3.3) or the more specific benign pattern seen in clear cell acanthoma where

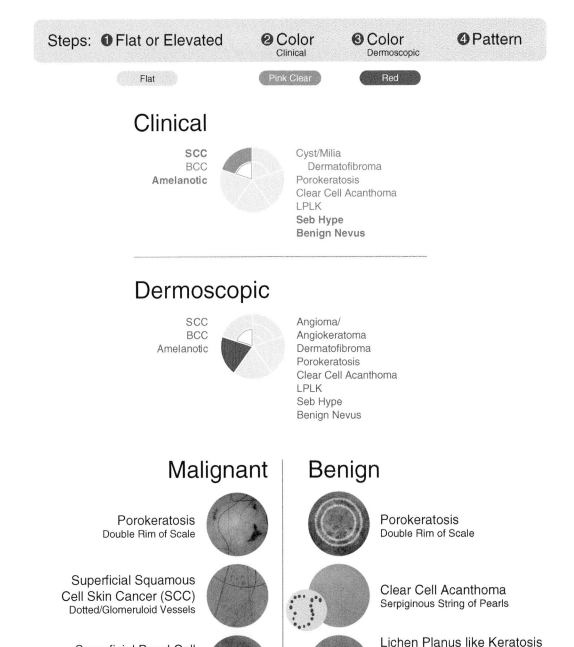

Steps: ❶ Flat or Elevated   ❷ Color   ❸ Color   ❹ Pattern
                                 Clinical   Dermoscopic

Flat   Pink Clear   Red

Clinical

SCC
BCC
Amelanotic

Cyst/Milia
    Dermatofibroma
Porokeratosis
Clear Cell Acanthoma
LPLK
Seb Hype
Benign Nevus

Dermoscopic

SCC
BCC
Amelanotic

Angioma/
Angiokeratoma
Dermatofibroma
Porokeratosis
Clear Cell Acanthoma
LPLK
Seb Hype
Benign Nevus

Malignant | Benign

Porokeratosis
Double Rim of Scale

Porokeratosis
Double Rim of Scale

Superficial Squamous
Cell Skin Cancer (SCC)
Dotted/Glomeruloid Vessels

Clear Cell Acanthoma
Serpiginous String of Pearls

Superficial Basal Cell
Skin Cancer (BCC)
Arborized Vessels & Pink-White

Lichen Planus like Keratosis
(LPLK) / Irritated Seborrheic
Keratosis (ISK)
Nonspecific Inflammation

FIGURE 3.2 Clinically flat lesions that are pink or skin-colored with a vascular dermoscopic pattern.

the red dots (vessels) form a serpiginous "string of pearls" pattern. Additionally, porokeratoses have a thick double-edged rim, and if a vascular pattern can be seen, it looks similar to a squamous cell. It will show diffuse red dots or diffuse glomeruloid vessels at the center of the double-rimmed lesion.

Flip to Chapter 1 for a more in-depth discussion on Patterns!

Malignant

Benign

BCC   VS   LPLK

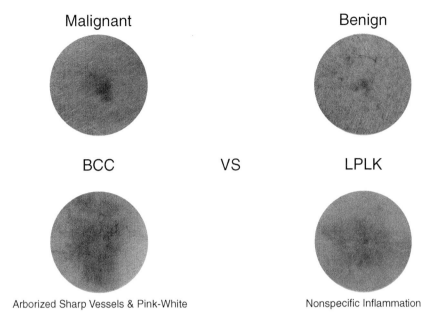

Arborized Sharp Vessels & Pink-White

Nonspecific Inflammation

FIGURE 3.3 In these flat lesions, the vascular pattern matters. Recognizing a specific pattern versus nonspecific inflammation.

Patterns of Basal Cell Skin Cancer

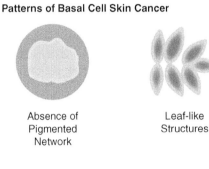

| Absence of Pigmented Network | Leaf-like Structures | Large Blue-Gray Ovoid Nests or Globular-like Structures | Arborizing (tree-like) Telangiectasias (sharp) |

Spoke Wheel Areas   Ulceration   Pink-White to White Shiny Areas   Crystalline Pattern

FIGURE 3.4 Illustrations of basal cell skin cancer patterns.

Patterns of Squamous Cell Skin Cancer

Pink-White
Shiny Area

White Reflective
Scaly Surface

Ulceration

Vascular

Dotted
Vessels

Glomeruloid/
Coiled Vessels

Keratinizing
Vessels

FIGURE 3.5 Illustrations of nonpigmented squamous skin cancer patterns.

Elevated/Pink-Clear/Red

Figure 3.6 shows an example of how we would evaluate clinically *elevated* lesions that are *pink-clear* clinically, are *red* dermoscopically, and have a *vascular dermoscopic* pattern.

Step 1: Is the lesion flat or raised? **Elevated**

Step 2: What color is the lesion on clinical assessment? **Pink-Clear**

Step 3: What is the dermoscopic color? **Red**

After cross-referencing the malignancies, we are considering SCC, BCC, +/− porokeratosis. We have now added the more advanced amelanotic melanoma, which is very concerning clinically and will often be biopsied without the need for further dermoscopic evaluation. Additionally, we are also considering Spitz nevi, which in adults are often treated like a malignancy and biopsied.

Remember we are now dealing with *elevated* lesions.

The benign lesions we are considering are similar: clear cell acanthoma, lichen planus, or irritated seborrheic keratosis, with the addition of intradermal nevi, and dermatofibromas.

Step 4: Is further elucidation needed to decide whether to biopsy or not? **Yes**

Is this a malignant or benign pattern?

Steps: ❶ Flat or Elevated   ❷ Color   ❸ Color   ❹ Pattern
                                      Clinical   Dermoscopic

Elevated   Pink Clear   Red

Clinical

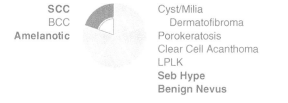

SCC
BCC
Amelanotic

Cyst/Milia
  Dermatofibroma
Porokeratosis
Clear Cell Acanthoma
LPLK
Seb Hype
Benign Nevus

Dermoscopic

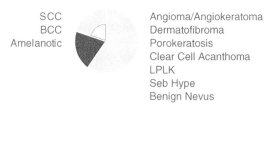

SCC
BCC
Amelanotic

Angioma/Angiokeratoma
Dermatofibroma
Porokeratosis
Clear Cell Acanthoma
LPLK
Seb Hype
Benign Nevus

Malignant | Benign

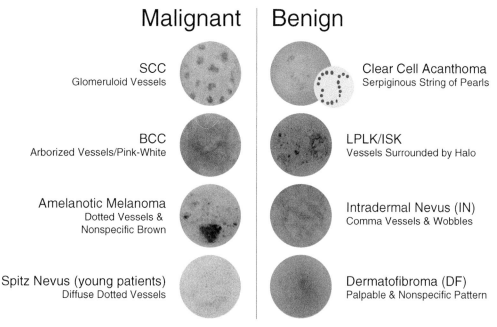

SCC
Glomeruloid Vessels

Clear Cell Acanthoma
Serpiginous String of Pearls

BCC
Arborized Vessels/Pink-White

LPLK/ISK
Vessels Surrounded by Halo

Amelanotic Melanoma
Dotted Vessels &
Nonspecific Brown

Intradermal Nevus (IN)
Comma Vessels & Wobbles

Spitz Nevus (young patients)
Diffuse Dotted Vessels

Dermatofibroma (DF)
Palpable & Nonspecific Pattern

FIGURE 3.6 Clinically elevated lesions that are pink or skin-colored with a vascular dermoscopic pattern.

Flat/Pink-Clear/Multicolored

Let's move on to some more colorful lesions. In Figure 3.7, we are considering *Flat*, clinically *pink-clear* lesions that are dermoscopically *multicolored*. Multicolored can include brown, yellow, and blue/gray, but not white.

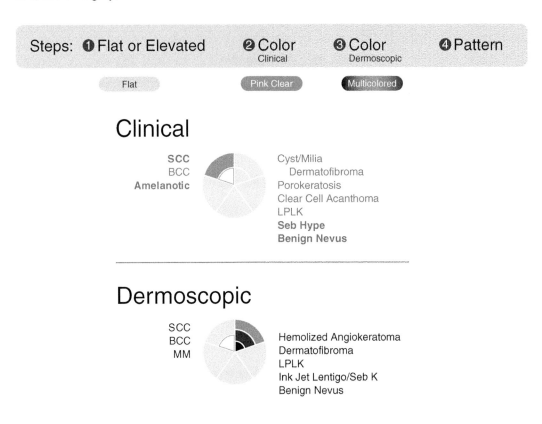

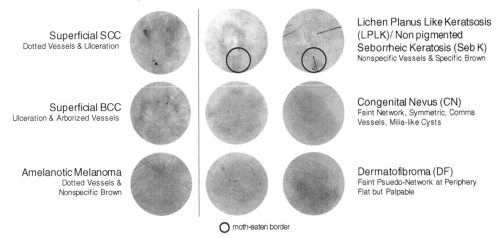

FIGURE 3.7 Clinically flat lesions that are pink or skin-colored with a multicolor dermoscopic pattern. Multiple colors can include brown, yellow, blue/gray, and/or a vascular pattern.

Step 1: Is the lesion flat or raised? **Flat**

Step 2: What color is the lesion on clinical assessment? **Pink-Clear**

Step 3: What is the dermoscopic color? **Multicolored**

Because our differential is still very similar, our malignant possibilities include superficial SCC, superficial BCC, and now amelanotic melanoma.

Our benign lesions include lichen planus–like keratosis/nonpigmented seborrheic keratosis as well as congenital nevi and flat-appearing dermatofibromas, which when touched, will still be palpable.

Step 4: Is further elucidation needed to decide whether to biopsy or not? **Yes**

Is this a malignant or benign pattern?

Looking at Figure 3.7, you can see that specific patterns will be useful to further distinguish between benign and malignant. In fact, in these flat multicolored lesions, you can see both vascular and pigment pattern matters. In Figures 3.8 to 3.10, you can see the important combination of a specific vascular pattern with nonspecific brown pigment indicative of malignancy. In contrast, nonspecific inflammation and a more specific pigment pattern are signs of a lesion that does not require a biopsy.

Additionally, the periphery is an important place to assess patterns. Figure 3.11 is a close-up of the lesions in Figure 3.9. When viewed dermoscopically, melanoma will always have a more asymmetric periphery, often with other malignant features. Again, the periphery of the benign DF has a specific pseudo-network that is regular and consistent. Figure 3.12 is a close-up of

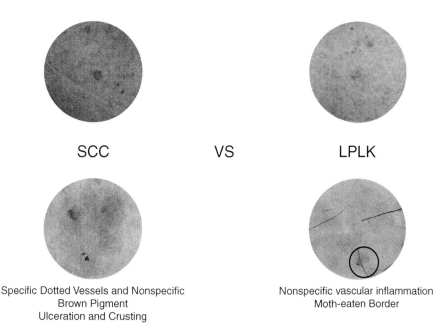

SCC   VS   LPLK

Specific Dotted Vessels and Nonspecific
Brown Pigment
Ulceration and Crusting

Nonspecific vascular inflammation
Moth-eaten Border

FIGURE 3.8 In these flat multicolored lesions, both vascular and pigment patterns matter. Recognizing a specific pattern versus nonspecific inflammation and or more specific pigment pattern is a sign of a lesion that does not require a biopsy, as opposed to a more malignant vascular pattern with a nonspecific pigment.

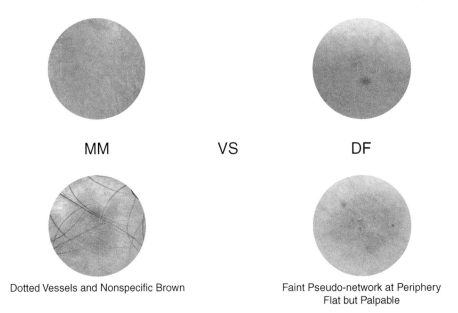

MM   VS   DF

Dotted Vessels and Nonspecific Brown   Faint Pseudo-network at Periphery
                                                      Flat but Palpable

FIGURE 3.9 In these flat multicolored lesions, both vascular and pigment pattern matter. Recognizing a specific pattern versus nonspecific inflammation and or more specific pigment pattern is a sign of a lesion that does not require a biopsy, as opposed to a more malignant vascular pattern with nonspecific pigment.

the periphery of the lesions in Figure 3.10. Again, we see the asymmetric border of the melanoma with additional malignant features, such as the polymorphous vessels and scar-like pattern. This is in comparison to the symmetric border of the congenital nevus without additional malignant features.

Because the flat/pink-clear/multicolored lesions include amelanotic melanoma on the differential, and these are aggressive and nondescript, **when in doubt, take it out!**

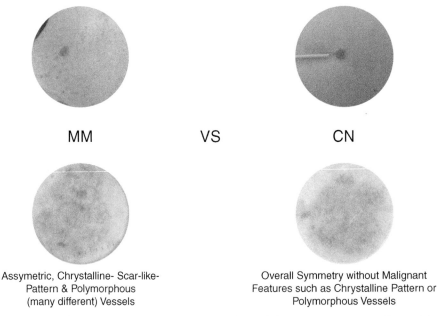

MM   VS   CN

Assymetric, Chrystalline- Scar-like-   Overall Symmetry without Malignant
Pattern & Polymorphous   Features such as Chrystalline Pattern or
(many different) Vessels   Polymorphous Vessels

FIGURE 3.10 In these flat multicolored lesions, both vascular and pigment pattern matter. Recognizing a specific pattern versus nonspecific inflammation and or more specific pigment pattern is a sign of a lesion that does not require a biopsy, as opposed to a more malignant vascular pattern with nonspecific pigment.

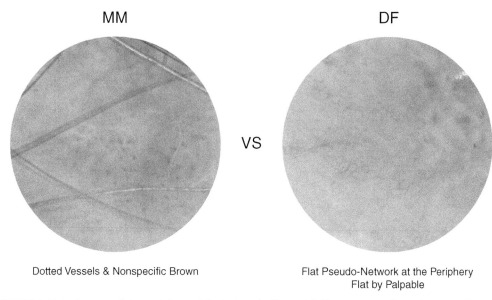

MM   VS   DF

Dotted Vessels & Nonspecific Brown

Flat Pseudo-Network at the Periphery
Flat by Palpable

FIGURE 3.11 A close-up of the periphery of the lesions in Figure 1.9. Dermoscopically, melanoma will always have a more asymmetric periphery that will often have malignant features, as opposed to similar-appearing benign lesions.

Elevated/Pink-Clear/Multicolored

When we elevate the clinically pink-clear, dermoscopically multicolored lesions, we change our differential and again will rely on the pattern for the final call. Let's take a look at Figure 3.13.

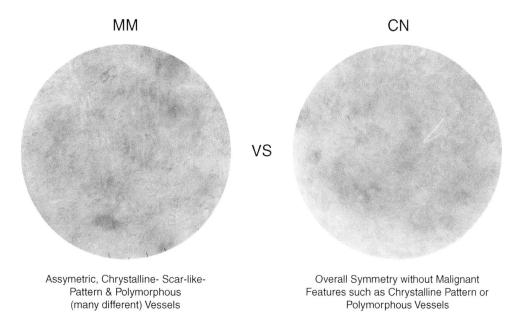

MM   VS   CN

Assymetric, Chrystalline- Scar-like-
Pattern & Polymorphous
(many different) Vessels

Overall Symmetry without Malignant
Features such as Chrystalline Pattern or
Polymorphous Vessels

FIGURE 3.12 A close-up of the periphery of the lesions in Figure 1.11. Dermoscopically, melanoma will always have a more asymmetric periphery that will often have malignant features, as opposed to similar-appearing benign lesions.

Steps: ❶ Flat or Elevated   ❷ Color   ❸ Color   ❹ Pattern
                                      Clinical   Dermoscopic

Elevated   Pink Clear   Multicolored

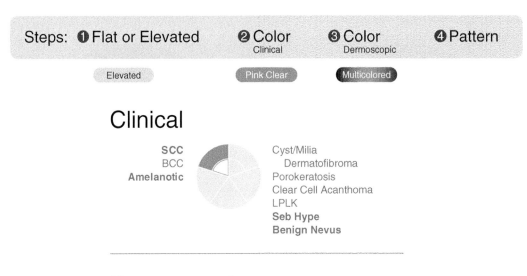

Clinical

SCC
BCC
Amelanotic

Cyst/Milia
Dermatofibroma
Porokeratosis
Clear Cell Acanthoma
LPLK
Seb Hype
Benign Nevus

Dermoscopic

SCC
BCC
MM

Hemolized Angiokeratoma
Dermatofibroma
LPLK
Ink Jet Lentigo/Seb K
Benign Nevus

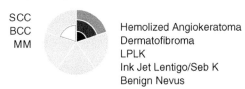

Malignant Benign

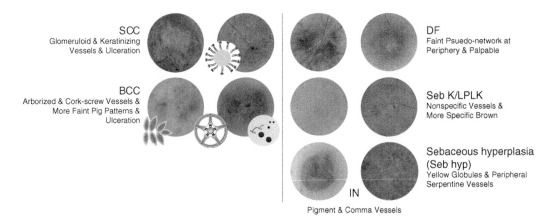

SCC
Glomeruloid & Keratinizing
Vessels & Ulceration

BCC
Arborized & Cork-screw Vessels &
More Faint Pig Patterns &
Ulceration

DF
Faint Psuedo-network at
Periphery & Palpable

Seb K/LPLK
Nonspecific Vessels &
More Specific Brown

**Sebaceous hyperplasia
(Seb hyp)**
Yellow Globules & Peripheral
Serpentine Vessels

IN
Pigment & Comma Vessels

FIGURE 3.13 Clinically elevated lesions that are pink or skin-colored with a multicolor dermoscopic pattern. Multiple colors can include brown, yellow, blue/gray, and/or a vascular pattern.

Step 1: Is the lesion flat or raised? **Elevated**

Step 2: What color is the lesion on clinical assessment? **Pink-Clear**

Step 3: What is the dermoscopic color? **Multicolored**

Importantly, amelanotic melanoma has come off our differential! The only two malignancies that we are now considering are SCC or BCC.

The benign lesions we are considering include dermatofibroma and seborrheic keratosis/lichen planus–like keratosis, and we have now added sebaceous hyperplasia. Remember that these are sebaceous hyperplasia that are multicolored and therefore can be irritated and more difficult to distinguish from SCC and BCC with ulceration. We will revisit this topic in Chapters 7 and 16.

Step 4: Is further elucidation needed to decide whether to biopsy or not? **Yes**

Is this a malignant or benign pattern?

We can use the color yellow in the setting of ulceration. Note in Figure 3.14 that the yellow is diffuse throughout the lesion, secondary to trauma. There is no other evidence of a malignant pattern, such as signs of blood vessels seen with the ulceration or a blue ovoid nest seen with a basal cell skin cancer. This is consistent with the benign patterns seen in a seborrheic keratosis and some skin-colored congenital nevi. An additional feature, such as peripheral crowing of vessels around yellow/white ball-like clusters, is also a feature of sebaceous hyperplasia. We will revisit this topic in Chapter 16.

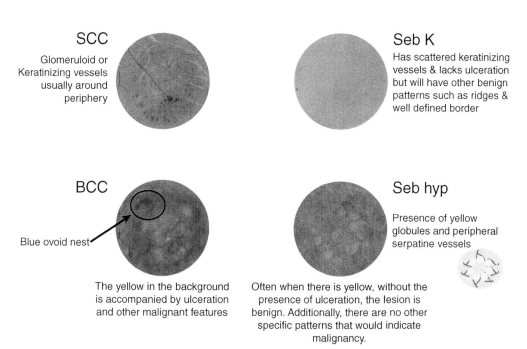

SCC
Glomeruloid or Keratinizing vessels usually around periphery

Seb K
Has scattered keratinizing vessels & lacks ulceration but will have other benign patterns such as ridges & well defined border

BCC
Blue ovoid nest
The yellow in the background is accompanied by ulceration and other malignant features

Seb hyp
Presence of yellow globules and peripheral serpatine vessels
Often when there is yellow, without the presence of ulceration, the lesion is benign. Additionally, there are no other specific patterns that would indicate malignancy.

FIGURE 3.14 When not associated with an ulceration, and when diffuse throughout the lesion, the color yellow indicates a benign lesion.

KEY POINTS

At this point, we want to bring up some critical reminders—when you get to pattern assessment, **do not lose the forest through the trees!**

1. Remember our goal is simply to determine between malignant or benign. As Figure 3.15 demonstrates, you do not need to differentiate between two malignant patterns. Knowing whether this is a SCC or amelanotic melanoma will not change the outcome—you will biopsy both of the lesions.

2. Do not forget the clinical history! As Figure 3.16 demonstrates, the pattern of a Spitz nevus and dermatofibroma may look alike; however, the clinical history and age of the patient will be the determining factor. Spitz nevi are often monitored in young patients.

3. There **will be lesions that stump you,** particularly benign elevated lesions that have become irritated. For example, in Figure 3.17, the irritation of these elevated lesions makes it difficult to differentiate malignant vascular patterns from benign. **Further, if no external cause is obvious, there can be a precancer or skin cancer causing the irritation. Sometimes, benign irritated seborrheic keratosis or lichen planus–like keratoses are benign and need to be biopsied.**

4. Finally, some lesions are too clinically obvious, are too thick or hyperkeratotic, and cannot be evaluated dermoscopically and therefore need to be biopsied. Figure 3.18 is an example of such a lesion. The dermatoscope is unable to visualize through the thick crust and therefore is not of use in such a situation.

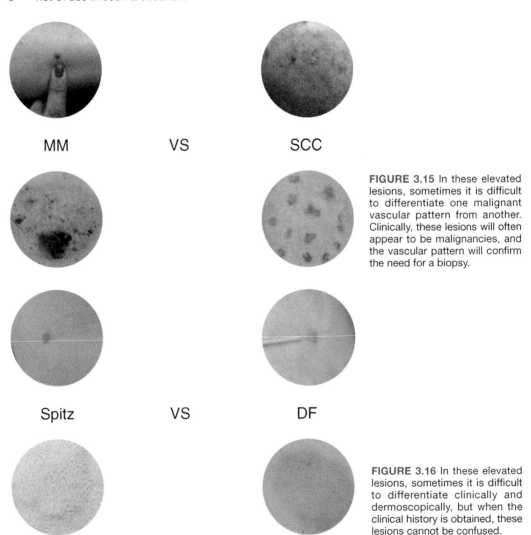

MM   VS   SCC

FIGURE 3.15 In these elevated lesions, sometimes it is difficult to differentiate one malignant vascular pattern from another. Clinically, these lesions will often appear to be malignancies, and the vascular pattern will confirm the need for a biopsy.

Spitz   VS   DF

FIGURE 3.16 In these elevated lesions, sometimes it is difficult to differentiate clinically and dermoscopically, but when the clinical history is obtained, these lesions cannot be confused.

MM 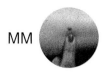   ISK

SCC 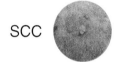 SCC

FIGURE 3.17 In these elevated lesions, sometimes it is difficult to differentiate malignant vascular patterns from benign. Irritated lesions may also appear malignant and often there can be a precancer or skin cancer causing the irritation. Sometimes benign irritated seborrheic keratosis or lichen planus–like keratosis are benign and need to be biopsied.

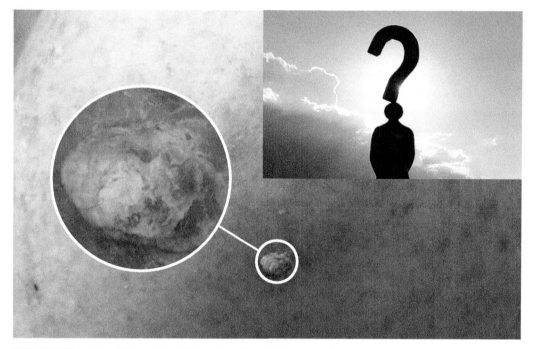

FIGURE 3.18 Lesions that are too thick or hyperkeratotic to show dermoscopy cannot be evaluated dermoscopically and therefore need to be biopsied. (Inset by Marco Bellucci; https://creativecommons.org/licenses/by/4.0/)

Reference

1. Grob JJ, Bonerandi JJ. The 'ugly duckling' sign: identification of the common characteristics of nevi in an individual as a basis for melanoma screening. *Arch Dermatol.* 1998;134(1):103–104.

Chapter 4 Flat/Pink-Clear/Red

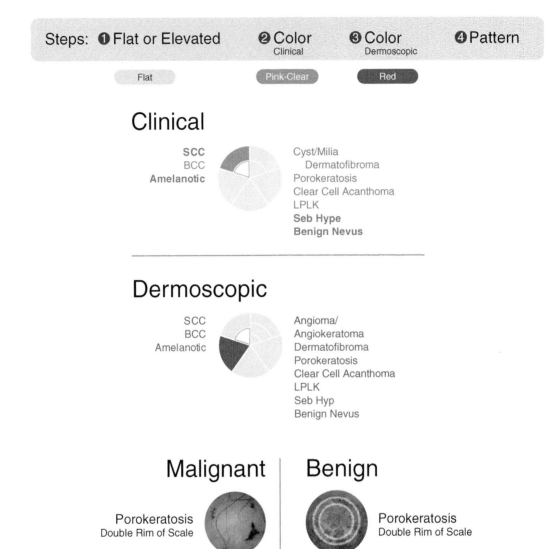

Steps: ❶ Flat or Elevated ❷ Color Clinical ❸ Color Dermoscopic ❹ Pattern

Flat   Pink-Clear   Red

Clinical

SCC
BCC
Amelanotic

Cyst/Milia
Dermatofibroma
Porokeratosis
Clear Cell Acanthoma
LPLK
Seb Hype
Benign Nevus

Dermoscopic

SCC
BCC
Amelanotic

Angioma/
Angiokeratoma
Dermatofibroma
Porokeratosis
Clear Cell Acanthoma
LPLK
Seb Hyp
Benign Nevus

Malignant

Porokeratosis
Double Rim of Scale

Superficial SCC
Dotted/Glomeruloid Vessels

Superficial BCC
Arborized Vessels & Pink-White

Benign

Porokeratosis
Double Rim of Scale

Clear Cell Acanthoma
Serpiginous String of Pearls

LPLK/ISK
Nonspecific Inflammation

FIGURE 4.1 Color wheel: flat/pink-clear/red.

Step 1: Is the lesion is flat or raised? **Flat**

Step 2: What color is the lesion on clinical assessment? **Pink/Clear**

Step 3: What is the dermoscopic color? **Red**

Step 4: Is further elucidation needed to decide whether to biopsy or not? **Yes**
Is this a malignant or benign pattern?

Take a look at the color wheel in Figure 4.1.
   Using the color wheel in Figure 4.1, we cross-reference the clinical and dermoscopic lists:
- Malignancies: squamous cell carcinoma (SCC), basal cell carcinoma (BCC), +/− porokeratosis
- Benign: benign porokeratosis, clear cell acanthoma, or lichen planus–like keratosis/irritated seborrheic keratosis, +/− porokeratosis

   Keep in mind that we are only considering *flat* lesions here, so dermatofibroma and intradermal nevi are not considered!

Benign Lesions

Porokeratosis

Pearls

- Flat/Pink-Clear/Red
  - A clinically and dermoscopically evident double rim of scale represents the cornea lamella on pathology.
  - While these lesions are considered benign, and do not change over time, squamous cell skin cancer can grow *within* these lesions; therefore, the lesions are usually treated/biopsied.
- **Step 4 Pattern:** On dermoscopy, a double rim of scale is visible, and if the lesion is not too thick, you can see a vascular pattern.
  - Diffuse dotted vessels
- **Bottom line: Benign, biopsy not necessary.**

Examples
Figure 4.2 shows a clinically flat, pink or skin-colored lesion with a dermoscopic red, vascular pattern. A double-rimmed scale is also evident. Diagnosis: Porokeratosis.
   Bottom line: Benign, biopsy not necessary.
   Figure 4.3 shows a clinically flat, pink or skin-colored lesion with a dermoscopic red, vascular pattern. A double-rimmed scale is also evident. The diffuse dotted vascular pattern is shown here. Diagnosis: Porokeratosis.
   Bottom line: Benign, biopsy not necessary.
   Figure 4.4 shows a clinically flat, pink/skin-colored lesion with a less obvious red/vascular pattern on dermoscopy. The double-rimmed scale is evident. Diagnosis: Porokeratosis.
   Bottom line: Benign, biopsy not necessary.

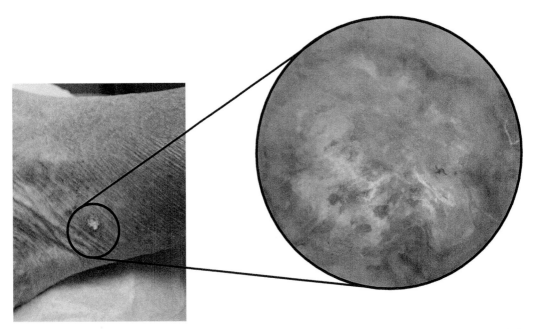

FIGURE 4.2 Clinically flat lesions that are pink or skin-colored with a vascular dermoscopic pattern. These clinical and dermoscopic examples of porokeratosis show a double-rimmed scale on dermoscopy.

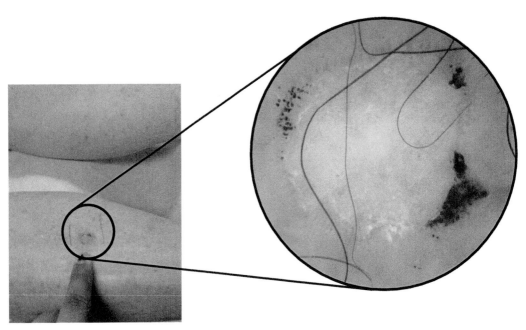

FIGURE 4.3 Clinically flat lesions that are pink or skin-colored with a vascular dermoscopic pattern. These clinical and dermoscopic examples of porokeratosis show a double-rimmed scale on dermoscopy.

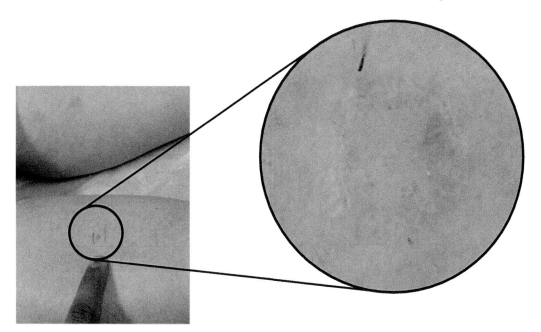

FIGURE 4.4 Clinically flat lesions that are pink or skin-colored with a vascular dermoscopic pattern. These clinical and dermoscopic examples of porokeratosis show a double-rimmed scale on dermoscopy.

Lichen Planus–Like Keratosis or Benign Lichenoid

Pearls

- Flat/Pink-Clear/Red
  - These lesions are often difficult to differentiate from malignant melanoma and nonmelanoma cancers.
- **Step 4 Pattern:** We will use the patterns described in Chapter 1 to look for benign features: sharp borders, moth-eaten borders, fingerprint patterns, milia-like cysts, comedo-like openings, and ridges.
  - These lesions are either solar lentigines undergoing regression or an inflammatory reaction or a seborrheic keratosis undergoing regression or inflammatory reaction.
  - The inflammatory nature of these lesions leads to a nonspecific vascular pattern.
- **Bottom line: Benign, biopsy not necessary.**

Examples

Figure 4.5 shows a clinically flat, pink lesion, with a faint red vascular dermoscopic pattern. The nonspecific inflammatory vascular pattern causes a crystalline, scar-like center and a faint peripheral pseudonetwork pattern. Diagnosis: Lichen planus–like keratosis.

Bottom line: Benign, biopsy not necessary.

Figure 4.6 shows clinically flat, pink lesions with nonspecific inflammation causing faint red vascular dermoscopic pattern. Diagnosis: Lichen planus–like keratosis.

Bottom line: Benign, biopsy not necessary.

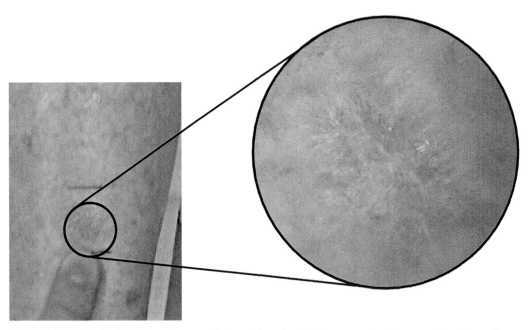

FIGURE 4.5 Clinically flat lesions that are pink or skin-colored with a vascular dermoscopic pattern. These clinical and dermoscopic examples of lichen planus–like keratosis show an inflammatory nonspecific vascular pattern, a crystalline scar-like center, and a faint peripheral pseudonetwork pattern.

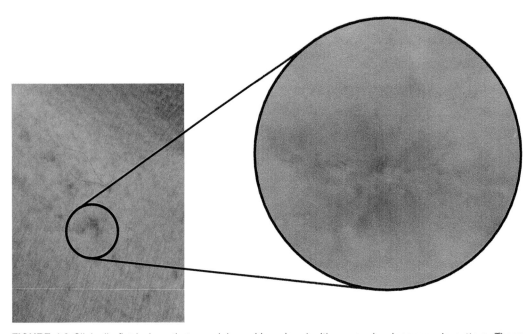

FIGURE 4.6 Clinically flat lesions that are pink or skin-colored with a vascular dermoscopic pattern. These clinical and dermoscopic examples of lichen planus–like keratosis show an inflammatory nonspecific vascular pattern.

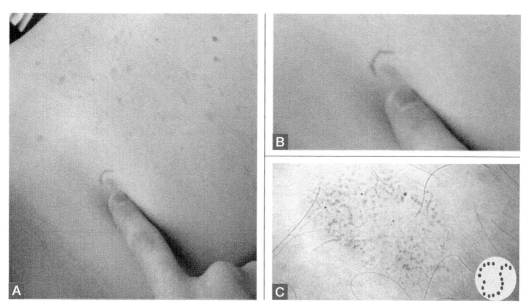

FIGURE 4.7 Clinically flat lesions that are pink or skin-colored with a vascular dermoscopic pattern. **A,B:** Clinical examples of clear cell acanthoma. **C:** A dermoscopic image of this lesion, showing a serpiginous, string-of-pearls-like pattern of vessels.

Clear Cell Acanthoma

Pearls

- Flat/Pink-Clear/Red
  - Can be flat or elevated
- **Step 4 Pattern:** Serpiginous patterns of diffuse red dots on dermoscopy
  - Often unnecessarily biopsied
- **Bottom line: Benign, biopsy not necessary.**

Example

Figure 4.7 shows a clinically flat, pink or skin-colored lesion with a dermoscopic red, vascular pattern. The dermoscopic image (Figure 4.7C) clearly demonstrates the hallmark serpiginous "string-of-pearls" pattern of vessels. Diagnosis: Clear cell acanthoma.

   Bottom line: Benign, biopsy not necessary.

Malignant Lesions

Squamous Cell Skin Cancer

Pearls

- Flat/Pink-Clear/Red
  - SCCs in this category are nonpigmented and superficial
- **Step 4 Pattern:** Don't forget your SCC patterns from Chapter 1! As a reminder, Figure 4.8 illustrates the classical SCC patterns.
  - Pink-white shiny area
  - White reflective scaly surface

(Continued)

- Ulceration
- Dotted vessels
- Glomeruloid/coiled vessels
- Keratinizing vessels
- Remember that the glomeruloid or dotted vessels can be seen in psoriasis and psoriasiform dermatitis, so don't forget to consider the clinical history!
- **Malignant** = Biopsy is necessary

Examples

Figure 4.9 shows a clinically flat, pink or skin-colored lesion with a dermoscopic red, vascular pattern. The dermoscopic image (Figure 4.9C) demonstrates the glomeruloid and dotted vessel pattern of an SCC. Diagnosis: Squamous cell skin cancer.

Bottom line: Potentially malignant, biopsy!

Figure 4.10 shows a clinically flat, pink or skin-colored lesion with a dermoscopic red, vascular pattern. The dermoscopic image (Figure 4.10C) demonstrates the glomeruloid and dotted vessel pattern of an SCC. Diagnosis: Squamous cell skin cancer.

Bottom line: Potentially malignant, biopsy!

Figure 4.11 shows a clinically flat, pink or skin-colored lesion with a dermoscopic red, vascular pattern. The dermoscopic image (Figure 4.11C) demonstrates the glomeruloid and dotted vessel pattern of an SCC. This is additionally a facial lesion with the class pink-white shiny area and white reflective scaly surface. Diagnosis: Squamous cell skin cancer.

Bottom line: Potentially malignant, biopsy!

Patterns of Squamous Cell Skin Cancer

Pink-White
Shiny Area

White Reflective
Scaly Surface

Ulceration

Vascular

Dotted
Vessels

Glomeruloid/
Coiled Vessels

Keratinizing
Vessels

FIGURE 4.8 Illustrations of nonpigmented squamous skin cancer patterns.

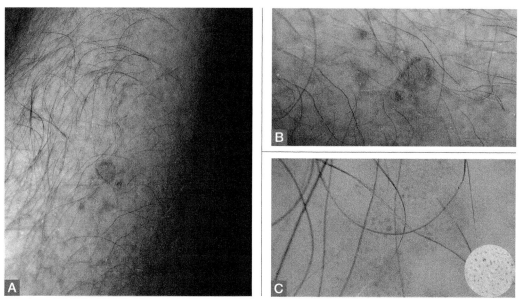

FIGURE 4.9 Clinically flat lesions that are pink or skin-colored with a vascular dermoscopic pattern. **A,B:** Clinical images of squamous cell skin cancer. **C:** The dermoscopic image of this lesion shows the glomeruloid/dotted vessels. This pattern can be seen in psoriasis and psoriasiform dermatitis; therefore, the clinical context of these lesions will be needed.

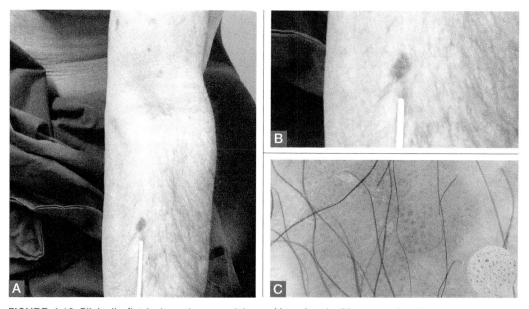

FIGURE 4.10 Clinically flat lesions that are pink or skin-colored with a vascular dermoscopic pattern. **A,B:** Clinical images of squamous cell skin cancer. **C:** The dermoscopic image of this lesion shows the glomeruloid/dotted vessels. This pattern can be seen in psoriasis and psoriasiform dermatitis; therefore, the clinical context of these lesions will be needed.

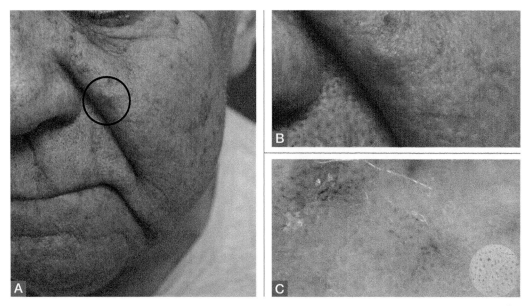

FIGURE 4.11 Clinically flat lesions that are pink or skin-colored with a vascular dermoscopic pattern. **A,B:** Clinical images of squamous cell skin cancer. **C:** The dermoscopic image of this lesion shows the glomeruloid/dotted vessels. This pattern can be seen in psoriasis and psoriasiform dermatitis; therefore, the clinical context of these lesions will be needed. This example is on a facial lesion and also has white hyperreflective scale.

Basal Cell Carcinoma

Pearls

- Flat/Pink-Clear/Red
  - BCCs at this stage will be superficial
- **Step 4 Pattern:** Don't forget your BCC patterns from Chapter 1! As a reminder, Figure 4.12 illustrates the classical BCC patterns.
  - Absence of pigmented network
  - Leaf-like structures
  - Large blue great ovoid nests or globular-like structures
  - Arborizing telangiectasias (sharply defined)
  - Spoke wheel areas
  - Ulceration
  - Pink-white to white-shiny areas
  - Crystalline pattern
- Leaf-like structures, large blue-gray ovoid nests or globular structures, and spoke wheel areas are typically seen in pigmented basal cells, so will not be seen here.
- **Malignant** = Biopsy is necessary

Examples

Figures 4.13 and 4.14 show a clinically flat, pink or skin-colored lesion with a dermoscopic red, vascular pattern. The dermoscopic image (Figure 4.14) demonstrates the thin, sharp arborizing telangiectasias specific for BCC. Additionally, there is an absence of any pigmented network. Diagnosis: Basal cell carcinoma.

Bottom line: Potentially malignant, biopsy!

Figure 4.15 shows a clinically flat, pink or skin-colored lesion with a dermoscopic red, vascular pattern. The dermoscopic image (Figure 4.15C) demonstrates the thin, sharp arborizing telangiectasias specific for BCC. Additionally, there is an absence of any pigmented network. Diagnosis: Basal cell carcinoma.

Bottom line: Potentially malignant, biopsy!

Patterns of Basal Cell Skin Cancer

Absence of
Pigmented
Network

Leaf-like
Structures

Large Blue-Gray
Ovoid Nests
or Globular-like
Structures

Arborizing
(tree-like)
Telengectasias
(sharp)

Spoke Wheel
Areas

Ulceration

Pink-White to
White Shiny
Areas

Crystalline
Pattern

FIGURE 4.12 Illustrations of basal cell skin cancer patterns.

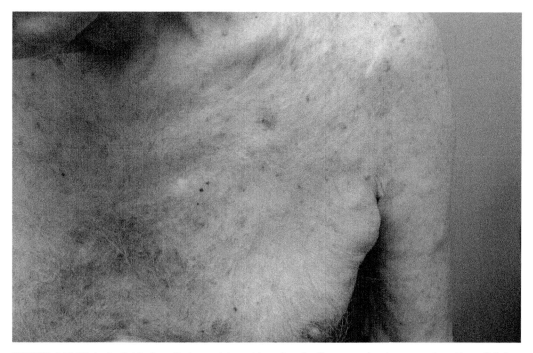

FIGURE 4.13 Clinically flat lesions that are pink or skin-colored with a vascular dermoscopic pattern. This is a clinical example of basal cell skin cancer.

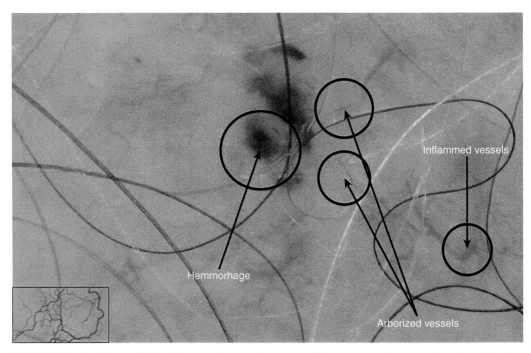

FIGURE 4.14 Clinically flat lesions that are pink or skin-colored with a vascular dermoscopic pattern. The dermoscopic example of the basal cell skin cancer seen in Figure 4.13 demonstrates different vascular patterns that are not specific to BCC, in addition to the specific pattern of arborized vessels.

Figure 4.16 shows a clinically flat, pink or skin-colored lesion with a dermoscopic red, vascular pattern. The dermoscopic image (Figure 4.16C) demonstrates the thin, sharp arborizing telangiectasias specific for BCC. Additionally, there is an absence of any pigmented network. Diagnosis: Basal cell carcinoma.

Bottom line: Potentially malignant, biopsy.

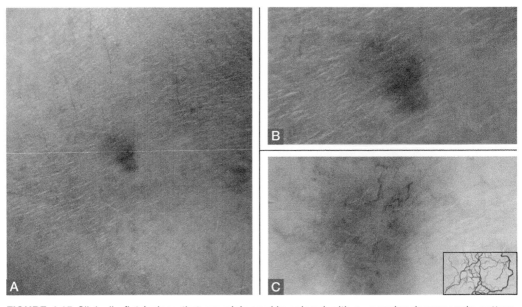

FIGURE 4.15 Clinically flat lesions that are pink or skin-colored with a vascular dermoscopic pattern. **A,B:** Clinical images of squamous cell skin cancer. **C:** The dermoscopic image shows the arborized vessels.

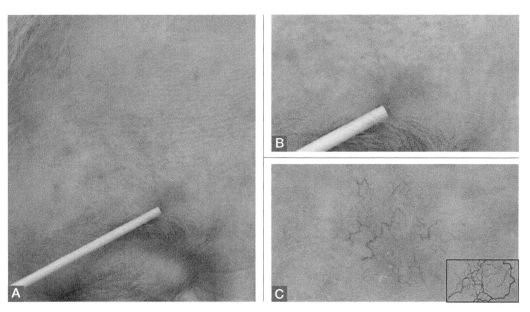

FIGURE 4.16 Clinically flat lesions that are pink or skin-colored with a vascular dermoscopic pattern. **A,B:** Clinical images of squamous cell skin cancer. **C:** The dermoscopic image shows the arborized vessels.

Figure 4.17 shows a clinically flat, pink or skin-colored lesion with a dermoscopic red, vascular pattern. The dermoscopic image (Figure 4.17C) demonstrates the thin, sharp arborizing telangiectasias specific for BCC. Additionally, there is an absence of any pigmented network; this is a clear example of the pink-white shiny areas. Diagnosis: Basal cell carcinoma.

Bottom line: Potentially malignant, biopsy.

Figure 4.18 shows a clinically flat, pink or skin-colored lesion with a dermoscopic red, vascular pattern. The dermoscopic image (Figure 4.18C) demonstrates the thin, sharp arborizing

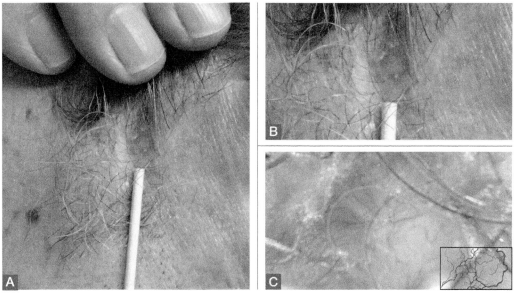

FIGURE 4.17 Clinically flat lesions that are pink or skin-colored with a vascular dermoscopic pattern. **A,B:** Clinical images of squamous cell skin cancer. **C:** The dermoscopic image shows the arborized vessels.

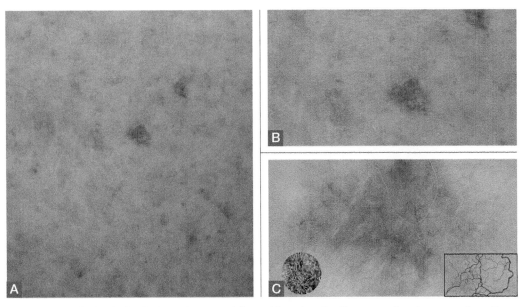

FIGURE 4.18 Clinically flat lesions that are pink or skin-colored with a vascular dermoscopic pattern. **A,B:** Clinical images of squamous cell skin cancer. **C:** The dermoscopic image shows the arborized vessels. Note the crystalline, scar-like pattern.

telangiectasias specific for BCC. Additionally, there is a faint crystalline pattern running through the lesion with an absence of any pigmented network. Diagnosis: Basal cell carcinoma.

Bottom line: Potentially malignant, biopsy.

Figure 4.19 shows a clinically flat, pink or skin-colored lesion with a dermoscopic red, vascular pattern. The dermoscopic image (Figure 4.19C) demonstrates the thin, sharp arborizing telangiectasias specific for BCC. Additionally, there is a faint crystalline pattern running through the lesion with an absence of any pigmented network. Diagnosis: Basal cell carcinoma.

Bottom line: Potentially malignant, biopsy.

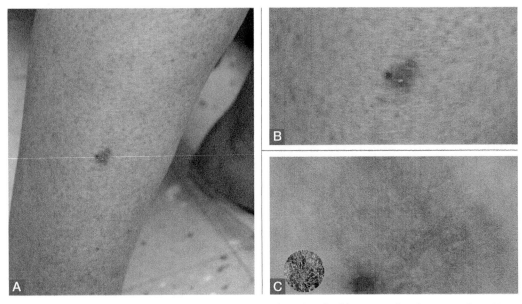

FIGURE 4.19 Clinically flat lesions that are pink or skin-colored with a vascular dermoscopic pattern. **A,B:** Clinical images of squamous cell skin cancer. **C:** The dermoscopic image shows the arborized vessels. Note the crystalline, scar-like pattern.

Chapter 5 Elevated/Pink-Clear/Red

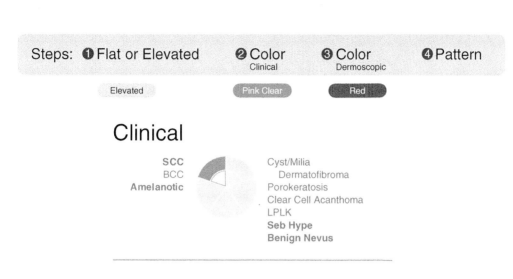

Steps: ❶ Flat or Elevated ❷ Color *Clinical* ❸ Color *Dermoscopic* ❹ Pattern

Elevated | Pink Clear | Red

Clinical

SCC
BCC
Amelanotic

Cyst/Milia
Dermatofibroma
Porokeratosis
Clear Cell Acanthoma
LPLK
Seb Hype
Benign Nevus

Dermoscopic

SCC
BCC
Amelanotic

Angioma/Angiokeratoma
Dermatofibroma
Porokeratosis
Clear Cell Acanthoma
LPLK
Seb Hype
Benign Nevus

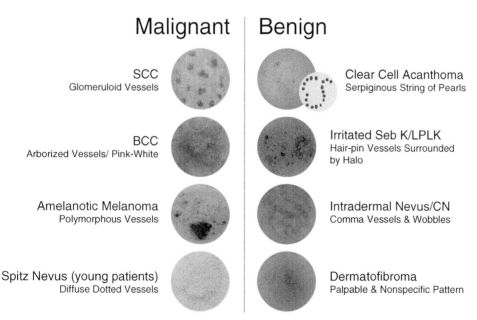

Malignant | Benign

SCC
Glomeruloid Vessels

Clear Cell Acanthoma
Serpiginous String of Pearls

BCC
Arborized Vessels/ Pink-White

Irritated Seb K/LPLK
Hair-pin Vessels Surrounded by Halo

Amelanotic Melanoma
Polymorphous Vessels

Intradermal Nevus/CN
Comma Vessels & Wobbles

Spitz Nevus (young patients)
Diffuse Dotted Vessels

Dermatofibroma
Palpable & Nonspecific Pattern

FIGURE 5.1 Color wheel: elevated/pink-clear/red.

Step 1: Is the lesion flat or raised? **Elevated**

Step 2: What color is the lesion on clinical assessment? **Pink/Clear**

Step 3: What is the dermoscopic color? **Red**

Step 4: Is further elucidation needed to decide whether to biopsy or not? **Yes**

Is this a malignant or benign pattern?

Take a look at the color wheel in Figure 5.1.

Using the color wheel in Figure 5.1, cross-reference the Clinical and Dermoscopic lists:
- Malignancies: Squamous cell carcinoma (SCC), basal cell carcinoma (BCC), amelanotic melanoma, Spitz nevus.
- Benign: Clear cell acanthoma, lichen planus–like keratosis/irritated seborrheic keratosis, intradermal/congenital nevus, and dermatofibroma.

When considering *elevated* lesions, this means that amelanotic melanomas, Spitz nevi, dermatofibroma, and intradermal nevi have entered the differential. There will be similar patterns to the flat lesions, but the elevation alone brings in a new set of lesions to consider.

Again, I want to stress the importance of a good clinical history; these new lesions should be clinically suspicious as well.

Benign Lesions

Intradermal Nevi (IN)/Congenital Nevi (CN)

Pearls
- Elevated/Pink-Clear/Red
  - Skin-colored papules that patients will have had for a long time; sometimes flat lesions can become neurotized or three dimensional, and patients may believe that they are new.
  - When IN or CNs are on the face, they can become irritated, making them clinically difficult to differentiate from BCCs.
  - Wobble: When moved, these lesions wobble back and forth.
- **Step 4 Pattern:** You may see some benign patterns such as coma-like vessels, faint pigmentation, or milia-like cysts. However, more importantly, you'll see a lack of the malignant features we covered in our patterns chapter of melanoma, SCC, or BCC.
- **Bottom line: Benign, biopsy is not necessary.**

Examples

Figure 5.2 shows the classic clinical (Figure 5.2A, B) and dermoscopic (Figure 5.2C) findings of an IN on the neck. We can clearly see the elevated, pink/fleshy-colored, "wobbly" looking lesion clinically. Dermoscopically, we see red comma-like vessels with no malignant patterns on dermoscopy. Diagnosis: Intradermal nevi (IN)/congenital nevi (CN).

   Bottom line: Benign, biopsy not necessary.

Figure 5.3 shows another example of the clinical (Figure 5.3A, B) and dermoscopic (Figure 5.3C) presentation of an IN. This elevated, pink/fleshy, protruding, wobbly lesion on the trunk shows no signs of malignancy, either clinically or dermoscopically. Again, we can see red comma-like vessels on dermoscopy. Diagnosis: Intradermal nevi (IN)/congenital nevi (CN).

   Bottom line: Benign, biopsy not necessary.

Figure 5.4 clearly depicts IN. They are elevated, fleshy/pink wobbly lesions clinically, with red comma-like vessels dermoscopically. Diagnosis: Intradermal nevi (IN)/congenital nevi (CN).

   Bottom line: Benign, biopsy not necessary.

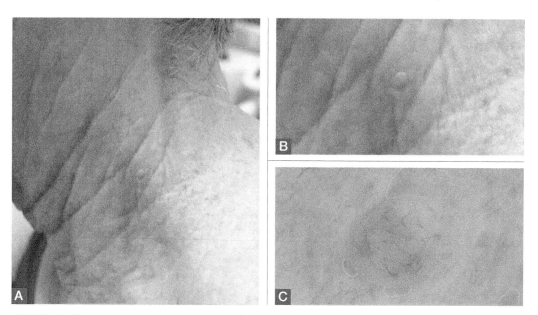

FIGURE 5.2 Clinically elevated lesions that are pink or skin-colored with a vascular/red dermoscopic pattern. **A** and **B** show a clinical example of an intradermal nevus. **C:** Dermoscopically, comma-like vessels are seen. Intradermal nevi wobble when moved back and forth with a contact dermatoscope.

Figure 5.5 shows clinically elevated, pink/skin-colored lesions with a red vascular dermoscopic pattern. Based on the clinical picture and dermoscopic finding, we are assured that this is an intradermal lesion with no malignant features, but rather, benign comma-like vessels on dermoscopy. Sometimes, you may see milia-like cysts and faint pigmentation, which are other benign features that we see here. Diagnosis: Intradermal nevi (IN)/congenital nevi (CN).

Bottom line: Benign, biopsy not necessary.

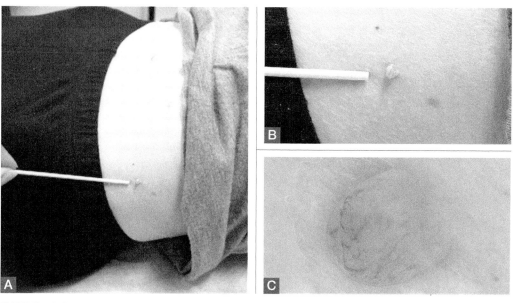

FIGURE 5.3 Clinically elevated lesions that are pink or skin-colored with a vascular/red dermoscopic pattern. **A** and **B** show a clinical example of an intradermal nevus. **C:** Dermoscopically, comma-like vessels are seen. Intradermal nevi wobble when moved back and forth with a contact dermatoscope.

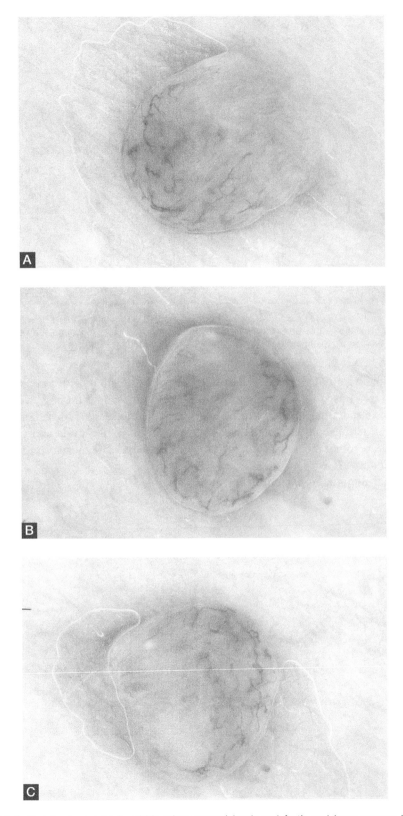

FIGURE 5.4 A–C: Intradermal nevi wobble when moved back and forth and have comma-like vessels. Sometimes you can see faint pigmentation.

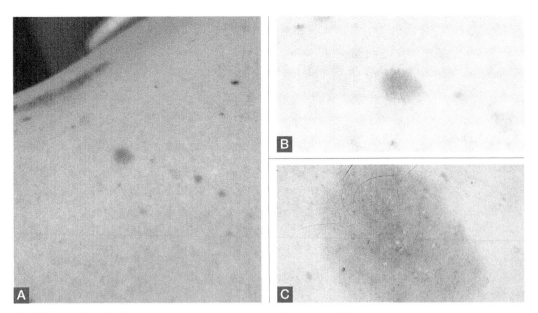

FIGURE 5.5 Clinically elevated lesions that are pink or skin-colored with a vascular/red dermoscopic pattern. **A** and **B** show a clinical example of a congenital nevus. **C:** The dermoscopic image shows comma-like vessels. Sometimes you see milia-like cysts and faint pigmentation.

Dermatofibroma

Pearls

- Elevated/Pink-Clear/Red
  - These raised and often palpable nodules can dimple on clinical exam.
  - Typically smooth and well circumscribed.
  - On dermoscopy, a faint pseudonetwork or fishnet-like network at the periphery of the lesion.
  - Sometimes, you can see diffuse dots, which you may recall can be seen in flat superficial squamous cells, but remember that dermatofibromas are elevated and palpable, whereas superficial SCCs are not.
  - These occur in an older patient population as a scar-like reaction, so you can sometimes see a scar-like pattern at the center of these lesions.
  - These can also show nonspecific inflammation on dermoscopy, but because they are elevated and firm/palpable, they are distinguished from malignant lesions.
- **Step 4 Pattern**: In some, you may see a scar-like pattern in the center with some faint pigmentation or a faint pseudonetwork at the periphery. Again, diffuse dots in these lesions are common and are not indicative of malignancy because of the elevation of the lesion. There is a lack of the malignant features we covered in our patterns chapter of melanoma, SCC, or BCC.
- **Bottom line: Benign, biopsy is not necessary.**

Examples

In Figure 5.6 we see a clinical and dermoscopic example of a dermatofibroma. We can see in parts Figure 5.6A and B that the lesion is elevated and pink; additionally, it will be firmly palpable. In part Figure 5.6C, we can see a nonspecific red vascular pattern/inflammation with a scar-like pattern at the center and faint pigmentation at the periphery of the lesion. Diagnosis: Dermatofibroma.

Bottom line: Benign, biopsy not necessary.

Figure 5.7 is another example of a clinically elevated, pink, and firmly palpable lesion. Dermoscopically, we see the nonspecific red inflammation, but again, we distinguish this from malignancy because this lesion is clinically elevated. Diagnosis: Dermatofibroma.

Bottom line: Benign, biopsy not necessary.

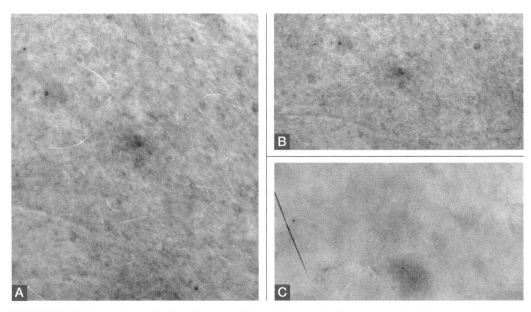

FIGURE 5.6 Clinically elevated lesions that are pink or skin-colored with a vascular/red dermoscopic pattern. **A,B:** Clinical examples of dermatofibromas. **C:** This dermoscopic image shows a nonspecific vascular pattern. Dermatofibromas are palpable and have a scar-like center, with a faint pigment or pseudonetwork at the periphery.

In Figure 5.8, we see an example of a dermatofibroma on the foot. Again, we see a clinically raised, pink lesion that will be firmly palpable. Dermoscopically, you can see faint pigmentation and a red diffuse dot pattern. This cannot be confused with flatter lesions with diffuse dots such as SCC or psoriasis because this lesion is elevated and palpable. Diagnosis: Dermatofibroma.

Bottom line: Benign, biopsy not necessary.

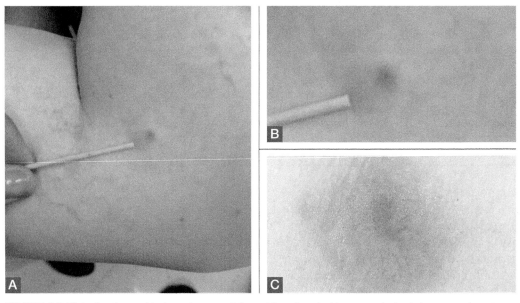

FIGURE 5.7 Clinically elevated lesions that are pink or skin-colored with a vascular/red dermoscopic pattern. **A,B:** Clinical examples of dermatofibromas. **C:** This dermoscopic image shows a nonspecific vascular pattern. Dermatofibromas are palpable.

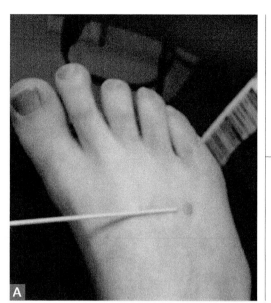
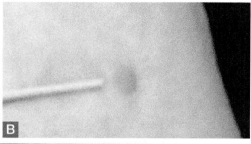

FIGURE 5.8 Clinically elevated lesions that are pink or skin-colored with a vascular/red dermoscopic pattern. **A,B:** Clinical examples of dermatofibromas. **C:** Dermoscopy shows diffuse red dots. Dermatofibromas are palpable and therefore should not be confused with flatter lesions that have diffuse red dots like SCC or psoriasis.

Clear Cell Acanthoma

Pearls

- Elevated/Pink-Clear/Red
  - These lesions are rarely diagnosed before biopsy, but are benign and can be distinguished from malignancy!
- **Step 4 Pattern**: Distinct serpiginous pattern of diffuse red dots on dermoscopy.
  - Can be either flat or elevated.
- **Bottom line: Benign, biopsy unnecessary.**

Example

In Figure 5.9, we see a clinically elevated and pink lesion. On dermoscopy, we see the classic red vascular pattern of a string of pearls. Diagnosis: Clear cell acanthoma.

Bottom line: Benign, biopsy not necessary.

Inflamed Seborrheic Keratosis

Pearls

- Elevated/Pink-Clear/Red.
  - These lesions are often difficult to differentiate from malignant melanoma and nonmelanoma cancers.
  - They can be either flat or elevated, as we saw in previous chapter.
- **Step 4 Pattern**: Use patterns from Chapter 1 to look for benign features: sharp borders, moth-eaten borders, fingerprint patterns, milia-like cysts, comedo-like openings, and ridges.
  - These lesions are either solar lentigines undergoing regression or inflammatory reaction OR a seborrheic keratosis undergoing regression or inflammatory reaction.
  - The inflammatory nature of these lesions leads to a nonspecific vascular pattern.
- **Bottom line: Benign, biopsy not necessary.**

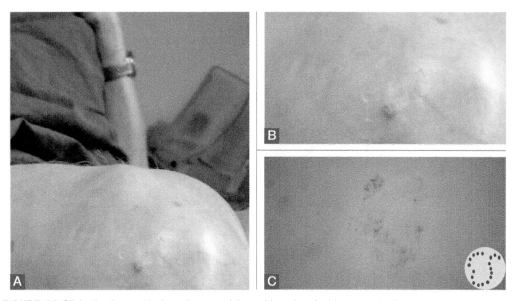

FIGURE 5.9 Clinically elevated lesions that are pink or skin-colored with a vascular/red dermoscopic pattern. **A,B:** Clinical examples of clear cell acanthoma. **C:** Dermoscopy shows a dotted vessel pattern that is serpiginous, like a string of pearls.

Examples

Figure 5.10 shows a dermoscopic image of an inflamed seborrheic keratosis. This lesion would have been clinically elevated and pink/flesh-colored. It may be difficult to pick out specific features of this lesion because of the inflammation, but you can identify looped-hairpin vessels,

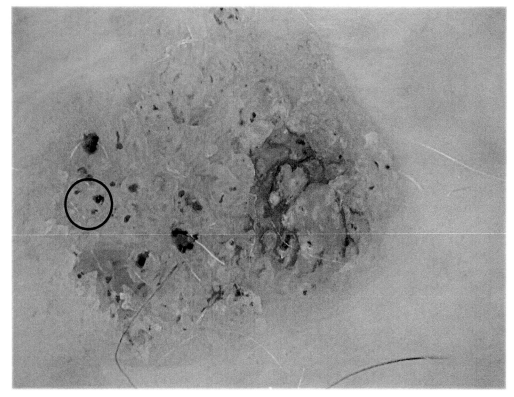

FIGURE 5.10 Clinically elevated lesions that are pink or skin-colored with a vascular/red dermoscopic pattern. Irritated seborrheic keratoses have hairpin-like vessels at the center of a white halo.

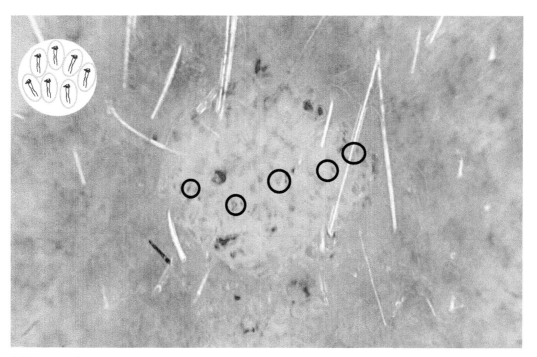

FIGURE 5.11 Clinically elevated lesions that are pink or skin-colored with a vascular/red dermoscopic pattern. Irritated seborrheic keratoses have hairpin-like vessels at the center of a white halo.

as well as vessels surrounded by a white halo. These are indicative of an inflamed seborrheic keratosis. Diagnosis: Inflamed seborrheic keratosis.

Bottom line: Benign, biopsy not necessary.

Figure 5.11 shows another dermoscopic example of an inflamed seborrheic keratosis. This lesion would have been clinically elevated and pink. Here, we can see multiple looped or hairpin red vasculature at the center of white halos. Diagnosis: Inflamed seborrheic keratosis.

Bottom line: Benign, biopsy not necessary.

Figure 5.12 shows a clinical example of an elevated pink lesion on the patient's forehead. Dermoscopically, we can appreciate the red vascular looped hairpin vessels. Additionally, we

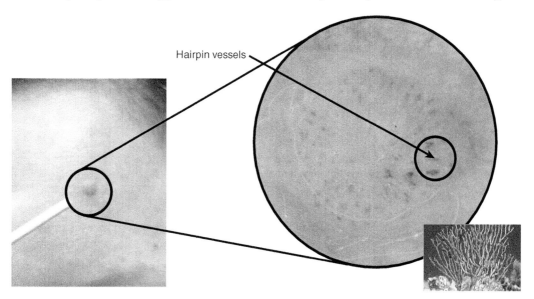

Hairpin vessels

FIGURE 5.12 Clinically elevated lesions that are pink or skin-colored with a vascular/red dermoscopic pattern. Irritated seborrheic keratoses have hairpin-like vessels at the center of a white halo.

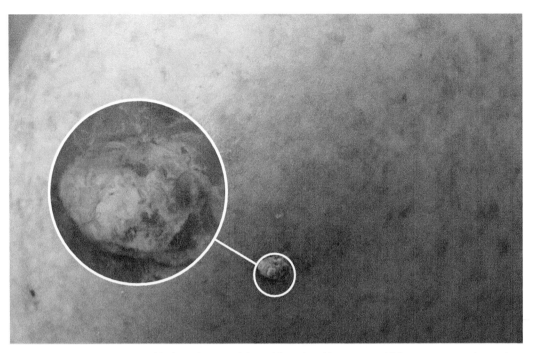

FIGURE 5.13 Clinically elevated lesions that are pink or skin-colored but are too thick to see a vascular pattern need to be biopsied, as you cannot tell if they are an irritated benign growth, like an irritated seborrheic keratosis, or a squamous cell skin cancer, or even amelanotic melanoma.

see another feature of seborrheic keratosis—ridges—like that of a coral reef along the periphery of the lesion. Diagnosis: Inflamed seborrheic keratosis.

Bottom line: Benign, biopsy not necessary.

***Note: If clinically elevated lesions that are pink or skin-colored are too thick to see a vascular pattern, you need to biopsy! You will not be able to determine if lesions like the one seen in Figure 5.13 is benign or malignant without a biopsy.**

Malignant Lesions

Amelanotic Melanoma

Pearls

- Elevated/Pink-Clear/Red
  - These are advanced lesions and will already be on your radar as clinically suspicious.
- **Step 4 Pattern**: Amelanotic melanomas are tricky, as they don't have any distinct features; rather they are typically characterized by polymorphous or erratic vasculature patterns.
- **Bottom line: Malignant, biopsy is necessary.**

Example

Figure 5.14 shows a clinically elevated and pink lesion that, on dermoscopy, has an erratic and polymorphous vasculature pattern. Diagnosis: Amelanotic melanoma.

Bottom line: Malignant, biopsy is necessary!

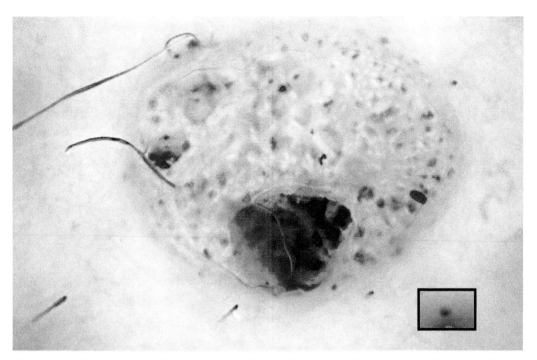

FIGURE 5.14 Clinically elevated lesions that are pink or skin-colored with a vascular/red dermoscopic pattern. Advanced amelanotic melanoma should be suspicious for biopsy clinically. Note the polymorphous/erratic vessels.

Nonpigmented Squamous Cell Skin Cancer

Pearls

- Elevated/Pink-Clear/Red
  - SCCs in this category are nonpigmented.
- **Step 4 Pattern**: Don't forget your SCC patterns from Chapter 1! Figure 5.15 illustrates the classic SCC patterns.
  - Pink-white shiny area
  - White reflective scaly surface
  - Ulceration
  - Dotted vessels
  - Glomeruloid/coiled vessels
  - Keratinizing vessels
- Remember that the glomeruloid or dotted vessels can be seen in psoriasis and psoriasiform dermatitis but cannot be confused with these benign lesions, as these will be elevated. Remember that dermatofibromas will be firmly palpable, whereas SCCs will not be.
- These will be clinically suspicious, because in order for SCCs to grow to an elevated level, they will have additional clinically suspicious findings, such as ulceration or crusting.
- **Bottom line: Malignant, biopsy is necessary!**

Examples

Figure 5.16 shows a clinical example of a nonpigmented SCC. We can see a clinically elevated, pink lesion with dermoscopy showing diffusely dotted vessels along with a central pink-white shiny area and reflective scaly surface—malignant features. Diagnosis: Nonpigmented squamous cell skin cancer.

   Bottom line: Malignant, biopsy is necessary!

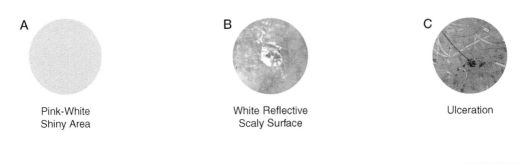

A
Pink-White
Shiny Area

B
White Reflective
Scaly Surface

C
Ulceration

Vascular

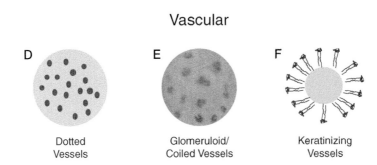

D
Dotted
Vessels

E
Glomeruloid/
Coiled Vessels

F
Keratinizing
Vessels

FIGURE 5.15 Illustrations of nonpigmented squamous skin cancer patterns. Nonpigmented squamous cells are much more common than pigmented squamous cells.

Figure 5.17 shows another example of a clinically elevated, pink lesion with dermoscopic findings consistent with SCC including white, reflective scaly surface, dotted, and glomeruloid vessels—malignant features. Diagnosis: Nonpigmented squamous cell skin cancer.

Bottom line: Malignant, biopsy is necessary!

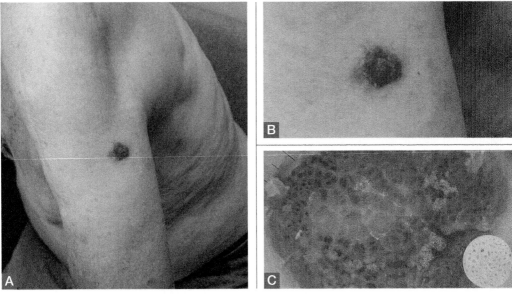

FIGURE 5.16 Clinically elevated lesions that are pink or skin-colored with a vascular dermoscopic pattern. **A,B:** Clinical examples of squamous cell skin cancer. **C:** Dermoscopy shows glomeruloid/dotted vessels. These elevated lesions are often clinically suspicious and are also less confused with other benign lesions, like psoriasis.

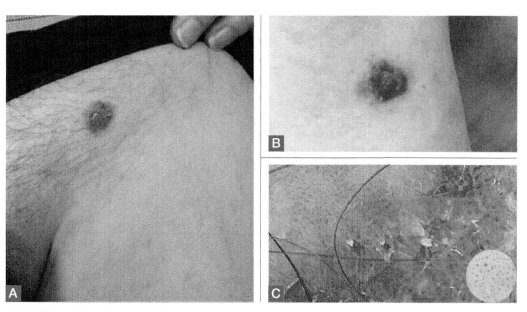

FIGURE 5.17 Clinically elevated lesions that are pink or skin-colored with a vascular dermoscopic pattern. **A,B:** Clinical examples of squamous cell skin cancer. **C:** Dermoscopy shows glomeruloid/dotted vessels. These elevated lesions are often clinically suspicious and are also less confused with other benign lesions, like psoriasis.

Figure 5.18 shows a clinically elevated, flesh-colored lesion with some visible crust. Dermoscopically, we see diffuse red dotted and glomeruloid vessels—malignant features. Again, this cannot be confused with dermatofibroma as it will not be firmly palpable, or with a benign lesion such as psoriasis, because it is elevated. Diagnosis: Nonpigmented squamous cell skin cancer.

Bottom line: Malignant, biopsy is necessary!

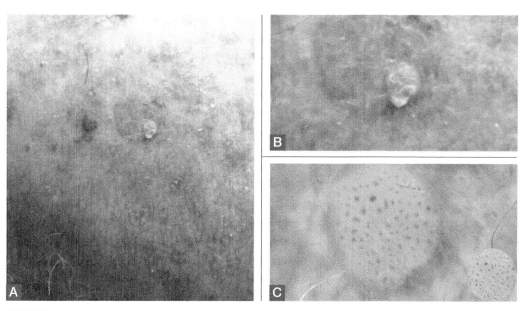

FIGURE 5.18 Clinically elevated lesions that are pink or skin-colored with a vascular dermoscopic pattern. **A,B:** Clinical examples of squamous cell skin cancer. **C:** Dermoscopy shows glomeruloid/dotted vessels. These elevated lesions are often clinically suspicious and are also less confused with other benign lesions, like psoriasis.

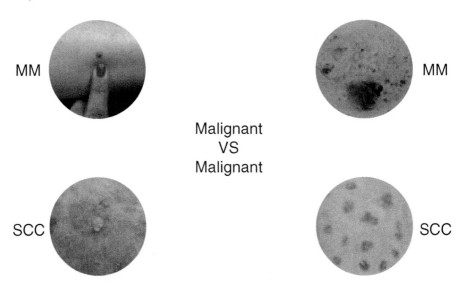

MM

MM

Malignant
VS
Malignant

SCC

SCC

FIGURE 5.19   Remember! You do not need to differentiate between two malignant patterns—knowing whether this is a SCC or a MM will not change the outcome. You will biopsy these lesions regardless.

> **KEY POINTS**
> Remember that your goal is not to distinguish between different malignancies—knowing whether the lesion is a SCC or a MM will not change your immediate outcome of biopsy. Rather, focus on distinguishing between benign and malignant. When dealing with elevated malignancies, it is critically important to remember the clinical picture. Elevated malignancies are by definition advanced lesions and will be clinically suspicious (Figure 5.19).

Basal Cell Carcinoma

Pearls

- Elevated/Pink-Clear/Red
- **Step 4 Pattern**: Don't forget your BCC patterns from Chapter 1! Figure 5.20 illustrates the classic BCC patterns.
  - Absence of pigmented network
  - Leaf-like structures
  - Large blue great ovoid nests or globular-like structures
  - Arborizing telangiectasias (sharply defined)
  - Spoke wheel areas
  - Ulceration
  - Pink-white to white-shiny areas
  - Crystalline pattern
- Remember that leaf-like structures, large blue-gray ovoid nests or globular structures, and spoke wheel areas are typically seen in pigmented basal cells and won't be seen here.
- **Bottom line: Malignant, biopsy is necessary.**

Examples

Figure 5.21A shows a clinically elevated, skin-colored lesion on the cheek. Figure 5.21B shows the dermoscopic image illustrating nonspecific vascular pattern as well as the specific sharp arborizing telangiectasias—a malignant feature. Diagnosis: Basal cell carcinoma.

   Bottom line: Malignant, biopsy is necessary!

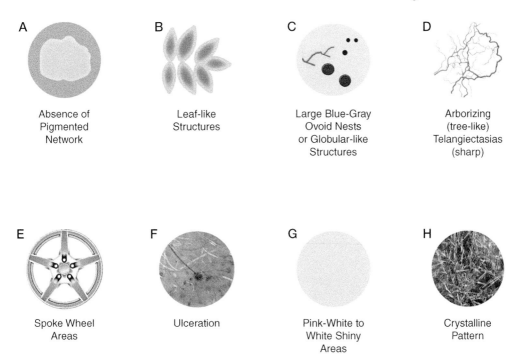

A — Absence of Pigmented Network

B — Leaf-like Structures

C — Large Blue-Gray Ovoid Nests or Globular-like Structures

D — Arborizing (tree-like) Telangiectasias (sharp)

E — Spoke Wheel Areas

F — Ulceration

G — Pink-White to White Shiny Areas

H — Crystalline Pattern

FIGURE 5.20 Illustrations of basal cell skin cancer patterns. Note that the features in **(B)**, **(C)**, and **(E)** are mainly seen in pigmented basal cell skin cancers.

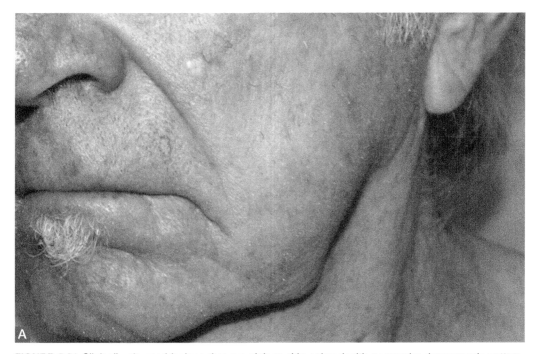

FIGURE 5.21 Clinically elevated lesions that are pink or skin-colored with a vascular dermoscopic pattern. **A:** Clinical example of basal cell skin cancer.

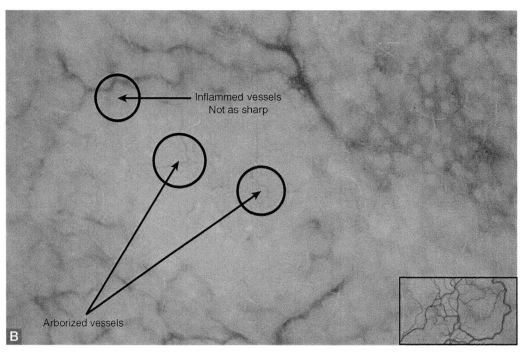

FIGURE 5.21 (*Continued*) **B:** The dermoscopic example of the basal cell skin cancer seen in Figure 5.20 demonstrating different vascular patterns that are not specific to BCC can also be seen in addition to the specific pattern of arborized vessels.

Figure 5.22 shows a clinically elevated, pink/skin-colored lesion with red vascular patterns seen dermoscopically. The lesion has a pink-white shiny background with sharp arborizing telangiectasias—malignant features. Diagnosis: Basal cell carcinoma.

Bottom line: Malignant, biopsy is necessary!

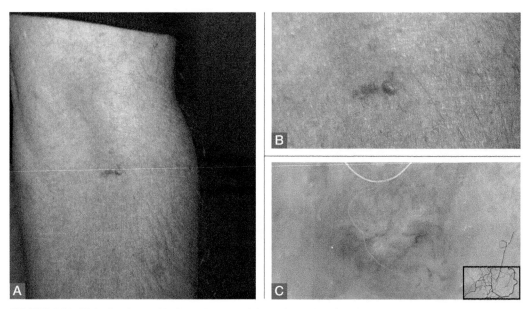

FIGURE 5.22 Clinically elevated lesions that are pink or skin-colored with a vascular dermoscopic pattern. **A, B:** Clinical examples of basal cell skin cancer. **C:** Dermoscopy shows arborized vessels. Note the pink-white shiny background

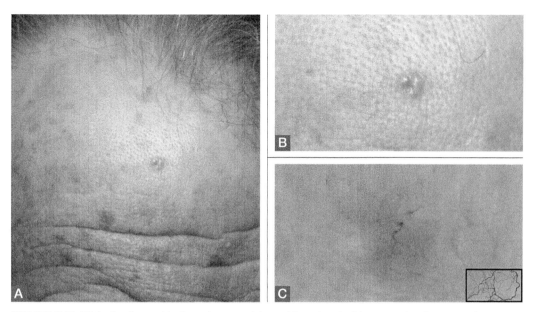

FIGURE 5.23 Clinically elevated lesions that are pink or skin-colored with a vascular dermoscopic pattern. **A, B:** Clinical examples of basal cell skin cancer. **C:** Dermoscopy shows arborized vessels. Note the pink-white shiny background

Figure 5.23 shows a clinically elevated, flesh-colored lesion, with red arborizing telangiectasias on dermoscopy—malignant features. Diagnosis: Basal cell carcinoma.

Bottom line: Malignant, biopsy is necessary!

Figure 5.24 shows a clinically elevated, flesh-colored lesion on the forehead with red colors on dermoscopy and malignant features. We see red, sharp arborizing telangiectasias on a white-shiny background and a crystalline scar-like pattern—a malignant feature. Diagnosis: Basal cell carcinoma.

Bottom line: Malignant, biopsy is necessary!

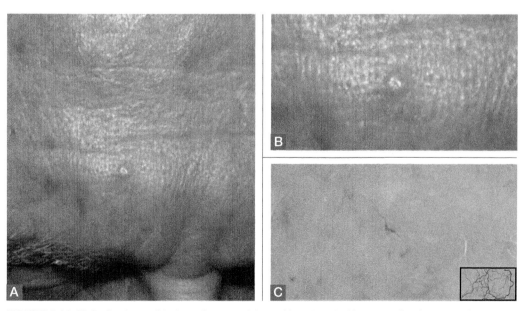

FIGURE 5.24 Clinically elevated lesions that are pink or skin-colored with a vascular dermoscopic pattern. **A, B:** Clinical examples of basal cell skin cancer. **C:** Dermoscopy shows arborized vessels. Note the pink-white shiny background

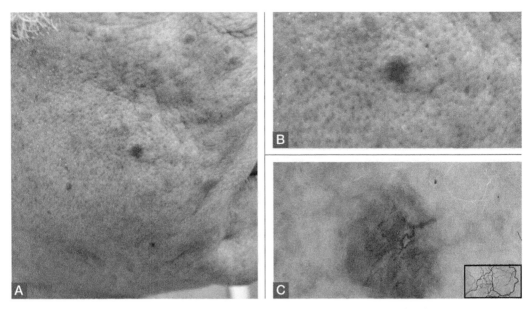

FIGURE 5.25 Clinically elevated lesions that are pink or skin-colored with a vascular dermoscopic pattern. **A, B:** Clinical examples of basal cell skin cancer. **C:** Dermoscopy shows arborized vessels. Note the pink-white shiny background

Figure 5.25 shows a clinically elevated, pink lesion with a red vascular dermoscopic pattern. You can see the arborizing telangiectasias—a malignant feature.

Bottom line: Malignant, biopsy is necessary!

Figure 5.26 shows a clinically elevated, pink lesion with a red vascular dermoscopic pattern. Again, we see the arborizing vessels on a pink-white shiny background. Diagnosis: Basal cell carcinoma.

Bottom line: Malignant, biopsy is necessary!

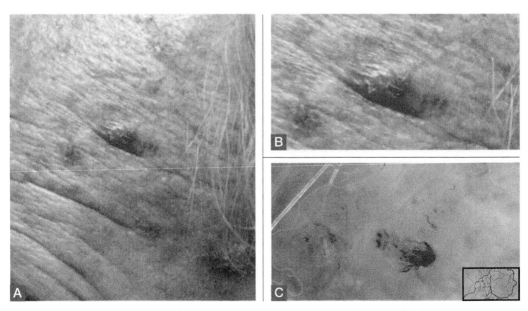

FIGURE 5.26 Clinically elevated lesions that are pink or skin-colored with a vascular dermoscopic pattern. **A, B:** Clinical examples of basal cell skin cancer. **C:** Dermoscopy shows arborized vessels. Note the pink-white shiny background

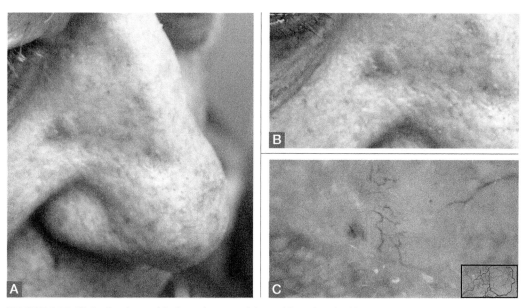

FIGURE 5.27 Clinically elevated lesions that are pink or skin-colored with a vascular dermoscopic pattern. **A, B:** Clinical examples of basal cell skin cancer. **C:** Dermoscopy shows arborized vessels. Note the pink-white shiny background

Figure 5.27 shows a clinically elevated, flesh-colored lesion on the nose with a red, vascular pattern on dermoscopy. We see arborizing telangiectasias, along with pink-white shiny areas indicative of BCC. Diagnosis: Basal cell carcinoma.

Bottom line: Malignant, biopsy is necessary!

Chapter 6 Flat/Pink-Clear/Multicolored

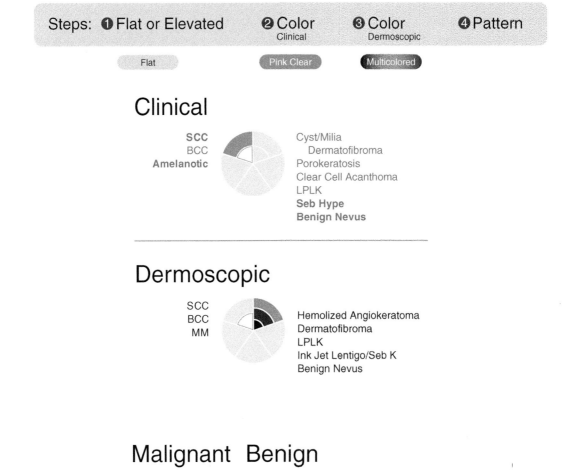

Steps: ❶ Flat or Elevated   ❷ Color
Clinical   ❸ Color
Dermoscopic   ❹ Pattern

Flat   Pink Clear   Multicolored

Clinical

SCC
BCC
Amelanotic

Cyst/Milia
Dermatofibroma
Porokeratosis
Clear Cell Acanthoma
LPLK
Seb Hype
Benign Nevus

Dermoscopic

SCC
BCC
MM

Hemolized Angiokeratoma
Dermatofibroma
LPLK
Ink Jet Lentigo/Seb K
Benign Nevus

Malignant Benign

Superficial SCC
Dotted Vessels & Ulceration

LPLK/Non pig Seb K
Nonspecific Vessels & Specific Brown

Superficial BCC
Ulceration & Arborized Vessels

CN
Faint Network, Symmetric, Comma
Vessels, Milia-like Cysts

Amelanotic Melanoma
Dotted Vessels &
Nonspecific Brown

DF
Faint Psuedo-Network at Periphery
Flat but Palpable

◯ moth-eaten border

FIGURE 6.1 Color wheel: flat/pink clear/multicolored.

Step 1: Is the lesion flat or raised? **Flat**

Step 2: What color is the lesion on clinical assessment? **Pink-Clear**

Step 3: What is the dermoscopic color? **Multicolored**—can include brown, yellow, or blue-gray, but not white.

Step 4: Is further elucidation needed to decide whether to biopsy or not? **Yes**

Is this a malignant or benign pattern?

Take a look at the color wheel in Figure 6.1.

Our differential is still very similar. Our malignant possibilities include superficial squamous cell carcinoma (SCC), superficial basal cell carcinoma (BCC), and amelanotic melanoma. Our benign lesions include lichen planus–like keratosis/nonpigmented seborrheic keratosis, congenital nevi, and flat-appearing dermatofibromas, which when touched will still be palpable.

Benign Lesions

Congenital Nevi

Pearls

- Flat/Pink-Clear/Multicolored
  - These will have been clinically present since childhood.
  - These are characteristically symmetrical lesions, especially at the periphery.
- **Step 4 Patterns:** Remember your benign patterns from Chapter 1. You can see all of the benign melanocytic patterns including reticular, globular/cobblestone, and homogenous. Less specific patterns include milia-like cysts and perifollicular hypopigmentation.
- **Bottom line: Benign, biopsy not necessary.**

Figure 6.2 shows a clinically flat, pink or skin-colored lesion with a multicolored (brown + pink) dermoscopic pattern. You can appreciate the symmetric pigmentation, especially at

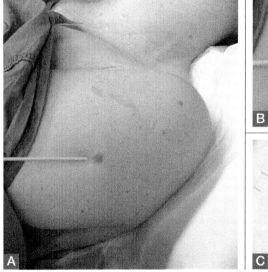
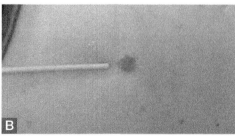

FIGURE 6.2 Clinically flat lesions that are pink or skin-colored, with a multicolored (brown + other = gray, pink, or yellow) dermoscopic pattern. **A,B:** Clinical examples of congenital nevi. **C:** Dermoscopy shows symmetric pigmentation with overall symmetry, especially at the periphery of the lesion.

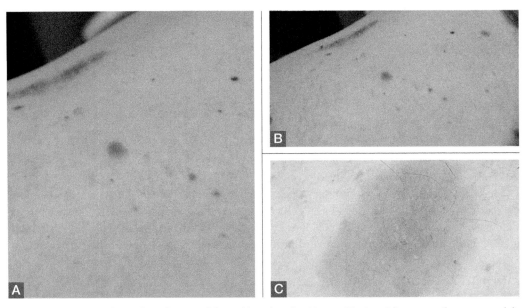

FIGURE 6.3 Clinically flat lesions that are pink or skin-colored, with a multicolored (brown + other = gray, pink, or yellow) dermoscopic pattern. **A,B:** Clinical examples of congenital nevi. **C:** Dermoscopy shows symmetric pigmentation with overall symmetry, especially at the periphery of the lesion. Note the benign milia-like cysts that can also be seen in other lesions, like BCCs Seb K's.

the periphery. There is a diffuse cobblestone pattern throughout with no malignant features. Diagnosis: Congenital nevi.

Bottom line: Benign, biopsy unnecessary.

Figure 6.3 shows a clinically flat, pink/skin-colored lesion with a multicolored (brown + pink) dermoscopic pattern. Again you can see symmetric pigmentation throughout and at the periphery of the lesion. Additionally, you can see milia-like cysts, a feature that can be seen in BCCs or seborrheic keratosis, but can be differentiated by remembering that we are dealing with flat lesions with multiple dermoscopic colors. Diagnosis: Congenital nevi.

Bottom line: Benign, biopsy unnecessary.

Dermatofibroma

Pearls

- Flat/Pink-Clear/Multicolored.
  - These "flat" dermatofibromas are typically found at an early stage, and while these may appear flat, they will be firmly palpable.
  - Characteristically smooth and well circumscribed.
- **Step 4 Patterns:** Remember your patterns from Chapter 1! Faint pseudonetwork-like periphery, pigmented network, central white patch, central vessels and erythema, globule-like/ring-like globules, and crystalline structures.
- **Bottom line: Benign, biopsy not necessary.**

Figure 6.4 shows a clinically flat, but palpable, pink lesion with a multicolored (brown + pink) dermoscopic pattern. You can see a faint pseudonetwork-like periphery. These are indicative of a dermatofibroma. Diagnosis: Dermatofibroma.

Bottom line: Benign, biopsy unnecessary.

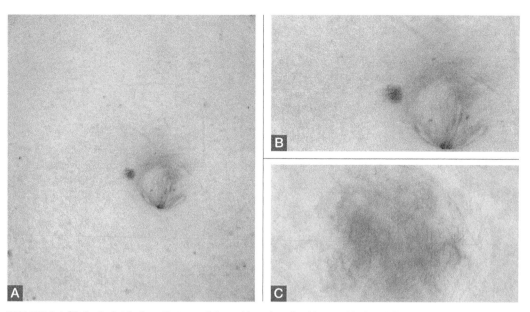

FIGURE 6.4 Clinically flat lesions that are pink or skin-colored, with a multicolored (brown + other = gray, pink, and/or yellow) dermoscopic pattern. **A,B:** Clinical examples of dermatofibromas. **C:** Dermoscopy shows a non-specific vascular pattern. Dermatofibromas are palpable. Note the faint pseudonetwork pattern.

Figure 6.5 shows a clinically flat, but palpable, pink/skin-colored lesion with a multicolored (brown + pink) dermoscopic pattern. Here you can see the central dotted vascular pattern with a faint pseudonetwork-like periphery. Diagnosis: Dermatofibroma.

Bottom line: Benign, biopsy unnecessary.

Figure 6.6 shows a clinically flat, but palpable, pink/skin-colored lesion with a multicolored (brown + pink + yellow) dermoscopic pattern. On dermoscopy, you can see the central

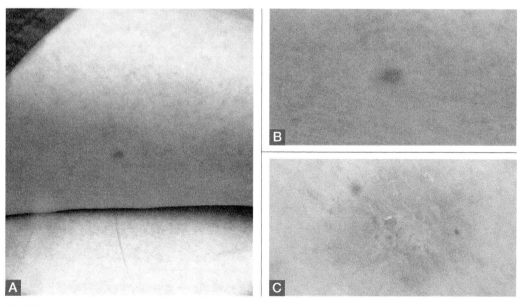

FIGURE 6.5 Clinically flat lesions that are pink or skin-colored, with a multicolored (brown + other = gray, pink, and/or yellow) dermoscopic pattern. **A,B:** Clinical examples of dermatofibromas. **C:** Dermoscopy shows a central dotted vascular pattern with a faint symmetric pseudonetwork pattern at the periphery. Dermatofibromas are palpable.

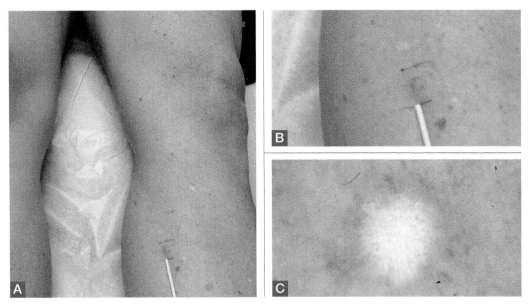

FIGURE 6.6 Clinically flat lesions that are pink or skin-colored, with a multicolored (brown + other = gray, pink, and/or yellow) dermoscopic pattern. **A,B:** Clinical examples of dermatofibromas. **C:** Dermoscopy shows a central crystalline scar-like pattern, with a faint symmetric pseudonetwork pattern at the periphery. Dermatofibromas are palpable.

crystalline scar-like pattern and a faint symmetric pseudonetwork-like pattern at the periphery. Diagnosis: Dermatofibroma.

Bottom line: Benign, biopsy unnecessary.

Figure 6.7 shows a clinically flat, but palpable, pink/skin-colored lesion with a multicolored (brown + pink + yellow) dermoscopic pattern. On dermoscopy, you can see the central

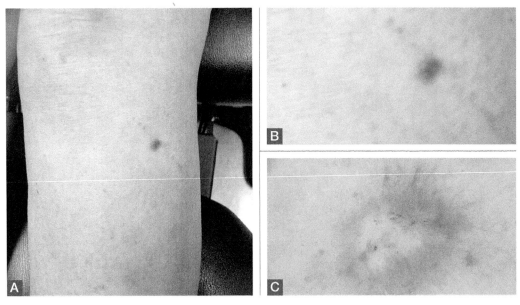

FIGURE 6.7 Clinically flat lesions that are pink or skin-colored, with a multicolored (brown + other = gray, pink, and/or yellow) dermoscopic pattern. **A,B:** Clinical examples of dermatofibromas. **C:** Dermoscopy shows a central crystalline scar-like pattern with a faint, slightly asymmetric pseudonetwork pattern at the periphery. Dermatofibromas are palpable.

crystalline scar-like pattern and a faint slightly asymmetric pseudonetwork-like pattern at the periphery. Diagnosis: Dermatofibroma.

Bottom line: Likely benign, but asymmetry makes it less obvious, so biopsy may be necessary.

Lichen planus–like Keratosis or Nonpigmented Seborrheic Keratosis

Pearls

- Flat/Pink-Clear/Multicolored
  - These lesions are often difficult to differentiate from malignant melanoma and nonmelanoma cancers because inflammation can often lead to a nonspecific vascular pattern.
- **Step 4 Pattern**: We will use patterns from Chapter 1 to look for benign features: sharp borders, moth-eaten borders, fingerprint patterns, milia-like cysts, comedo-like openings, and ridges.
  - These lesions are either solar lentigines undergoing regression or inflammatory reactions or a seborrheic keratosis undergoing regression or an inflammatory reaction.
- **Bottom line: Likely benign, but if no obvious benign pattern, biopsy may be necessary.**

Figure 6.8 shows a clinically flat, pink/skin-colored lesion with a multicolored (brown + pink + yellow) dermoscopic pattern. The nonspecific vascular pattern is due to the inflammation, but you can still pick out some benign characteristics, such as a moth-eaten border and milia-like cysts. Diagnosis: Lichen planus–like keratosis or nonpigmented seborrheic keratosis.

Bottom line: Benign, biopsy unnecessary.

Figure 6.9 shows a clinically flat, pink/skin-colored lesion with a multicolored (brown + pink) dermoscopic pattern. There is a nonspecific vascular pattern, but you can identify a crystalline scar-like pattern with a sharp border—ultimately signs of a benign lesion.

Diagnosis: Lichen planus–like keratosis or nonpigmented seborrheic keratosis.

Bottom line: benign, biopsy unnecessary.

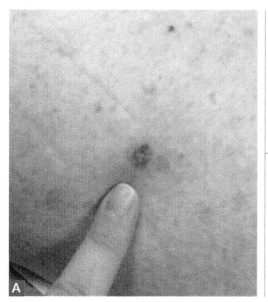
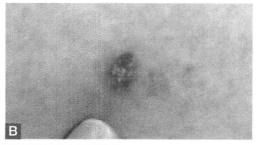
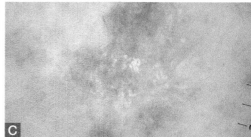

FIGURE 6.8 Clinically flat lesions that are pink or skin-colored with a multicolored (brown + other = gray, pink, and/or yellow) dermoscopic pattern. **A,B:** Clinical examples of lichen planus–like keratosis. **C:** Dermoscopy shows a nonspecific vascular pattern with a moth-eaten border at the periphery. Note how clinically inflamed lesion appears.

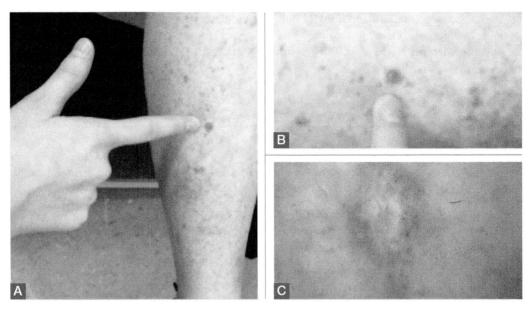

FIGURE 6.9 Clinically flat lesions that are pink or skin-colored, with a multicolored (brown + other = gray, pink, and/or yellow) dermoscopic pattern. **A,B:** Clinical examples of lichen planus–like keratosis. **C:** Dermoscopy shows a nonspecific vascular pattern, crystalline scar-like pattern with a sharp border.

Figure 6.10 shows a clinically flat, pink/skin-colored lesion with a multicolored (brown + pink + gray) dermoscopic pattern. Again, we see nonspecific inflammation; however, we can also see a localized gray granularity and moth-eaten border—indicative of a lichen planus–like keratosis. Diagnosis: Lichen planus–like keratosis or nonpigmented seborrheic keratosis.

Bottom line: Benign, biopsy unnecessary.

Figure 6.11 shows an example of a clinical lesion that is flat and pink/flesh-colored. From this description, we are starting to think of a few options, including seborrheic keratosis and squamous cell carcinoma. Diagnosis: Lichen planus–like keratosis or nonpigmented seborrheic keratosis.

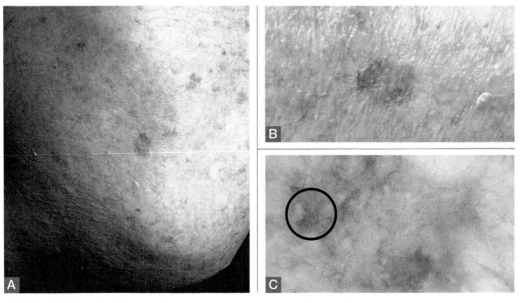

FIGURE 6.10 Clinically flat lesions that are pink or skin-colored, with a multicolored (brown + other = gray, pink, and/or yellow) dermoscopic pattern. **A,B:** Clinical examples of lichen planus–like keratosis. **C:** Dermoscopy shows a nonspecific vascular pattern, with localized gray granularity circled in black and a moth-eaten border.

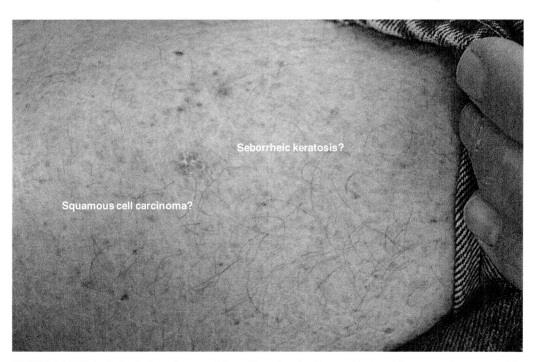

FIGURE 6.11 Clinically flat lesions that are pink or skin-colored, with a multicolored (brown + other = gray, pink, and/or yellow) dermoscopic pattern.

Bottom line: Benign, biopsy unnecessary.

Figure 6.12 shows the multicolored dermoscopic pattern (brown + pink + yellow) present in this lesion. We also can see a faint reticular pattern with thin lines, moth-eaten borders,

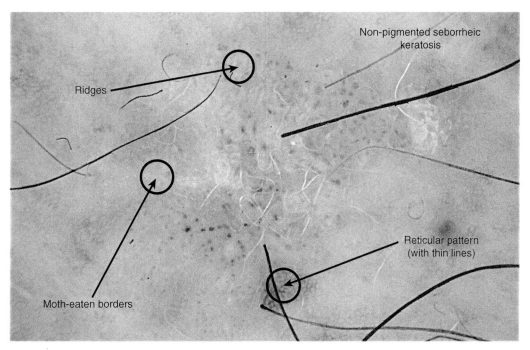

FIGURE 6.12 Clinically flat lesions that are pink or skin-colored, with a multicolored (brown + other = gray, pink, and/or yellow) dermoscopic pattern. The clinical differential of an isolate pink scaly patch can be narrowed down by the dermoscopic pattern shown in Figure 6.10, with moth-eaten borders, ridges, and a reticular pattern with thin lines seen in a nonpigmented seborrhea keratosis.

and ridges—all indicative of a seborrheic keratosis. Diagnosis: Lichen planus–like keratosis or nonpigmented seborrheic keratosis.

Bottom line: Benign, biopsy unnecessary.

Malignant Lesions

Squamous Cell Skin Cancer

Pearls
- Flat/Pink-Clear/Multicolored
- **Step 4 Pattern**: Remember your SCC patterns from Chapter 1! Figure 6.13 illustrates the classic SCC patterns.
  - Pink-white shiny area
  - White reflective scaly surface
  - Ulceration
  - Dotted vessels
  - Glomeruloid/coiled vessels
  - Keratinizing vessels
- **Bottom line: Malignant, biopsy is necessary.**

Figure 6.14A shows a clinically flat, scalp lesion that is pink/flesh-colored. Figure 6.14B shows its corresponding dermoscopic image showing multiple colors (brown + pink + yellow). We can see areas of ulceration, white reflective shiny areas, and glomeruloid vessels. Diagnosis: Squamous cell skin cancer.

Bottom line: Malignant, biopsy.

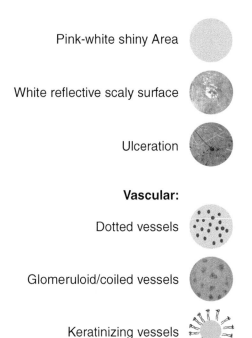

Pink-white shiny Area

White reflective scaly surface

Ulceration

Vascular:

Dotted vessels

Glomeruloid/coiled vessels

Keratinizing vessels

FIGURE 6.13 Squamous cell carcinoma patterns.

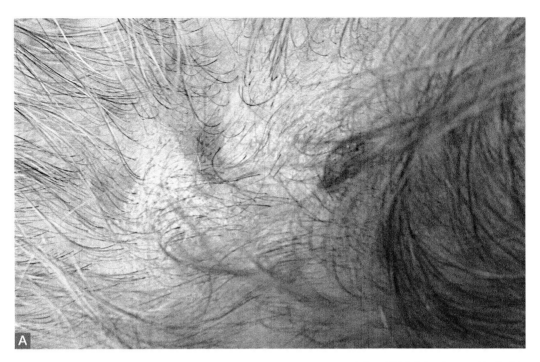

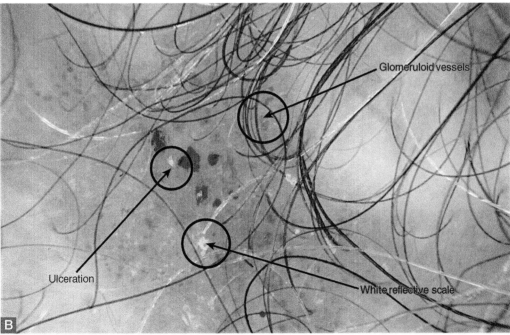

FIGURE 6.14 A: Clinically flat lesions that are pink or skin-colored, with a multicolored (brown + other = gray, pink, and/or yellow) dermoscopic pattern. **B:** The dermoscopic pattern shows ulceration, glomeruloid vessels, and white hyperreflective scale narrowing consistent with SCC.

Figure 6.15 shows a clinically flat, pink/flesh-colored lesion with a multicolored (brown + pink + yellow + red) dermoscopic pattern. Additionally, we see the characteristic keratinizing vascular pattern of hairpin vessels surrounding central ulceration, all surrounded by a halo at the periphery. Diagnosis: Squamous cell skin cancer.

Bottom line: Malignant, biopsy.

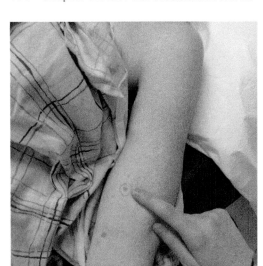
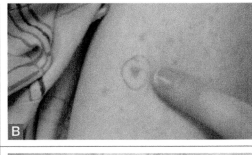
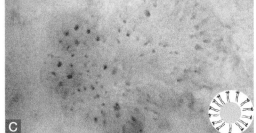

FIGURE 6.15 Clinically flat lesions that are pink or skin-colored, with a multicolored (brown + other = gray, pink, and/or yellow) dermoscopic pattern. **A,B:** Clinical examples of squamous cell skin cancers. **C:** Dermoscopy shows the keratinizing vascular pattern of a hairpin vessel surrounded by a halo all around the periphery and central ulceration similar to the illustration.

Figure 6.16 shows a clinically flat, pink/skin-colored lesion with a multicolored (brown + pink + yellow) dermoscopic pattern. We can see an area of central ulceration with hairpin vessels surrounding its periphery. Diagnosis: Squamous cell skin cancer.

Bottom line: Malignant, biopsy.

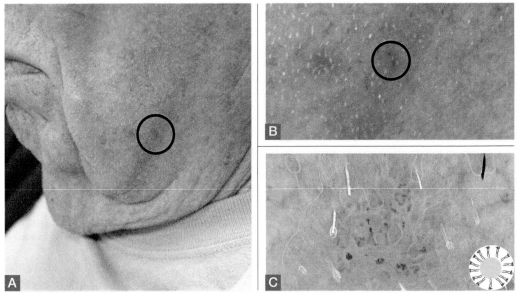

FIGURE 6.16 Clinically flat lesions that are pink or skin-colored, with a multicolored (brown + other = gray, pink, and/or yellow) dermoscopic pattern. **A,B:** Clinical examples of squamous cell skin cancer. **C:** Dermoscopy shows the keratinizing vascular pattern of a hairpin vessel surrounded by a halo all around the periphery and central ulceration similar to the illustration.

Basal Cell Carcinoma

Pearls

- Flat/Pink-Clear/Multicolored
- **Step 4 Pattern**: Remember your BCC patterns from Chapter 1! Figure 6.17 illustrates the classic BCC patterns.
  - Absence of pigmented network
  - Leaf-like structures
  - Large blue great ovoid nests or globular-like structures
  - Arborizing telangiectasias (sharply defined)
  - Spoke wheel areas
  - Ulceration
  - Pink-white to white-shiny areas
  - Crystalline pattern
- Remember that leaf-like structures, large blue-gray ovoid nests or globular structures, and spoke wheel areas are typically seen in pigmented basal cells and won't be seen here.
- **Bottom line: Malignant, biopsy is necessary.**

Figure 6.18A shows a clinically flat, pink/skin-colored lesion. Figure 6.18B shows the dermoscopy of this lesion, multicolored (brown + pink + yellow) with malignant patterns, including localized ulceration, arborizing vessels, and crystalline patterns. Diagnosis: Basal cell carcinoma.

   Bottom line: Malignant, biopsy.

   Figure 6.19 shows another clinically flat, pink/skin-colored lesion with a multicolored (brown + pink) dermoscopic pattern. You can clearly see the crystalline scar-like pattern, with a pink-white shiny background and localized ulceration on dermoscopy. Diagnosis: Basal cell carcinoma.

   Bottom line: Malignant, biopsy.

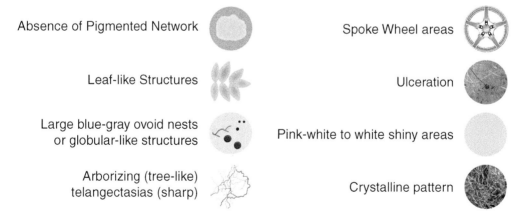

FIGURE 6.17 Basal cell carcinoma patterns.

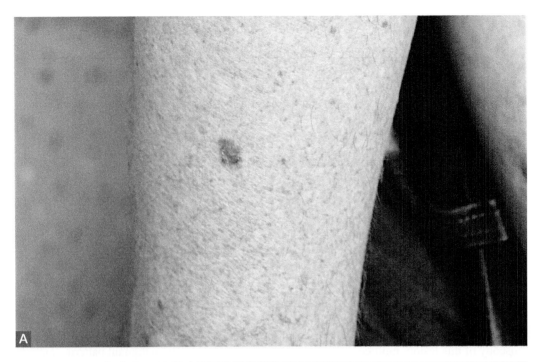

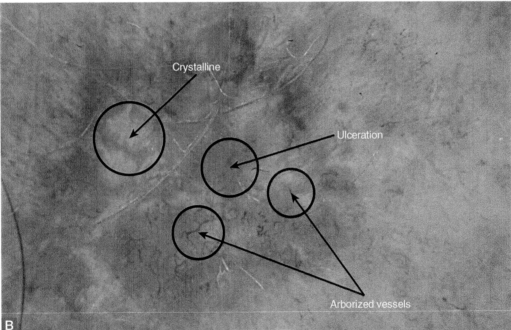

FIGURE 6.18 A: Clinically flat lesions that are pink or skin-colored, with a multicolored (brown + other = gray, pink, and/or yellow) dermoscopic pattern. **B:** The dermoscopic pattern shows ulceration, arborized vessels crystalline pattern, and localized ulceration consistent with basal cell skin cancer.

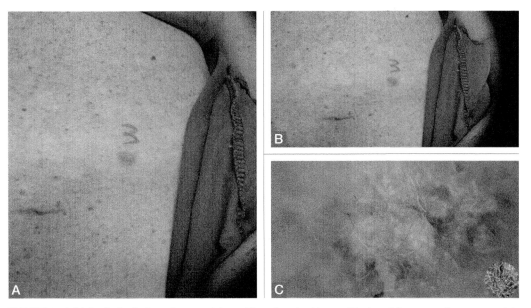

FIGURE 6.19 Clinically flat lesions that are pink or skin-colored, with a multicolored (brown + other = gray, pink, and/or yellow) dermoscopic pattern. **A,B:** Clinical examples of basal cell skin cancer. **C:** Dermoscopy shows a crystalline scar-like pattern, pink-white shiny background, and localized ulceration.

Figure 6.20 shows a clinically flat, pink/skin-colored lesion with a multicolored (brown + pink + yellow) dermoscopic pattern. You can appreciate the crystalline pattern with a pink-white shiny background, as well as an absence of pigmented network. Diagnosis: Basal cell carcinoma.

Bottom line: Malignant, biopsy.

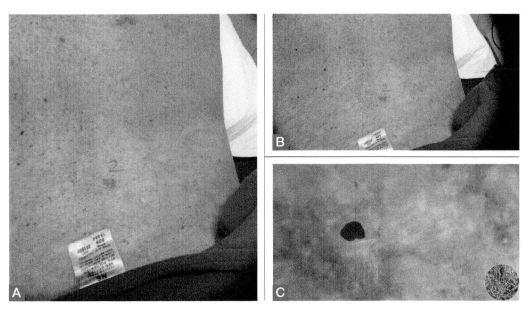

FIGURE 6.20 Clinically flat lesions that are pink or skin-colored, with a multicolored (brown + other = gray, pink, and/or yellow) dermoscopic pattern. **A,B:** Clinical examples of basal cell skin cancer. **C:** Dermoscopy shows a crystalline scar-like pattern, pink-white shiny background, and localized ulceration.

Early Amelanotic Melanoma

Pearls

- Flat/Pink-Clear/Multicolored
- **Step 4 Pattern**: Early amelanotic melanomas in this category may have
  - Irregular, faint pigmentation
  - Diffuse dotted vessels
  - Polymorphous vessels
- They may also show some other malignant features such as:
  - Crystalline scar-like pattern
  - Radial streak
  - Peripheral pseudopods
  - Blue-gray dots and granules
- **Bottom line: Malignant, Biopsy is necessary.**

Figure 6.21 shows a new clinically flat lesion that is clinically pink/skin-colored. Figure 6.22 shows the dermoscopy; you can see the multicolored (brown + pink + red + gray) dermoscopic pattern with additional malignant characteristics. We can see polymorphous vessels, a crystalline scar-like pattern, a few blue-gray dots, and faint nonspecific, irregular pigmentation. Diagnosis: Early amelanotic melanoma.

Bottom line: Malignant, biopsy necessary!

Figure 6.23 shows three lesions, all clinically flat and pink/skin-colored. Figure 6.24 shows their corresponding dermoscopic images—all multicolored, consisting of brown and pink. They all share diffuse dotted and polymorphous vessels, as well as faint nonspecific, irregular pigmentation. Diagnosis: Early amelanotic melanoma.

Bottom line: Malignant, biopsy necessary!

Recent pink patch

FIGURE 6.21 Clinically flat lesions that are pink or skin-colored, with a multicolored (brown + other = gray, pink, and/or yellow) dermoscopic pattern. The diagnosis is early amelanotic melanoma.

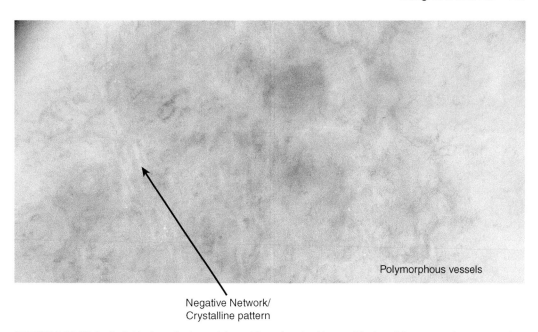

Polymorphous vessels

Negative Network/
Crystalline pattern

FIGURE 6.22 Clinically flat lesions that are pink or skin-colored, with a multicolored (brown + other = gray, pink, and/or yellow) dermoscopic pattern. The dermoscopic pattern shows polymorphous vessels, a crystalline scar-like pattern, and faint, nonspecific pigmentation. The diagnosis is early amelanotic melanoma, with minimal dermal involvement associated with the scar-like pattern.

Test Yourself!

Figure 6.25 shows four clinically flat, pink/skin-colored lesions. Figure 6.26 shows their dermoscopic counterparts—all multicolored lesions. Can you pick out their patterns?

A: Pattern: Diffuse glomeruloid vessels = malignant feature, likely SCC. **Biopsy!**

B: Pattern: Dotted/glomeruloid vessels in a serpiginous string-of-pearls pattern, likely clear cell acanthoma. **No Biopsy**.

C: Pattern: Hairpin vessels, ridges, moth-eaten border, and thin reticular pattern, likely seborrheic keratosis. **No Biopsy**.

D: Pattern: Dotted diffuse vessels with faint, nonspecific, irregular pigment, likely amelanotic melanoma. **Biopsy**.

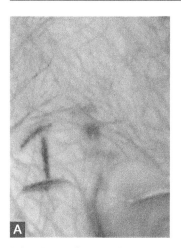
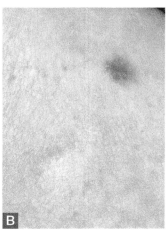
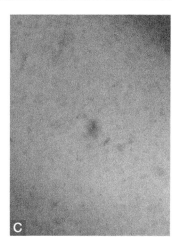

FIGURE 6.23 Clinically flat lesions that are pink or skin-colored, with a multicolored (brown + other = gray, pink, and/or yellow) dermoscopic pattern. These are examples of three early melanotic melanomas.

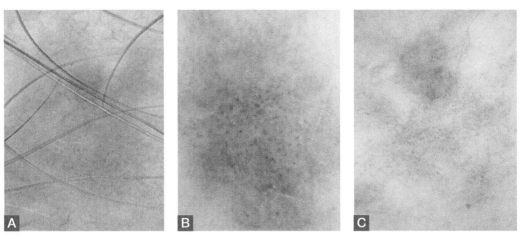

FIGURE 6.24 The dermoscopic pattern of the corresponding figures A, B, and C from Figure 6.23 with polymorphous/dotted vessels and faint nonspecific pigmentation. These are examples of three early melanotic melanomas.

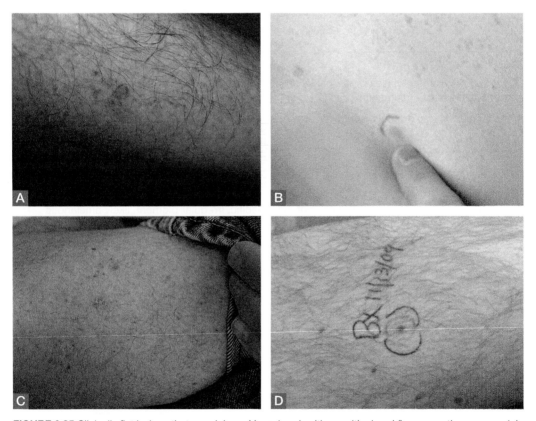

FIGURE 6.25 Clinically flat lesions that are pink or skin-colored, with a multicolored (brown + other = gray, pink, and/or yellow) dermoscopic pattern.

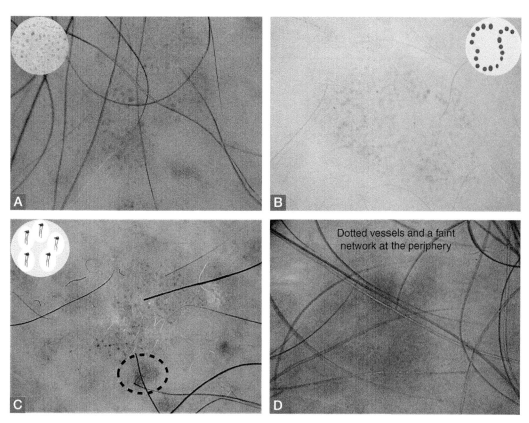

FIGURE 6.26 The dermoscopic pattern of the corresponding figures **A–D** from Figure 6.24. **A:** Diffuse glomeruloid vessels show a diagnosis of SCC. **B:** The dotted/glomeruloid vessels in a serpiginous string-of-pearl pattern show a diagnosis of clear cell acanthoma. **C:** Hairpin vessels, ridges, moth-eaten borders, and a thin reticular pattern all demonstrate a diagnosis of Seb K. **D:** Dotted vessels with a faint nonspecific pigment pattern indicate a diagnosis of amelanotic melanoma.

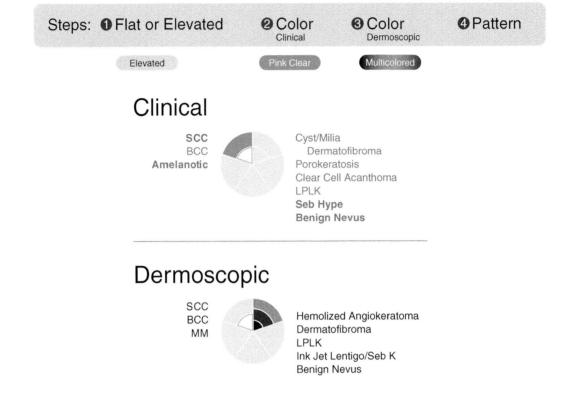

Steps: ❶ Flat or Elevated   ❷ Color
Clinical   ❸ Color
Dermoscopic   ❹ Pattern

Elevated   Pink Clear   Multicolored

Clinical

SCC
BCC
Amelanotic

Cyst/Milia
Dermatofibroma
Porokeratosis
Clear Cell Acanthoma
LPLK
Seb Hype
Benign Nevus

Dermoscopic

SCC
BCC
MM

Hemolized Angiokeratoma
Dermatofibroma
LPLK
Ink Jet Lentigo/Seb K
Benign Nevus

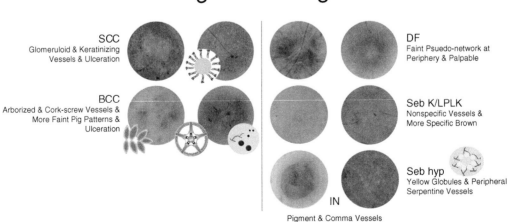

Malignant Benign

SCC
Glomeruloid & Keratinizing
Vessels & Ulceration

BCC
Arborized & Cork-screw Vessels &
More Faint Pig Patterns &
Ulceration

DF
Faint Psuedo-network at
Periphery & Palpable

Seb K/LPLK
Nonspecific Vessels &
More Specific Brown

Seb hyp
Yellow Globules & Peripheral
Serpentine Vessels

IN
Pigment & Comma Vessels

FIGURE 7.1 Color wheel: elevated/pink-clear/multicolored.

Step 1: Is the lesion flat or raised? **Elevated**

Step 2: What color is the lesion on clinical assessment? **Pink-Clear**

Step 3: What is the dermoscopic color? **Multicolored**—can include brown, yellow, or blue-gray, but not white

Step 4: Is further elucidation needed to decide whether to biopsy or not? **Yes** Is this a malignant or benign pattern?

Take a look at the color wheel in Figure 7.1.

Our differential is still very similar to the Flat/Pink-Clear/Multicolored ones, but, with a few differences in patterns you may see additionally, amelanotic melanoma is *off* our differential—you can breathe a sigh of relief! However, our malignant possibilities still include squamous cell carcinoma (SCC) and basal cell carcinoma (BCC).

Our benign lesions include dermatofibroma, seborrheic keratosis/lichen planus–like keratosis, intradermal nevi, and seborrheic hyperplasia.

Benign Lesions

Nonpigmented (Pink) Seborrheic Keratoses

Pearls

- Elevated/Pink-Clear/Multicolored.
  - We saw these in our Flat/Pink-Clear/Multicolored differential, but they can also be elevated.
  - These can be difficult to differentiate from SCC, but look for pattern clues to help you!
- **Step 4 Patterns**: Moth-eaten or sharp borders, fingerprint patterns, ridges, comedo-like openings, and milia-like cysts.
- **Bottom line: Benign, biopsy not necessary.**

Examples

Figure 7.2 shows a clinically slightly elevated, pink or skin-colored lesion with a multicolored (brown + pink + yellow) dermoscopic pattern (Figure 7.3). This presentation can be difficult to differentiate from a SCC. Pay close attention to the patterns. You can appreciate the diffuse yellow pigmentation, ridges, and moth-eaten and sharp border. These clues will lead you to consider a nonpigmented SK, rather than an SCC. Diagnosis: Nonpigmented (pink) seborrheic keratoses.

Bottom line: Benign, biopsy unnecessary.

Figure 7.4 shows a clinically elevated, pink/skin-colored lesion (A, B) with a multicolored (brown + yellow) dermoscopic pattern (C). We see very clear demarcated, sharp borders, with a diffuse yellow pigmentation, as opposed to a focal yellow spot. Additionally, this is a great example of the clear ridges and fissure, which is a classic presentation for seborrheic keratosis. Diagnosis: Nonpigmented (pink) seborrheic keratoses.

Bottom line: Benign, biopsy unnecessary.

Figure 7.5 shows a clinically slightly elevated, pink or skin-colored lesion (Figure 7.5A, B) with a multicolored (brown + pink + yellow) dermoscopic pattern (Figure 7.5C). The inflammation of this lesion makes it an "ugly" lesion, and you may be tempted to think of malignancy at first glance, but pay close attention to the patterns. You will see diffuse yellow pigmentation, ridges, and a sharp border. Diagnosis: Nonpigmented (pink) seborrheic keratoses.

Bottom line: Benign, biopsy unnecessary.

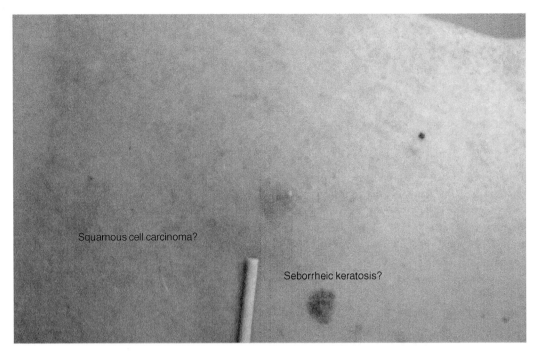

FIGURE 7.2 Clinically elevated lesions that are pink or skin-colored, with a multicolored (brown + other = gray, pink, and/or yellow) dermoscopic pattern.

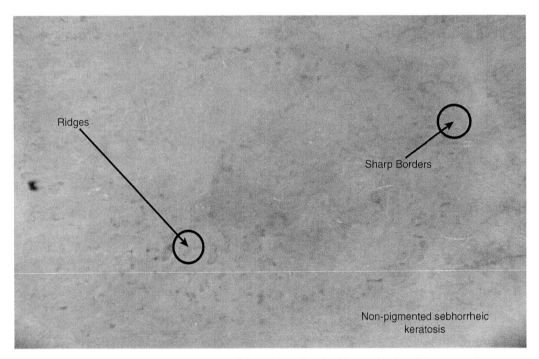

FIGURE 7.3 Clinically elevated lesions that are pink or skin-colored, with a multicolored (brown + other = gray, pink and/or yellow) dermoscopic pattern. Here, you can see the dermoscopic pattern of Figure 7.2 with moth-eaten borders and ridges and a diffuse (rather than the localized) yellow pattern seen in malignancies such as SCC and BCC. Diagnosis is a nonpigmented seborrheic keratosis.

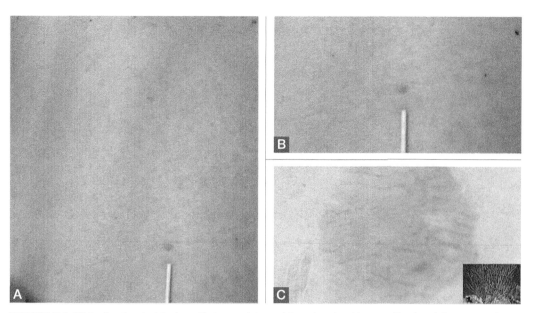

FIGURE 7.4 Clinically elevated lesions that are pink or skin-colored, with a multicolored (brown + other = gray, pink, and/or yellow) dermoscopic pattern. **A,B:** Clinical examples of nonpigmented seborrheic keratosis. **C:** Dermoscopy shows ridges, sharp borders, and a diffuse (rather than the localized) yellow pattern seen in malignancies such as SCC and BCC.

Figure 7.6 shows a clinically elevated, pink/skin-colored lesion (Figure 7.6A, B) with a multicolored (brown + yellow) dermoscopic pattern (Figure 7.6C). This lesion could easily be mistaken for an SCC. However, we can see very clear demarcated, sharp borders, clear ridges and fissures, as well as milia-like cysts and comedo-like openings. Diagnosis: Nonpigmented (pink) seborrheic keratoses.

Bottom line: Benign, biopsy unnecessary.

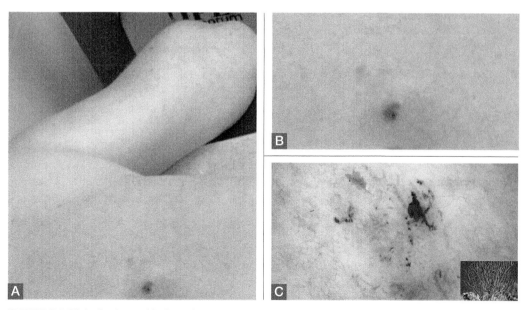

FIGURE 7.5 Clinically elevated lesions that are pink or skin-colored, with a multicolored (brown + other = gray, pink, and/or yellow) dermoscopic pattern. **A,B:** Clinical examples of an irritated nonpigmented seborrheic keratosis. **C:** Dermoscopy shows ridges, sharp borders, and some evidence of inflammation seen as blood spots.

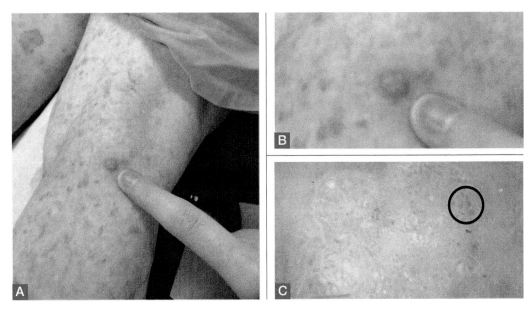

FIGURE 7.6 Clinically elevated lesions that are pink or skin-colored, with a multicolored (brown + other = gray, pink, and/or yellow) dermoscopic pattern. **A,B:** Clinical examples of a nonpigmented seborrheic keratosis. **C:** Dermoscopy shows ridges, sharp borders, milia-like cysts, and comedo-like openings circled in black.

Dermatofibroma

Pearls

- Elevated/Pink-Clear/Multicolored
  - These raised, palpable nodules often dimple clinically.
  - Characteristically smooth and well circumscribed.
  - These scar-like reactions are often seen in older patient populations. You may see a scar-like pattern on dermoscopy.
- **Step 4 Patterns: See Figure 7.7**. Remember your patterns from Chapter 1: faint pseudonetwork-like periphery, pigmented network, central white patch, central vessels and erythema, globule-like/ring-like globules, and crystalline structures.
  - Also, remember that they can sometimes appear as diffuse dots and resemble a superficial SCC on dermoscopy, but DFs are firmly palpable and raised and therefore cannot be a superficial SCC.
- **Bottom line: Benign, biopsy not necessary.**

Figure 7.8 shows a clinically elevated, palpable, pink lesion (Figure 7.8A, B) with a multicolored (brown + pink) dermoscopic pattern (Figure 7.8C). There is a clear central crystalline scar-like pattern with a faint symmetric pseudonetwork pattern at the periphery. Diagnosis: Dermatofibroma.

Bottom line: Benign, biopsy unnecessary.

Figure 7.9 shows a clinically elevated, palpable, pink/skin-colored lesion (Figure 7.9A, B) with a multicolored (brown + pink) dermoscopic pattern (Figure 7.9C). You can see the central crystalline scar-like pattern with a faint pseudonetwork pattern at the periphery. Additionally, there are little rosettes circled in black that can often be seen in more elevated or thicker lesions. Diagnosis: Dermatofibroma.

Bottom line: benign, biopsy unnecessary.

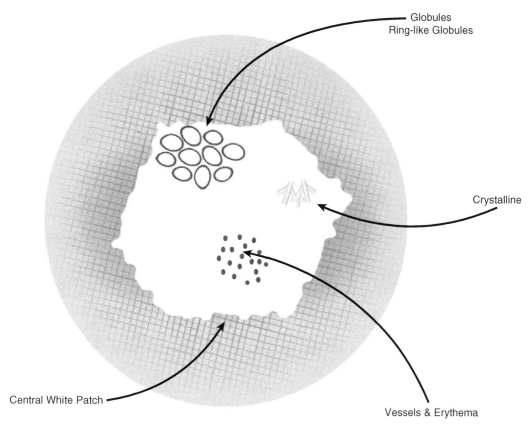

FIGURE 7.7 An illustration of dermatofibromas that have pigmented network–like structures at the periphery, a central white patch, a crystalline pattern, ring-like globules, and/or vessels and erythema at the center.

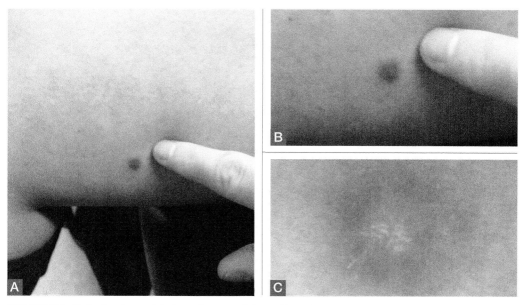

FIGURE 7.8 Clinically elevated lesions that are pink or skin-colored, with a multicolored (brown + other = gray, pink, and/or yellow) dermoscopic pattern. **A,B:** Clinical examples of dermatofibromas. **C:** Dermoscopy shows a central crystalline scar-like pattern with a faint symmetric pseudonetwork pattern at the periphery. Dermatofibromas are palpable.

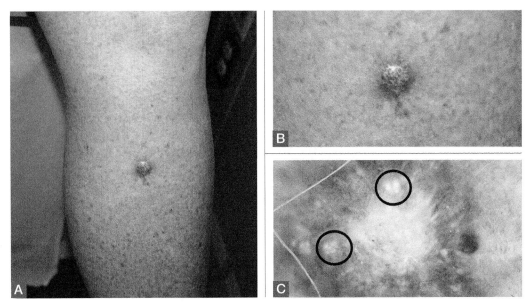

FIGURE 7.9 Clinically elevated lesions that are pink or skin-colored, with a multicolored (brown + other = gray, pink, and/or yellow) dermoscopic pattern. **A,B:** Clinical examples of dermatofibromas. **C:** Dermoscopy shows a central crystalline scar-like pattern with a faint symmetric pseudonetwork pattern at the periphery. Note the rosettes circled in black are often seen with more elevated and thicker lesions. Dermatofibromas are palpable.

Figure 7.10 shows a clinically elevated, palpable, pink/skin-colored lesion (Figure 7.10A, B) with a multicolored (brown + pink + red) dermoscopic pattern (Figure 7.10C). On dermoscopy, you can see a smaller central crystalline scar-like pattern and a more prominent symmetric pseudonetwork-like pattern at the periphery. Additionally, you can see some erythema. Diagnosis: Dermatofibroma.

Bottom line: Benign, biopsy unnecessary.

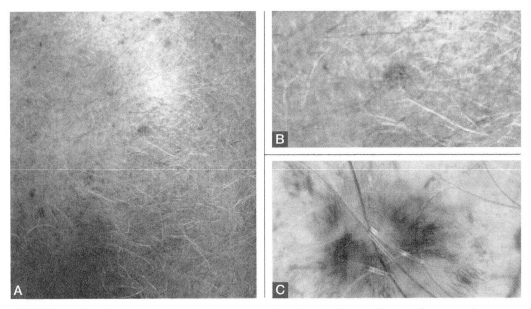

FIGURE 7.10 Clinically elevated lesions that are pink or skin-colored, with a multicolored (brown + other = gray, pink, and/or yellow) dermoscopic pattern. **A,B:** Clinical examples of dermatofibromas. **C:** Dermoscopy shows a central crystalline scar-like pattern with a network-like pattern at the periphery. Dermatofibromas are palpable.

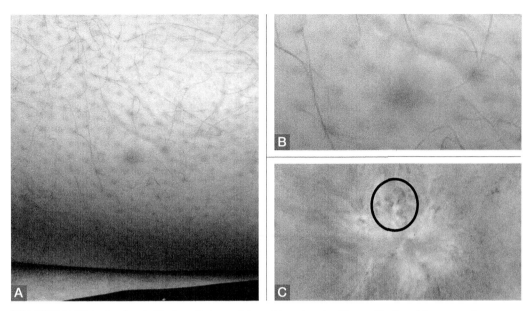

FIGURE 7.11 Clinically elevated lesions that are pink or skin-colored, with a multicolored (brown + other = gray, pink, and/or yellow) dermoscopic pattern. **A,B:** Clinical examples of dermatofibromas. **C:** Dermoscopy shows a central crystalline scar-like pattern with a faint network-like pattern at the periphery. Note the globule-like structures circled in black. Dermatofibromas are palpable.

Figure 7.11 shows a clinically elevated, palpable, pink/skin-colored lesion (Figure 7.11A, B) with a multicolored (brown + pink + yellow) dermoscopic pattern (Figure 7.11C). On dermoscopy, you can see a large central crystalline scar-like pattern with a faint pseudonetwork-like pattern at the periphery. Additionally, we see globule-like structures circled in black. Diagnosis: Dermatofibroma.

Bottom line: Benign, biopsy unnecessary.

Sebaceous Hyperplasia

Pearls

- Elevated/Pink-Clear/Multicolored
  - These pink or skin-colored papules often have a central dell or depression.
  - They often have a yellow color on dermoscopy that can sometimes be appreciated clinically; we will revisit SHs in Chapter 16.
  - Irritated sebaceous hyperplasia can clinically look like BCCs and will be important to distinguish with patterns.
- **Step 4 Patterns**: Sebaceous hyperplasia characteristically has yellow-white lobular structures resembling popcorn that appear with serpentine radial vessels resembling a crown. These radial vessels typically do not cross the midline.
- **Bottom line: Benign, biopsy not necessary.**

Figure 7.12 shows a clinically elevated, pink/skin-colored lesion with an appreciable depression in the center clinically. Figure 7.13 shows the multicolored (brown + pink + yellow) dermoscopic pattern. We see the yellow lobular, popcorn-like structures with serpentine, crowning vessels not crossing the midline. Diagnosis: Sebaceous hyperplasia.

Bottom line: Benign, biopsy unnecessary.

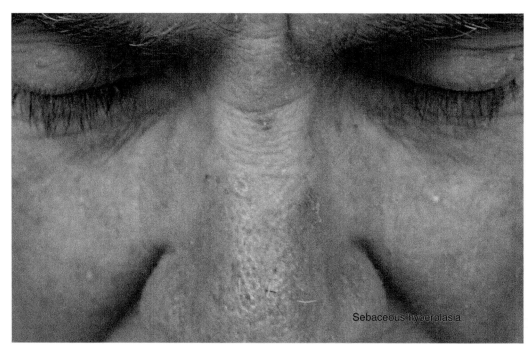

Sebaceous hyperplasia

FIGURE 7.12 Clinically elevated lesions that are pink or skin-colored, with a multicolored (brown + other = gray, pink, and/or yellow) dermoscopic pattern.

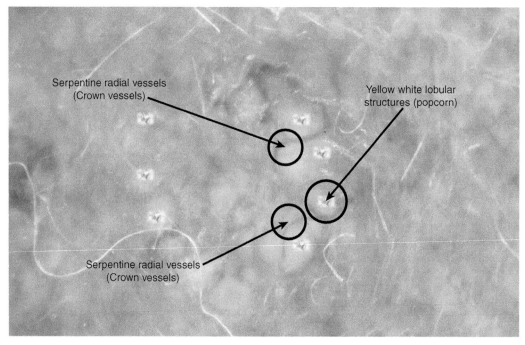

Serpentine radial vessels
(Crown vessels)

Yellow white lobular
structures (popcorn)

Serpentine radial vessels
(Crown vessels)

FIGURE 7.13 Sebaceous hyperplasia. Clinically elevated lesions that are pink or skin-colored, with a multi-colored (brown + other = gray, pink, and/or yellow) dermoscopic pattern. Here, you can see the dermoscopic pattern of Figure 7.11, with yellow-white lobular structures that resemble popcorn and serpentine radial vessels that resemble a crown; they usually do not cross the midline.

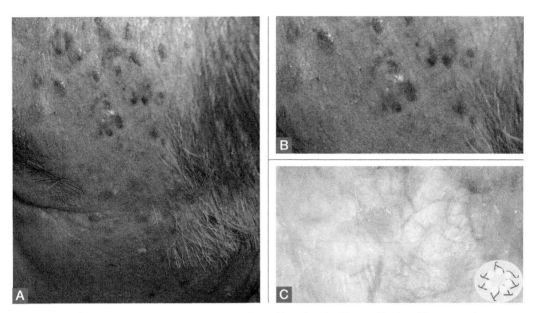

FIGURE 7.14 Clinically elevated lesions that are pink or skin-colored with a multicolored (brown + other = gray, pink, and/or yellow) dermoscopic pattern. **A,B:** Clinical examples of sebaceous hyperplasia. **C:** Dermoscopy shows yellow-white lobular structures that resemble popcorn and serpentine radial vessels that resemble a crown; they usually do not cross the midline. Note the central dell visible in this lesion.

Figure 7.14 shows a clinically elevated, pink/skin-colored lesion with a clinically appreciable central depression (Figure 7.14A, B) with a multicolored (brown + pink) dermoscopic pattern (Figure 7.14C). Again, you see the yellow-white lobular, popcorn-like structures with serpentine, crowning vessels. The vessels are not crossing the midline. Diagnosis: Sebaceous hyperplasia.

Bottom line: Benign, biopsy unnecessary.

Figure 7.15 shows a clinically elevated, pink/skin-colored lesion (Figure 7.15A, B) with a multicolored (brown + pink) dermoscopic pattern (Figure 7.15C). Here, you see the entire

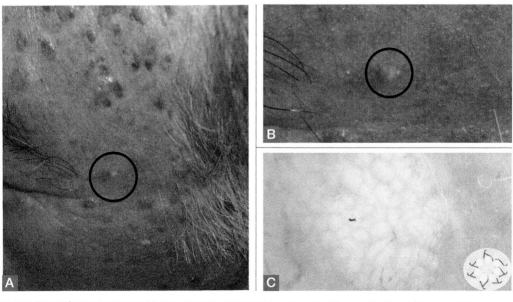

FIGURE 7.15 Clinically elevated lesions that are pink or skin-colored, with a multicolored (brown + other = gray, pink, and/or yellow) dermoscopic pattern. Review these clinical and dermoscopic examples of a sebaceous hyperplasia. **A,B:** Clinical example. **C:** The dermoscopic example shows yellow-white lobular structures that resemble popcorn and serpentine radial vessels that resemble a crown; they usually do not cross the midline. Note the central dell visible in this lesion.

Clinical Pink-Clear

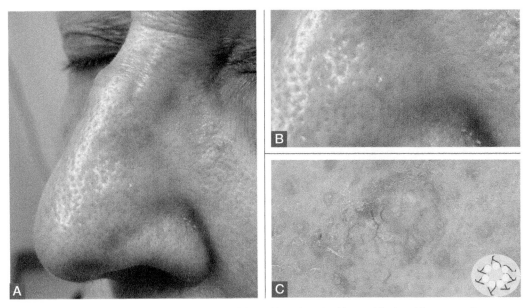

FIGURE 7.16 Clinically elevated lesions that are pink or skin-colored, with a multicolored (brown + other = gray, pink, and/or yellow) dermoscopic pattern. Review these clinical and dermoscopic examples of a sebaceous hyperplasia. **A,B:** Clinical examples. **C:** The dermoscopic example shows yellow-white lobular structures that resemble popcorn and serpentine radial vessels that resemble a crown; they usually do not cross the midline. Note the central dell visible in this lesion.

lesion is a yellow-white lobular, popcorn-like structure with just a couple of serpentine, crowning vessels. The vessels are not crossing the midline. Diagnosis: Sebaceous hyperplasia.

Bottom line: Benign, biopsy unnecessary.

Figure 7.16 shows a clinically elevated, pink/skin-colored lesion with a clinically appreciable central depression (Figure 7.16A, B) with a multicolored (brown + pink) dermoscopic pattern (Figure 7.16C). Here, we see less of the yellow-white lobular, popcorn-like structures, with more of the serpentine, crowning vessels. The vessels are not crossing the midline. Diagnosis: Sebaceous hyperplasia.

Bottom line: Benign, biopsy unnecessary.

Figure 7.17 shows two clinically elevated, pink/skin-colored lesions (1, 2) with multicolored (brown + pink +yellow) dermoscopic colors. Here, we can see how sebaceous hyperplasia can resemble basal cell carcinomas. (1) is a BCC—we can see blue-gray globules, with arborizing vessels. (2) is a sebaceous hyperplasia—we see the yellow-white lobular, popcorn-like structures with more of the serpentine, crowning vessels. The vessels are not crossing the midline. Diagnosis: Sebaceous hyperplasia.

Bottom line: Benign, biopsy unnecessary.

Intradermal Nevi (IN)/Congenital Nevi (CN)

Pearls

- Elevated/Pink-Clear/Multicolored
  - Skin-colored papules that patients will have had for a long time; however, sometimes flat lesions can become neurotized, or three dimensional, and patients may believe they are new.
  - When IN or CNs are on the face, they can become irritated, making them clinically difficult to differentiate from BCCs.
  - Wobble: When you move them, they wobble back and forth. Malignancies do not demonstrate this.

(Continued)

- **Step 4 Pattern**: You may see some benign patterns such as coma-like vessels, faint pigmentation, or milia-like cysts. However, more importantly, you'll see a lack of the malignant features we covered in our pattern chapter of melanoma, SCC, or BCC.
- **Bottom line: Benign, biopsy is not necessary.**

Examples

Figure 7.18 shows the clinically elevated lesions that are pink or skin-colored. Figure 7.18A is a BCC and Figure 7.18B is a traumatized intradermal nevi. Figure 7.19 demonstrates the dermoscopic findings for each lesion; (Figure 7.19A) the BCC and (Figure 7.19B) the IN. Both lesions

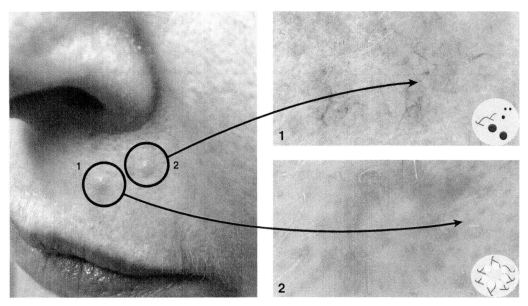

FIGURE 7.17 Clinically elevated lesions that are pink or skin-colored, with a multicolored (brown + other = gray, pink, and/or yellow) dermoscopic pattern. Review clinical *1* and *2* with corresponding dermoscopic examples. *1* is a basal cell skin cancer with blue-gray globules and *2* is a sebaceous hyperplasia/milia, with yellow/white lobular structures that resemble popcorn and serpentine radial vessels that resemble a crown.

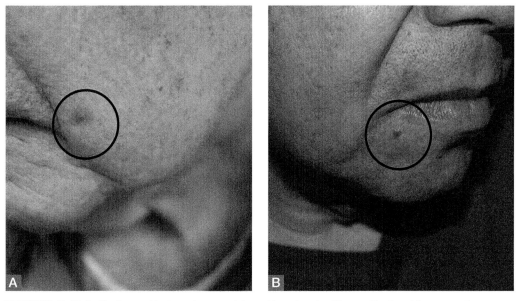

FIGURE 7.18 Clinically elevated lesions that are pink or skin-colored, with a multicolored (brown + other = gray, pink, and/or yellow) dermoscopic pattern. **A:** Basal cell skin cancer. **B:** A traumatized benign intradermal nevus.

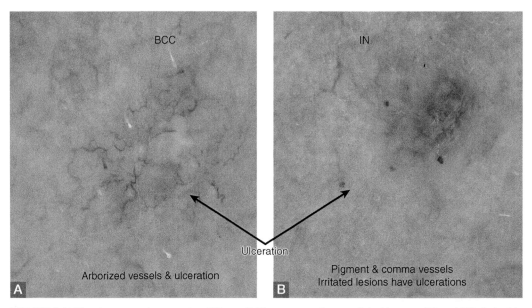

FIGURE 7.19 The dermoscopic example of Figure 7.18 corresponding to clinical images **(A)** and **(B)**. **A:** In this lesion, note that in the BCC, the yellow ulceration is localized. **B:** In this lesion, note the traumatized intradermal nevus where the yellow is diffuse throughout the lesion secondary to trauma; there are no other findings. When not associated with an ulceration, yellow is also an indication of a benign lesion.

are multicolored dermoscopically (brown + yellow + pink). We can see that in image A there is an area of localized yellow ulceration, whereas in image B, the yellow is diffuse throughout. The BCC has clear arborizing, sharp telangiectasias. The traumatized IN has few other findings, such as pigment and comma vessels. Diagnosis: Intradermal nevi (IN)/congenital nevi (CN).

Bottom line: Benign, biopsy not necessary.

Figure 7.20 shows an example of clinically elevated, wobbly, pink/skin-colored lesion (Figure 7.20A, B) with a multicolored (brown + pink + yellow) dermoscopy (Figure 7.20C).

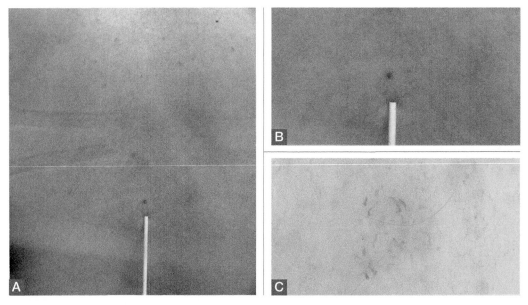

FIGURE 7.20 Clinically elevated lesions that are pink or skin-colored, with a multicolored (brown + other = gray, pink, and/or yellow) dermoscopic pattern. Review these clinical and dermoscopic examples of an intradermal nevus. **A,B:** Clinical examples. **C:** This dermoscopic example shows comma-like vessels with background homogeneous pigmentation. These lesions are soft and pedunculated and wobble back and forth with a contact dermatoscope.

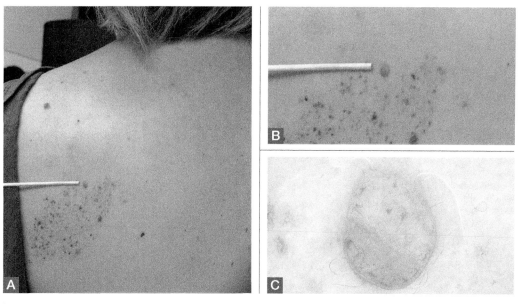

FIGURE 7.21 Clinically elevated lesions that are pink or skin-colored, with a multicolored (brown + other = gray, pink, and/or yellow) dermoscopic pattern. Review these clinical and dermoscopic examples of an intradermal nevus. **A,B:** Clinical examples. **C:** This dermoscopic example shows comma-like vessels with background homogeneous pigmentation. These lesions are soft and pedunculated and wobble back and forth with a contact dermatoscope.

We can see comma-like vessels on a homogenous background of faint pigmentation. Check for the wobble! Diagnosis: Intradermal nevi (IN)/congenital nevi (CN).

Bottom line: Benign, biopsy not necessary.

Figure 7.21 shows an example of clinically elevated, wobbly, pink/skin-colored lesions (Figure 7.21A, B) with a multicolored (brown + pink + yellow) dermoscopy (Figure 7.21C). Again, we see comma-like vessels on a homogenous background of faint pigmentation. Check for the wobble! Diagnosis: Intradermal nevi (IN)/congenital nevi (CN).

Bottom line: Benign, biopsy not necessary.

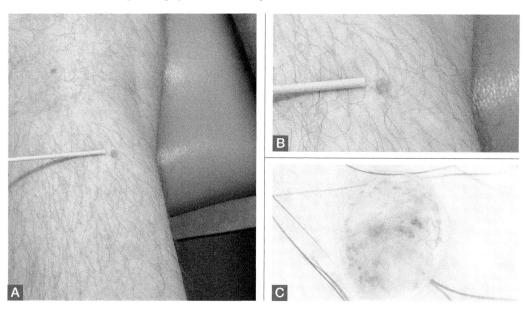

FIGURE 7.22 Clinically elevated lesions that are pink or skin-colored, with a multicolored (brown + other = gray, pink, and/or yellow) dermoscopic pattern. Review these clinical and dermoscopic examples of an intradermal nevus. **A,B:** Clinical examples. **C:** This dermoscopic example shows comma-like vessels with background homogeneous pigmentation. These lesions are soft and pedunculated and wobble back and forth with a contact dermatoscope.

Figure 7.22 shows an example of clinically elevated, wobbly, pink/skin-colored lesions (Figure 7.22A, B) with a multicolored (brown + pink + yellow) dermoscopy (Figure 7.22C). We can see comma-like vessels on the periphery of a symmetrical, homogenous background of faint pigmentation. Check for the wobble! Figures 7.23A and B show the change seen when the lesion is moved from side to side. Diagnosis: Intradermal nevi (IN)/congenital nevi (CN).

Bottom line: Benign, biopsy not necessary.

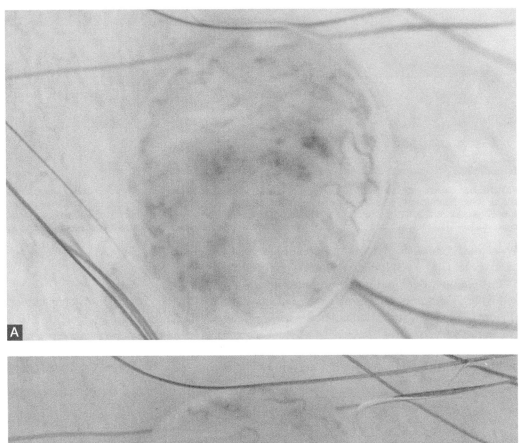

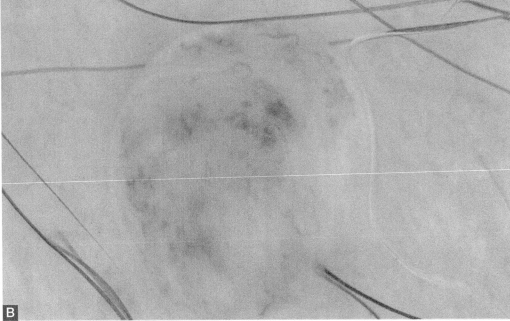

FIGURE 7.23 **A:** This dermoscopic image from Figure 7.22A shows one direction of wobbling. **B:** This dermoscopic image from Figure 7.22B shows another direction of wobbling.

Malignant Lesions

Squamous Cell Skin Cancer—Keratoacanthoma Type

Pearls

- Elevated/Pink-Clear/Multicolored
  - KA-type SCCs are rapidly growing keratocytic epithelial tumors, almost exclusively found on sun-damaged skin—face, neck, chest, hands, arms, and legs.
  - They appear as nodular, erythematous lesions that are either dome-shaped early on or crater-like later on in development.
  - They tend to be firm to palpation with central crusting as they enlarge or develop and can reach up to 3 cm in size. Additionally, patients describe them as being tender.
  - Along with the traditional SCC patterns, KA types often demonstrate white circles, evident keratin, and blood spots.
- **Step 4 Pattern**: Remember your SCC patterns from Chapter 1! Figure 7.24 illustrates the classic SCC patterns.
  - Pink-white shiny area
  - White reflective scaly surface
  - Ulceration
  - Dotted vessels
  - Glomeruloid/coiled vessels
  - Keratinizing vessels
- **Bottom line: Malignant, biopsy is necessary.**

Examples

Figure 7.25A shows a clinically elevated, pink/skin-colored lesion. Figure 7.25B shows the dermoscopic multicolored pattern (brown + pink + red). This is an example of an SCC—

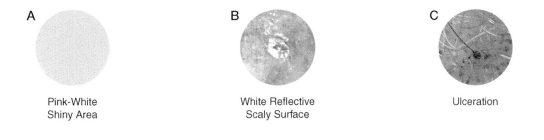

A — Pink-White Shiny Area

B — White Reflective Scaly Surface

C — Ulceration

Vascular

D — Dotted Vessels

E — Glomeruloid/ Coiled Vessels

F — Keratinizing Vessels

FIGURE 7.24 Illustrations of nonpigmented squamous skin cancer patterns. Nonpigmented squamous cells are much more common than pigmented squamous cells.

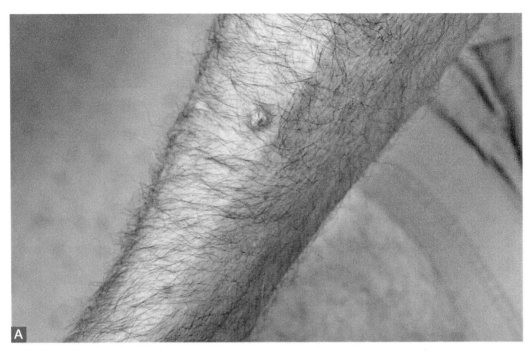

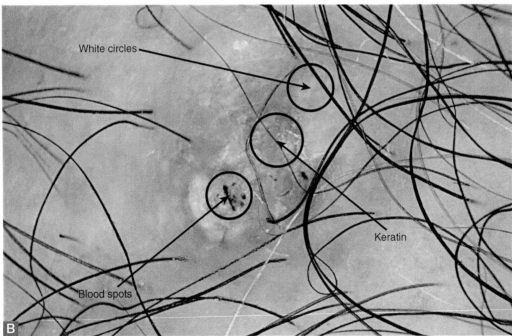

FIGURE 7.25 A: Clinically elevated lesions that are pink or skin-colored, with a multicolored (brown + other = gray, pink, and/or yellow) dermoscopic pattern. This is an example of squamous cell skin cancer, the keratoacanthoma type. **B:** The dermoscopic image of Figure 7.20. Note the keratin, white circles, and blood spots. This is an example of squamous cell skin cancer, the keratoacanthoma type.

keratoacanthoma type. You can see the thick keratin and blood spots in the center. Additionally, you can see white circles on the flatter, nonkeratinized part of the lesion. You can still see features of SCC—a clear pink-white shiny area with dotted vessels and keratinizing vessels around the periphery of the lesion. Diagnosis: Squamous cell skin cancer—keratoacanthoma type.

Bottom line: Malignant, biopsy is necessary.

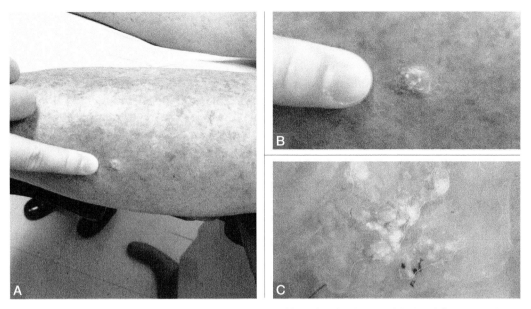

FIGURE 7.26 Clinically elevated lesions that are pink or skin-colored, with a multicolored (brown + other = gray, pink, and/or yellow) dermoscopic pattern. Review these clinical and dermoscopic examples of an irritated seborrheic keratosis. **A,B:** Clinical examples. **C:** The dermoscopic example shows similar findings to keratoacanthoma of white circles, keratin, and blood spots. These benign irritated masqueraders need to be biopsied because at times they contain ACC or precancers to SCC-actinic keratosis.

Figure 7.26 shows a clinically elevated, pink/flesh colored lesion (Figure 7.26A, B) with a multicolored (brown + pink + yellow + red) dermoscopic pattern (Figure 7.26C). This is a benign inflamed seborrheic keratosis. We can see milia-like cysts on the periphery, but the central white scaly keratin, white circles, and blood spots raise a red flag. Often these masqueraders need to be biopsied; at times they contain SCC or precancers growing within them. Diagnosis: Squamous cell skin cancer—keratoacanthoma type.

Bottom line: Questionable, biopsy is necessary.

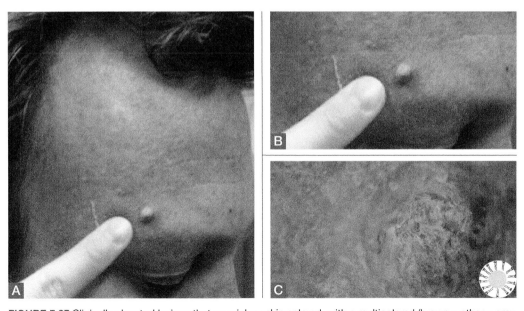

FIGURE 7.27 Clinically elevated lesions that are pink or skin colored, with a multicolored (brown + other = gray, pink and/or yellow) dermoscopic pattern. **A,B:** Clinical examples of Keratoacanthoma. **C:** The dermoscopic example shows white circles, keratin and blood spots. Note the peripheral keratinizing vessels.

Figure 7.27 shows a clinically elevated, pink/skin-colored lesion (A, B) with a multicolored (brown + pink + yellow) dermoscopic pattern (C). We can see an area of central ulceration with keratinizing vessels surrounding its periphery. Additionally, we can see white circles, keratin, and blood spots. Diagnosis: Squamous cell skin cancer—keratoacanthoma type.

Bottom line: Malignant, biopsy is necessary.

Figure 7.28 shows a clinically elevated, pink/skin-colored lesion (Figure 7.28A, B) with a multicolored (brown + pink + yellow) dermoscopic pattern (Figure 7.28C). We can see an area of central ulceration, with keratinizing vessels surrounding its periphery. Additionally, we can see white-shiny areas with white circles, keratin, and blood spots. Diagnosis: Squamous cell skin cancer—keratoacanthoma type.

Bottom line: Malignant, biopsy is necessary.

Figure 7.29 shows a clinically elevated, pink/skin-colored lesion (Figure 7.29A, B) with a multicolored (brown + pink + yellow) dermoscopic pattern (Figure 7.29C). We can see an area of central yellow ulceration and white-shiny surface. Additionally, we can see white circles, keratin, and blood spots. Diagnosis: Squamous cell skin cancer—keratoacanthoma type.

Bottom line: Malignant, biopsy is necessary.

Figure 7.30 shows a clinically elevated, pink/skin-colored lesion (Figure 7.30A, B) with a multicolored (brown + pink + yellow) dermoscopic pattern (Figure 7.30C). Here, we see an example of a non–KA-type elevated SCC. We see a classic central ulceration, with keratinizing vessels around the periphery. Diagnosis: Squamous cell skin cancer—keratoacanthoma type.

Bottom line: Malignant, biopsy is necessary.

Figure 7.31 shows a clinically elevated, pink/skin-colored lesion (Figure 7.31A, B) with a multicolored (brown + pink + yellow) dermoscopic pattern (Figure 7.31C). Here, we see an example of a non–KA-type elevated SCC. We see an area of white-shiny reflective scaly surface with keratinizing vessels around the periphery and additionally some glomeruloid/coiled vessels. Diagnosis: Squamous cell skin cancer—keratoacanthoma type.

Bottom line: Malignant, biopsy is necessary.

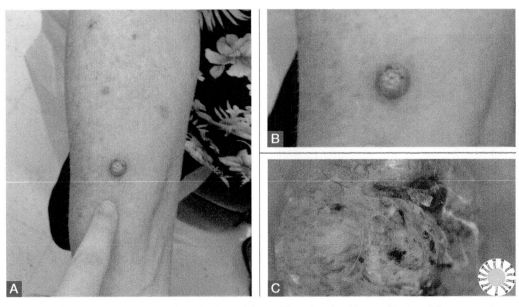

FIGURE 7.28 Clinically elevated lesions that are pink or skin-colored, with a multicolored (brown + other = gray, pink, and/or yellow) dermoscopic pattern. Review these clinical and dermoscopic examples of keratoacanthoma. **A,B:** Clinical examples. **C:** The dermoscopic examples show white circles, keratin, and blood spots. Note the peripheral keratinizing vessels.

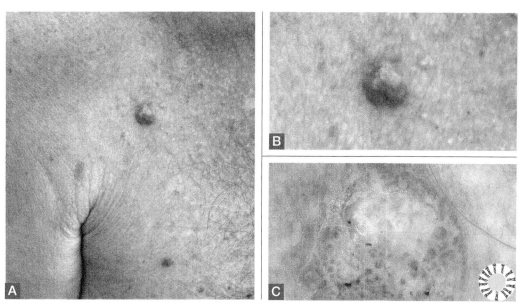

FIGURE 7.29 Clinically elevated lesions that are pink or skin-colored, with a multicolored (brown + other = gray, pink, and/or yellow) dermoscopic pattern. Review these clinical and dermoscopic examples of keratoacanthoma. **A,B:** Clinical examples. **C:** The dermoscopic example shows white circles, keratin, and blood spots. Note the peripheral keratinizing vessels.

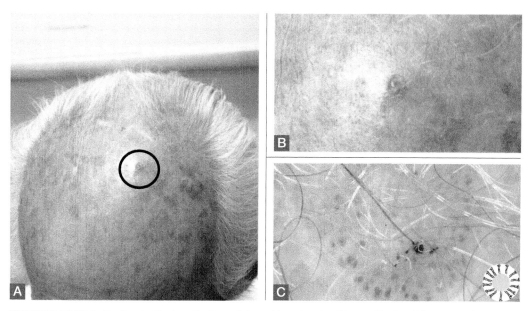

FIGURE 7.30 Clinically elevated lesions that are pink or skin-colored, with a multicolored (brown + other = gray, pink, and/or yellow) dermoscopic pattern. Review these clinical and dermoscopic examples of squamous cell skin cancer. **A,B:** Clinical examples. **C:** The dermoscopic example shows peripheral keratinizing vessels.

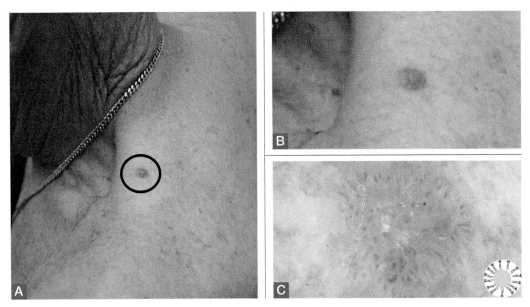

FIGURE 7.31 Clinically elevated lesions that are pink or skin-colored, with a multicolored (brown + other = gray, pink, and/or yellow) dermoscopic pattern. Review these clinical and dermoscopic examples of squamous cell skin cancer. **A,B:** Clinical examples. **C:** The dermoscopic example shows peripheral keratinizing vessels. Note the white hyperreflective scale.

Basal Cell Carcinoma

Pearls

- Elevated/Pink-Clear/Multicolored
- **Step 4 Pattern**: Remember your BCC patterns from Chapter 1! Figure 7.32 illustrates the classic BCC patterns.
  - Absence of pigmented network
  - Leaf-like structures
  - Large blue great ovoid nests or globular-like structures
  - Arborizing telangiectasias (sharply defined)
  - Spoke wheel areas
  - Ulceration
  - Pink-white to white-shiny areas
  - Crystalline pattern
- Remember that leaf-like structures, large blue-gray ovoid nests or globular structures, and spoke wheel areas are typically seen in pigmented basal cells.
- **Bottom line: Malignant, biopsy is necessary.**

Examples

Figure 7.33 shows a clinically elevated, pink/skin-colored lesion (Figure 7.33A, B) with a multicolored (brown + pink + yellow) dermoscopy pattern (Figure 7.33C). You can see a handful of malignant patterns, including localized ulceration, arborizing vessels, blue-gray ovoid nests, and globular-like structures. Diagnosis: Basal cell carcinoma.

    Bottom line: Malignant, biopsy is necessary.

    Figure 7.34 shows a clinically elevated, pink/skin-colored lesion (Figure 7.34A, B) with a multicolored (brown + pink + yellow) dermoscopy pattern (Figure 7.34C). You can see an asymmetric pink-white shiny area with some arborizing vessels and small blue-gray ovoid nests. Diagnosis: Basal cell carcinoma.

    Bottom line: Malignant, biopsy is necessary.

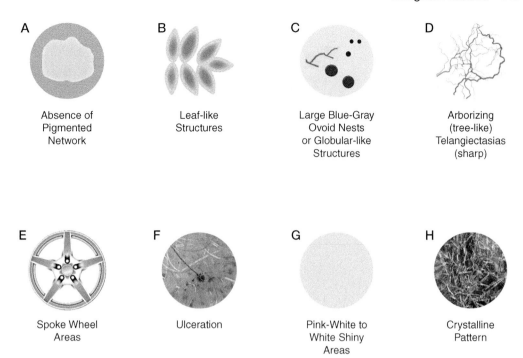

FIGURE 7.32 Illustrations of basal cell skin cancer patterns. Note that the features in **(B)**, **(C)**, and **(E)** are mainly seen in pigmented basal cell skin cancers.

Figure 7.35 shows a clinically elevated, pink/skin-colored lesion (Figure 7.35A, B) with a multicolored (brown + pink + yellow) dermoscopy pattern (Figure 7.35C). In this lesion, we see sharp arborizing vessels with blue-gray ovoid nests and a prominent globular-like structure. Diagnosis: Basal cell carcinoma.

Bottom line: Malignant, biopsy is necessary.

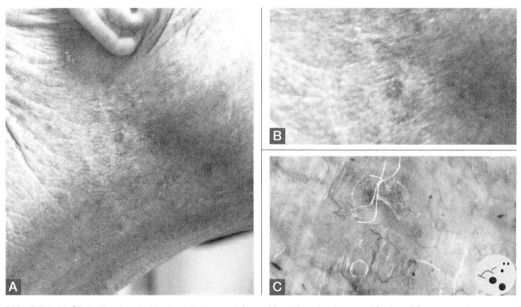

FIGURE 7.33 Clinically elevated lesions that are pink or skin-colored, with a multicolored (brown + other = gray, pink, and/or yellow) dermoscopic pattern. Review these clinical and dermoscopic examples of basal cell skin cancer. **A,B:** Clinical examples. **C:** The dermoscopic example shows arborized vessels and blue-gray ovoid nests and globular-like structures.

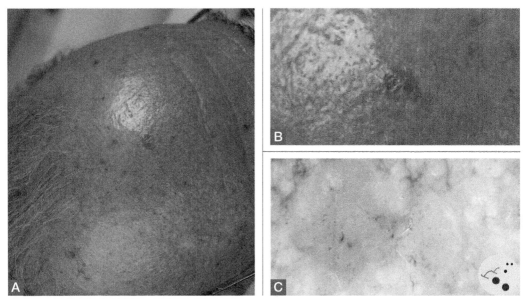

FIGURE 7.34 Clinically elevated lesions that are pink or skin-colored, with a multicolored (brown + other = gray, pink, and/or yellow) dermoscopic pattern. Review these clinical and dermoscopic examples of basal cell skin cancer. **A,B:** Clinical examples. **C:** The dermoscopic example shows arborized vessels and blue-gray ovoid nests and globular-like structures.

Figure 7.36 shows a clinically elevated, pink/skin-colored lesion (Figure 7.36A, B) with a multicolored (brown + pink + yellow) dermoscopy pattern (Figure 7.36C). Here, we see an asymmetric lesion with arborizing, sharp vessels and a few blue-gray ovoid nests. Diagnosis: Basal cell carcinoma.

Bottom line: Malignant, biopsy is necessary.

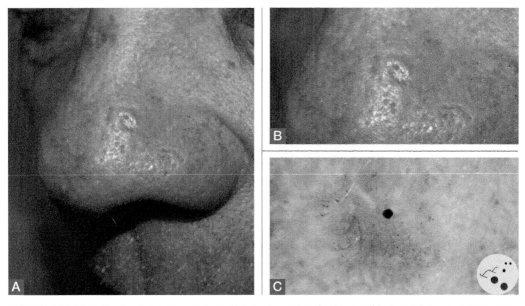

FIGURE 7.35 Clinically elevated lesions that are pink or skin-colored, with a multicolored (brown + other = gray, pink, and/or yellow) dermoscopic pattern. Review these clinical and dermoscopic examples of basal cell skin cancer. **A,B:** Clinical examples. **C:** The dermoscopic example shows arborized vessels and blue-gray ovoid nests and globular-like structures.

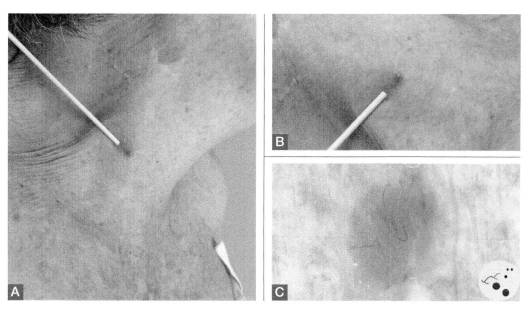

FIGURE 7.36 Clinically elevated lesions that are pink or skin-colored, with a multicolored (brown + other = gray, pink, and/or yellow) dermoscopic pattern. Review these clinical and dermoscopic examples of basal cell skin cancer. **A,B:** Clinical examples. **C:** The dermoscopic example shows arborized vessels and blue-gray ovoid nests and globular-like structures.

Figure 7.37 shows a clinically elevated, pink/skin-colored lesion (Figure 7.37A, B) with a multicolored (brown + pink + yellow) dermoscopy pattern (Figure 7.37C). Here, we see some ash leaf–like structures at the periphery of the asymmetric lesion. Small, sharp arborizing vessels, blue-gray ovoid nests, and globular-like structures are also apparent. Diagnosis: Basal cell carcinoma. **Bottom line: Malignant, biopsy is necessary.**

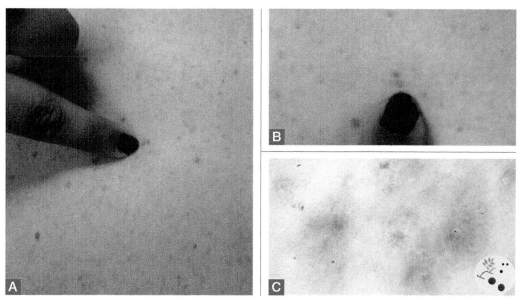

FIGURE 7.37 Clinically elevated lesions that are pink or skin-colored, with a multicolored (brown + other = gray, pink, and/or yellow) dermoscopic pattern. Review these clinical and dermoscopic examples of basal cell skin cancer. **A,B:** Clinical examples. **C:** The dermoscopic example shows arborized vessels, blue-gray ovoid nests, and globular-like structures as well as some ash leaf–like structures at the periphery.

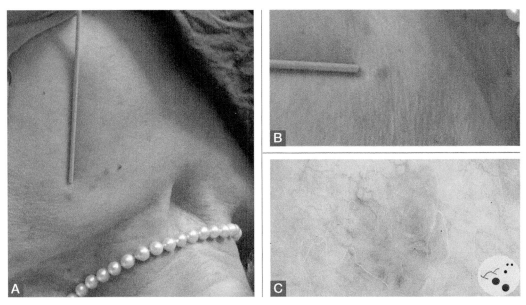

FIGURE 7.38 Clinically elevated lesions that are pink or skin-colored, with a multicolored (brown + other = gray, pink, and/or yellow) dermoscopic pattern. Review these clinical and dermoscopic examples of basal cell skin cancer. **A,B:** Clinical examples. **C:** The dermoscopic example shows arborized vessels, blue-gray ovoid nests, and globular-like structures.

Figure 7.38 shows a clinically elevated, pink-/skin-colored lesion (Figure 7.38A, B) with a multicolored (brown + pink + yellow) dermoscopy pattern (Figure 7.38C). Clear, sharp arborizing telangiectasias, faint blue-gray ovoid nests, and globular structures are evident. A very faint crystalline pattern can just be made out in the center. Diagnosis: Basal cell carcinoma.

Bottom line: Malignant, biopsy is necessary.

Figure 7.39 shows a clinically elevated, pink/skin-colored lesion (Figure 7.39A, B) with a multicolored (brown + pink) dermoscopy pattern (Figure 7.39C). Blue-gray ovoid nests, globu-

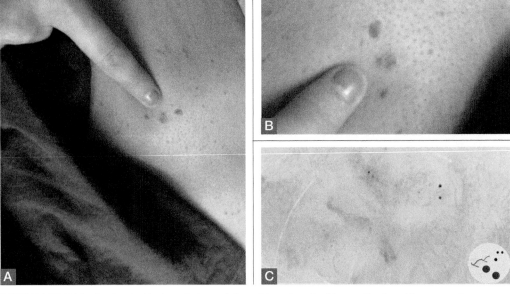

FIGURE 7.39 Clinically elevated lesions that are pink or skin-colored, with a multicolored (brown + other = gray, pink, and/or yellow) dermoscopic pattern. Review these clinical and dermoscopic examples of basal cell skin cancer. **A,B:** Clinical examples. **C:** The dermoscopic example shows arborized vessels, blue-gray ovoid nests, and globular-like structures.

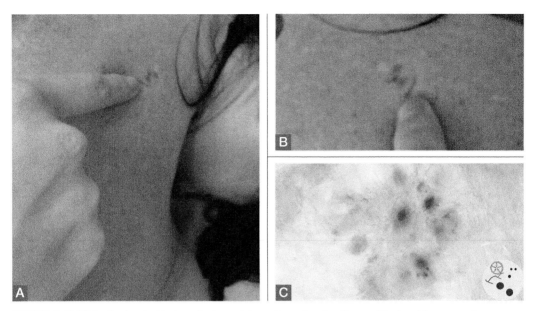

FIGURE 7.40 Clinically elevated lesions that are pink or skin-colored, with a multicolored (brown + other = gray, pink, and/or yellow) dermoscopic pattern. Review these clinical and dermoscopic example of basal cell skin cancer. **A,B:** Clinical examples. **C:** The dermoscopic example shows arborized vessels, blue-gray ovoid nests, and globular-like structures. Note the spoke wheel–like structures.

lar-like vessels, and faint arborizing vessels are very faint on this pigmented networkless lesion. Diagnosis: Basal cell carcinoma.

Bottom line: Malignant, biopsy is necessary.

Figure 7.40 shows a clinically elevated, pink/skin-colored lesion (Figure 7.40A, B) with a multicolored (brown + pink + yellow) dermoscopy pattern (Figure 7.40C). Pink-white shiny areas, with crystalline patterns are evident, along with arborizing vessels, blue-gray ovoid nests, globular-like structures, and spoke wheel structures. Diagnosis: Basal cell carcinoma.

Bottom line: Malignant, biopsy is necessary.

Figure 7.41 shows a clinically elevated, pink/skin-colored lesion (Figure 7.41A, B) with a multicolored (brown + pink + yellow) dermoscopy pattern (Figure 7.41C). This erythematous lesion has blue-gray ovoid nests and globular-like structures, as well as some white shiny areas. These vessels appear more corkscrew-shaped, which some BCCs have; however, the arborizing vessels seen in previous examples are defining for BCC. Diagnosis: Basal cell carcinoma.

Bottom line: Malignant, biopsy is necessary.

Figure 7.42 shows a clinically elevated, pink/skin-colored lesion (Figure 7.42A, B) with a multicolored (brown + pink + yellow) dermoscopy pattern (Figure 7.42C). In this lesion, we can see white hyperreflective scaly areas, as well as ulceration and arborizing vessels. We would consider this a basosquamous cell—as it has features of both lesions. But don't lose the forest through the trees! Diagnosis: Basal cell carcinoma.

Bottom line: Malignant, biopsy is necessary.

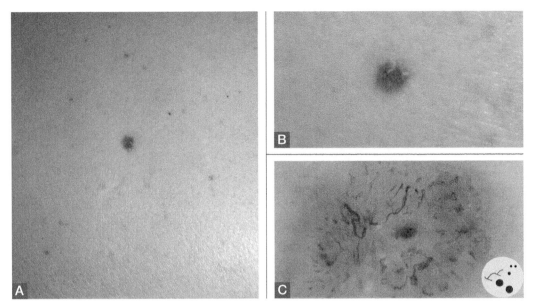

FIGURE 7.41 Clinically elevated lesions that are pink or skin-colored, with a multicolored (brown + other = gray, pink, and/or yellow) dermoscopic pattern. Review these clinical and dermoscopic examples of basal cell skin cancer. **A,B:** Clinical examples. **C:** The dermoscopic example shows arborized vessels, blue-gray ovoid nests, and globular-like structures. Some BCCs have corkscrew-like vessels, but arborized vessels are defining for basal cell skin cancer.

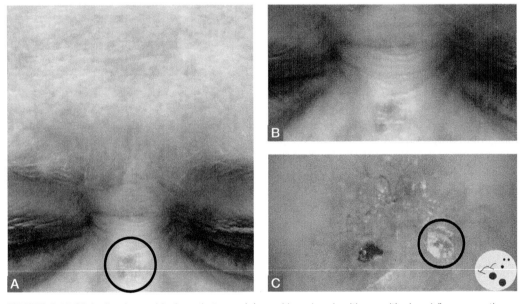

FIGURE 7.42 Clinically elevated lesions that are pink or skin-colored, with a multicolored (brown + other = gray, pink, and/or yellow) dermoscopic pattern. Review these clinical and dermoscopic examples of basosquamous cell skin cancer. **A,B:** Clinical examples. **C:** The dermoscopic example shows arborized vessels with white hyperreflective scales in a black circle and ulceration. In this basosquamous lesion, you can see essential features of both BCC and SCC.

Chapter 8 Flat/Pale Brown/Brown

Steps: ❶ Flat or Elevated ❷ Color Clinical ❸ Color Dermoscopic ❹ Pattern

Flat Pale Brown Brown

Clinical

MM
Pigmented Bowens

MM
Lentigo/Seb K
Dermatofibroma
Benign Nevus

Dermoscopic

Dermatofibroma
Benign Nevi
Lentigo/Seb K
MM
Benign Nevus

Malignant   Benign

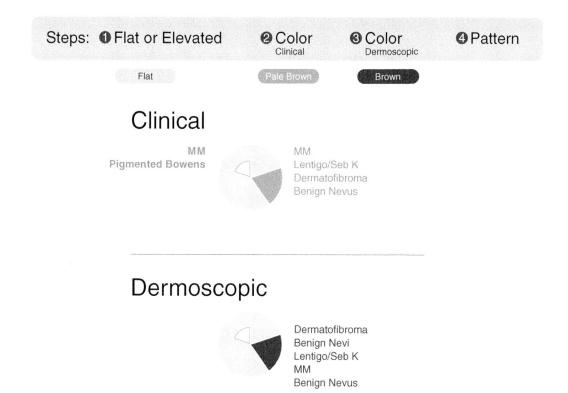
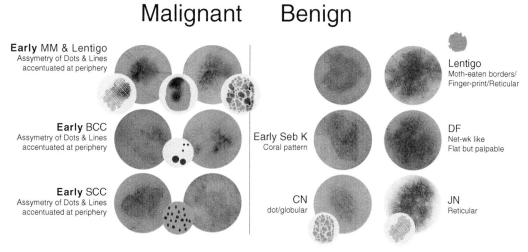

Early MM & Lentigo
Assymetry of Dots & Lines
accentuated at periphery

Early BCC
Assymetry of Dots & Lines
accentuated at periphery

Early SCC
Assymetry of Dots & Lines
accentuated at periphery

Early Seb K
Coral pattern

CN
dot/globular

Lentigo
Moth-eaten borders/
Finger-print/Reticular

DF
Net-wk like
Flat but palpable

JN
Reticular

FIGURE 8.1 Color wheel: flat/pale brown/brown.

Step 1: Is the lesion flat or raised? **Flat**

Step 2: What color is the lesion on clinical assessment? **Pale Brown**

Step 3: What is the dermoscopic color? **Brown**

Step 4: Is further elucidation needed to decide whether to biopsy or not? **Yes**

Is this a malignant or benign pattern?

Take a look at the color wheel in Figure 8.1.

We've moved into the world of brown! When we are looking at flat, clinically pale brown, dermoscopically brown lesions, we have to consider malignancies that are *early* in their development, and this is good, because we want to catch them early! Early malignant melanoma (MM) and lentigo maligna, early basal cell carcinoma (BCC), and early squamous cell carcinoma (SCC) are in our differential. Our benign lesions include early dermatofibroma, early seborrheic keratosis, congenital and junctional nevi, and lentigo.

Benign Lesions

Solar Lentigo

Pearls

- Flat/Pale Brown/Brown
  - In lay terms, usually referred to as "sun spots" or "freckles."
  - These benign lesions can have any of the benign melanocytic patterns from Chapter 1.
- **Step 4 Patterns:** Fingerprint pattern, reticular network pattern, diffuse globular pattern, diffuse light brown structureless area, and moth-eaten or sharply demarcated borders
- **Bottom line: Benign, biopsy not necessary.**

Examples

Figures 8.2 to 8.4 show clinically flat, pale brown lesions (A, B) that are dermoscopically brown (C). In all three images, you can appreciate a clear fingerprint pattern with a moth-eaten border. Diagnosis: Solar lentigo.

Bottom line: Benign, biopsy unnecessary.

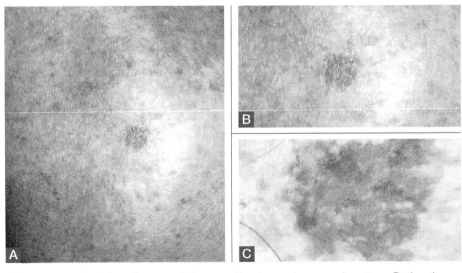

FIGURE 8.2 Clinically flat lesions that are pale brown, with a brown dermoscopic pattern. Review these clinical and dermoscopic example of lentigo (sun spot). **A,B:** Clinical examples. **C:** The dermoscopic example shows a fingerprint pattern and moth-eaten borders.

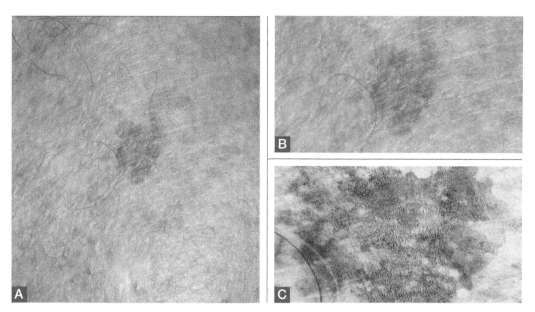

Clinical Pale Brown

FIGURE 8.3 Clinically flat lesions that are pale brown, with a brown dermoscopic pattern. Review these clinical and dermoscopic examples of lentigo (sun spot). **A,B:** Clinical examples. **C:** The dermoscopic example shows a fingerprint pattern and moth-eaten borders.

Figures 8.5 to 8.8 show clinically flat, pale brown lesions (A, B) that are dermoscopically brown (C). In all three, you can appreciate a homogeneous pattern with a moth-eaten border. Diagnosis: Solar lentigo.

Bottom line: Benign, biopsy unnecessary.

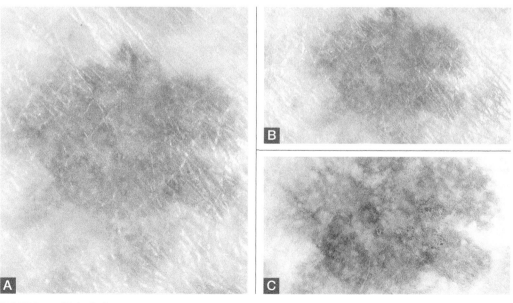

FIGURE 8.4 Clinically flat lesions that are pale brown, with a brown dermoscopic pattern. Review these clinical and dermoscopic examples of lentigo (sun spot). **A,B:** Clinical examples. **C:** The dermoscopic example shows a fingerprint pattern and moth-eaten borders.

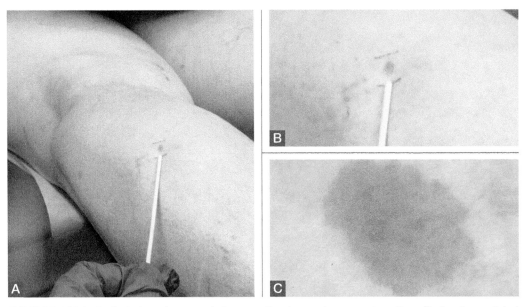

FIGURE 8.5 Clinically flat lesions that are pale brown, with a brown dermoscopic pattern. Review these clinical and dermoscopic examples of lentigo (sun spot). **A,B:** Clinical examples. **C:** The dermoscopic example shows a homogeneous pattern and moth-eaten borders.

Junctional Nevi

Pearls

- Flat/Pale Brown/Brown
  - Deeper lesions than lentigines, but it is sometimes difficult to differentiate between the two.
  - These benign lesions can also have any of the benign melanocytic nevi patterns from Chapter 1.
- **Step 4 Patterns:** homogeneous pattern, reticular network pattern, and diffuse globular pattern
- **Bottom line: Benign, biopsy not necessary.**

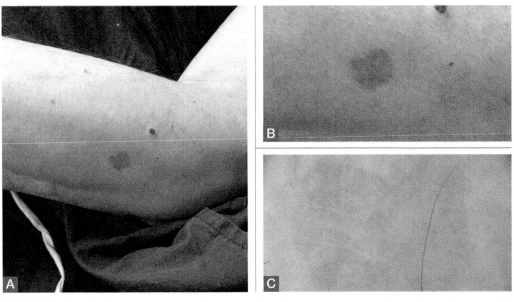

FIGURE 8.6 Clinically flat lesions that are pale brown, with a brown dermoscopic pattern. Review these clinical and dermoscopic examples of lentigo (sun spot). **A,B:** Clinical examples. **C:** The dermoscopic example shows a homogeneous pattern and moth-eaten borders.

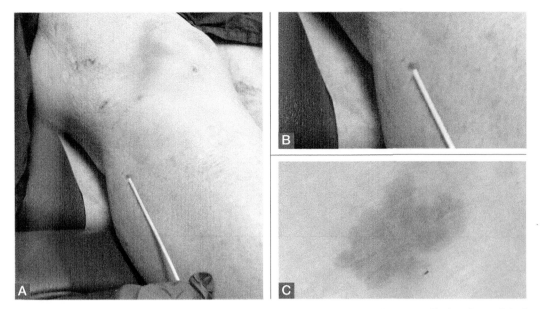

FIGURE 8.7 Clinically flat lesions that are pale brown, with a brown dermoscopic pattern. Review these clinical and dermoscopic examples of lentigo (sun spot). **A,B:** Clinical examples. **C:** The dermoscopic example shows a homogeneous pattern and moth-eaten borders.

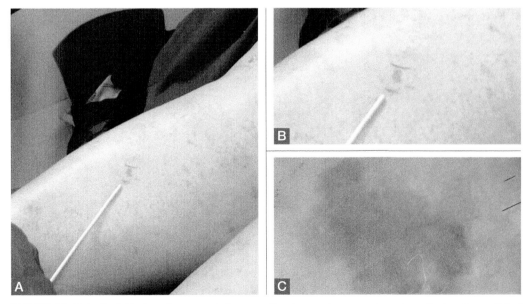

FIGURE 8.8 Clinically flat lesions that are pale brown, with a brown dermoscopic pattern. Review these clinical and dermoscopic examples of lentigo (sun spot). **A,B:** Clinical examples. **C:** The dermoscopic example shows a homogeneous pattern and moth-eaten borders.

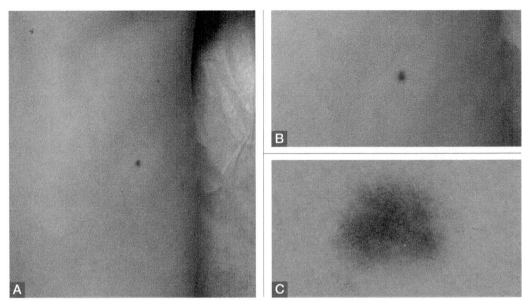

FIGURE 8.9 Clinically flat lesions that are pale brown, with a brown dermoscopic pattern. Review these clinical and dermoscopic examples of junctional nevi. **A,B:** Clinical examples. **C:** The dermoscopic example shows a symmetric reticular network pattern.

Figures 8.9 and 8.10 show clinically flat, pale brown lesions (A, B) that are dermoscopically brown (C). These lesions are characteristic of junctional nevi with a symmetric reticular network pattern. Diagnosis: Junctional nevi.

   Bottom line: Benign, biopsy unnecessary.

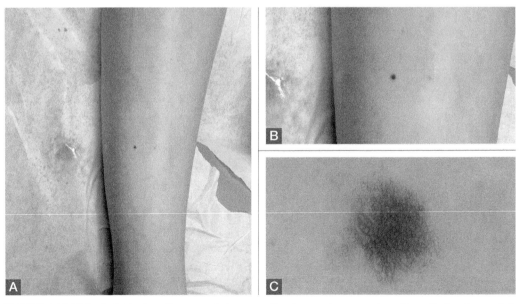

FIGURE 8.10 Clinically flat lesions that are pale brown, with a brown dermoscopic pattern. Review these clinical and dermoscopic example of junctional nevi. **A,B:** Clinical examples. **C:** The dermoscopic examples show a symmetric reticular network pattern.

Early Seborrheic Keratoses

Pearls

- Flat/Pale Brown/Brown
- **Step 4 Patterns:** The dermoscopic features of evolving seborrheic keratosis can overlap with those of solar lentigines. In both lesions, you can see
  - Fingerprinting
  - Moth-eaten borders
  - Focal thickening of networks
  - Broken interrupted lines
  - Few comedo-like openings, ridges, milia-like cysts, and fissures
- **Bottom line: Benign, biopsy not necessary.**

Examples

Figure 8.11 shows a clinically flat, pale brown lesion (Figure 8.11A, B) that is dermoscopically brown (Figure 8.11C). The coral-like early ridge pattern is characteristic of an early seborrheic keratosis. Diagnosis: Early seborrheic keratoses.

Bottom line: Benign, biopsy unnecessary.

Figure 8.12 shows a clinically flat, pale brown lesion (Figure 8.12A, B) that is dermoscopically brown (Figure 8.12C). We can appreciate the dermoscopic ridges of a seborrheic keratosis with the moth-eaten border of a solar lentigo. This is characteristic of an early seborrheic keratosis evolving from a solar lentigo. Diagnosis: Early seborrheic keratoses.

Bottom line: Benign, biopsy unnecessary.

Figure 8.13 shows a clinically flat, pale brown lesion (Figure 8.13A, B) that is dermoscopically brown (Figure 8.13C). We can see dermoscopic ridges, milia-like cysts, and the sharp borders of a seborrheic keratosis. Additionally, we see the peripheral fingerprint pattern of a lentigo circled in black. This is characteristic of an early seborrheic keratosis evolving from a solar lentigo. Diagnosis: Early seborrheic keratoses.

Bottom line: Benign, biopsy unnecessary.

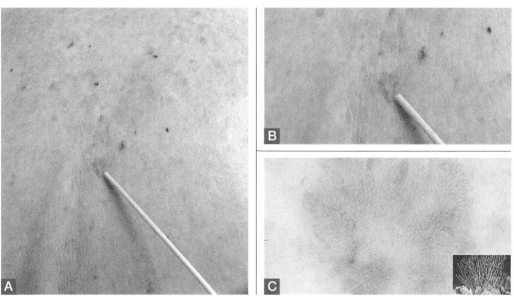

FIGURE 8.11 Clinically flat lesions that are pale brown, with a brown dermoscopic pattern. Review these clinical and dermoscopic examples of junctional nevi. **A,B:** Clinical examples. **C:** The dermoscopic examples show a coral-like early ridge pattern.

Clinical Pale Brown

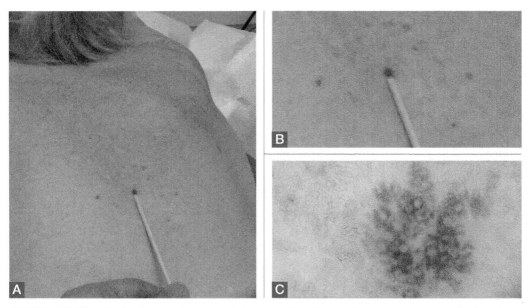

FIGURE 8.12 Clinically flat lesions that are pale brown, with a brown dermoscopic pattern. Review these clinical and dermoscopic examples of an early seborrheic keratosis evolving from a lentigo. **A,B:** Clinical examples. **C:** The dermoscopic example shows ridges of a seborrheic keratosis, with the moth-eaten border of a lentigo.

Figure 8.14 shows a clinically flat, pale brown lesion (Figure 8.14A, B) that is dermoscopically brown (Figure 8.14C). Circled in black, we can see the dermoscopic ridges of a seborrheic keratosis, but we still see the moth-eaten border of a lentigo. This is characteristic of an early seborrheic keratosis evolving from a solar lentigo. Diagnosis: Early seborrheic keratoses.

Bottom line: Benign, biopsy unnecessary.

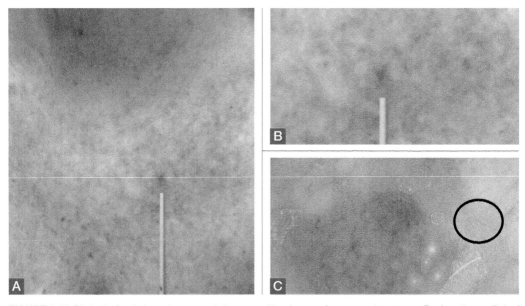

FIGURE 8.13 Clinically flat lesions that are pale brown, with a brown dermoscopic pattern. Review these clinical and dermoscopic examples of an early seborrheic keratosis evolving from a lentigo. **A,B:** Clinical examples. **C:** The dermoscopic example shows ridges, milia-like cysts, and the sharp borders of a seborrheic keratosis, with the peripheral fingerprint pattern of a lentigo circled in black.

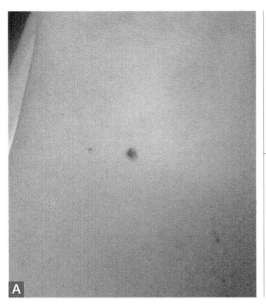
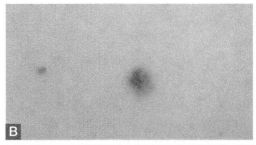
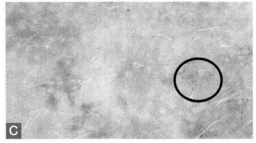

FIGURE 8.14 Clinically flat lesions that are pale brown, with a brown dermoscopic pattern. Review these clinical and dermoscopic examples of an early seborrheic keratosis evolving from a lentigo. **A,B:** Clinical examples. **C:** The dermoscopic example shows ridges circled in black seen in a seborrheic keratosis, with the moth-eaten border of a lentigo.

Early Dermatofibroma

Pearls

- Flat/Pale Brown/Brown
  - These "flat" dermatofibromas are typically found at an early stage.
  - Flat, but firmly palpable.
  - Characteristically smooth and well circumscribed.
- **Step 4 Patterns:** Remember your patterns from Chapter 1!
  - Faint pseudo network-like/lace-like network pattern
  - Faint pigmented network
  - Central white/depigmentation scar-like patch.
- **Bottom line: Benign, biopsy not necessary.**

Examples

Figure 8.15 shows a clinically flat, pale brown lesion (Figure 8.15A, B) that is dermoscopically brown (Figure 8.15C). Dermoscopically, we see a fine network-like pattern. Clinically, this lesion is palpable. Diagnosis: Early dermatofibroma.

    Bottom line: Benign, biopsy unnecessary.

Figure 8.16 shows a clinically flat, pale brown lesion (Figure 8.16A, B) that is dermoscopically brown (Figure 8.16C). Dermoscopically, we see a fine network-like pattern and a central white scar-like area. Clinically, this lesion is palpable. Diagnosis: Early dermatofibroma.

    Bottom line: Benign, biopsy unnecessary.

Figure 8.17 shows a clinically flat, pale brown lesion (Figure 8.17A, B) that is dermoscopically brown (Figure 8.17C). Dermoscopically, we see a fine network-like pattern. Clinically, this lesion is palpable. Diagnosis: Early dermatofibroma.

    Bottom line: Benign, biopsy unnecessary.

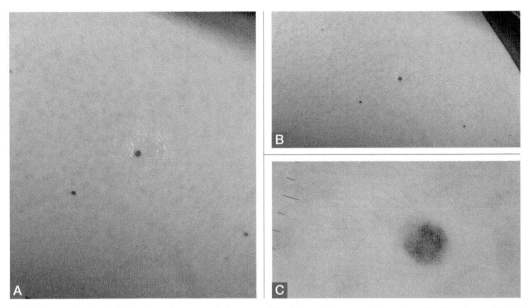

FIGURE 8.15 Clinically flat lesions that are pale brown, with a brown dermoscopic pattern. Review these clinical and dermoscopic examples of dermatofibroma. **A,B:** Clinical examples. **C:** The dermoscopic example shows a fine network-like structure. A dermatofibroma is palpable.

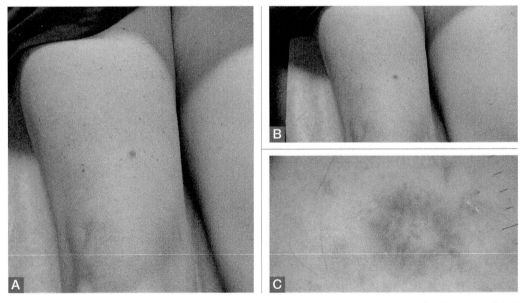

FIGURE 8.16 Clinically flat lesions that are pale brown, with a brown dermoscopic pattern. Review these clinical and dermoscopic examples of dermatofibroma. **A,B:** Clinical examples. **C:** The dermoscopic example shows a peripheral fine network-like structure and a central white scar-like area. A dermatofibroma is palpable.

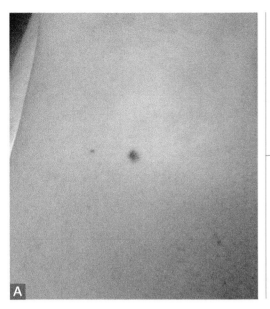
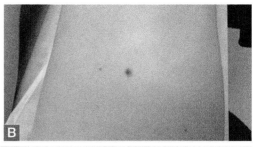
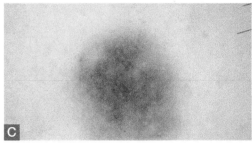

FIGURE 8.17 Clinically flat lesions that are pale brown, with a brown dermoscopic pattern. Review these clinical and dermoscopic examples of dermatofibroma. **A,B:** Clinical examples. **C:** The dermoscopic example shows a fine network-like structure. A dermatofibroma is palpable.

Malignant Lesions

Early Pigmented BCC

Pearls

- Flat/Pale Brown/Brown
- **Step 4 Patterns:** Remember your patterns from Chapter 1!
  - Irregular pigmentation
  - Speckled asymmetric globular pattern
  - Gray/blue ovoid structures
- Bottom line: Malignant, biopsy necessary

Examples

Figure 8.18 shows a clinically flat, pale brown lesion (Figure 8.18A, B) that is dermoscopically brown (Figure 8.18C). Dermoscopically, we see globular-like structures resembling a spoke wheel. Remember that it is the overall asymmetry of these lesions that distinguishes them as malignant. This is an example of an early, pigmented BCC. Diagnosis: Early pigmented BCC.

Bottom line: Malignancy, biopsy!

Figure 8.19 shows a clinically flat, pale brown lesion (Figure 8.19A, B) that is dermoscopically brown (Figure 8.19C). Dermoscopically, we see globular-like structures in an asymmetric distribution. This is an example of an early, pigmented BCC. Diagnosis: Early pigmented BCC.

Bottom line: Malignancy, biopsy!

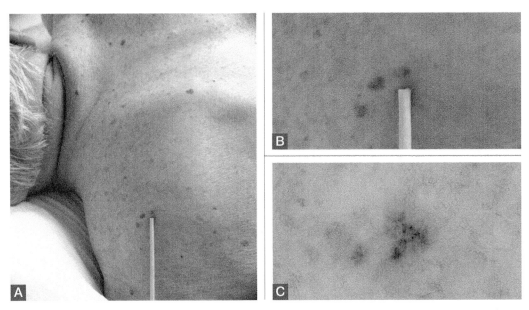

FIGURE 8.18 Clinically flat lesions that are pale brown, with a brown dermoscopic pattern. Review these clinical and dermoscopic examples of an early pigmented basal cell skin cancer. **A,B:** Clinical examples. **C:** The dermoscopic example shows globular-like structures resembling a spoke wheel. Remember it is the overall asymmetry of these lesions that distinguishes malignant from benign.

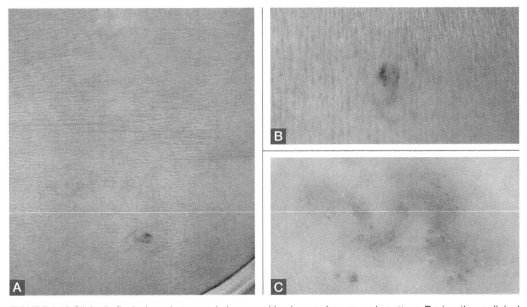

FIGURE 8.19 Clinically flat lesions that are pale brown, with a brown dermoscopic pattern. Review these clinical and dermoscopic examples of an early pigmented basal cell skin cancer. **A,B:** Clinical examples. **C:** The dermoscopic example shows globular-like structures. Remember it is the overall asymmetry of these lesions that distinguishes malignant from benign.

Early Superficial Spreading Melanoma

Pearls

- Flat/Pale Brown/Brown
  - This is the **most common** presentation of malignant melanoma (MM) that you will encounter.
- **Step 4 Patterns: Remember your patterns from Chapter 1**!
  - Irregular pigmentation
  - Asymmetry of homogeneous, globular, and reticular patterns.
  - Streaks, radial streaming, and pseudopods at the periphery.
- **Bottom line: Malignant, biopsy!**

Examples

Figure 8.20 shows a clinically flat, pale brown lesion (Figure 8.20A, B) that is dermoscopically brown (Figure 8.20C). Dermoscopically, we see focal pseudopods and radial streaming circled in black. Additionally, this lesion appears overall asymmetric, especially at the periphery. This is an early superficial MM. Diagnosis: Early superficial spreading melanoma.

Bottom line: Malignancy, biopsy!

Figure 8.21 shows a clinically flat, pale brown lesion (Figure 8.21A, B) that is dermoscopically brown (Figure 8.21C). Dermoscopically, we see focal pseudopods and radial streaming circled in black. Additionally, this lesion appears to have an overall asymmetric, globular pattern. The asymmetry is also particularly evident at the periphery. This is an early superficial MM. Diagnosis: Early superficial spreading melanoma.

Bottom line: Malignancy, biopsy!

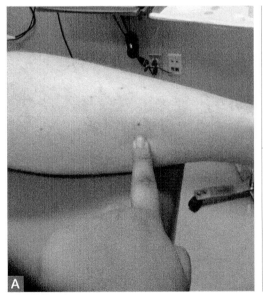
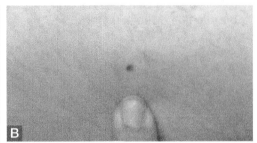
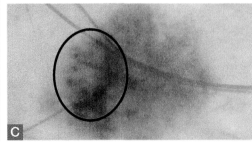

FIGURE 8.20 Clinically flat lesions that are pale brown, with a brown dermoscopic pattern. Review these clinical and dermoscopic examples of an early malignant melanoma. **A,B:** Clinical examples. **C:** The dermoscopic example shows focal pseudopods and radial streaming circled in black, as well as overall asymmetry, especially at the periphery of the lesion. Remember it is the overall asymmetry of these lesions that distinguishes malignant from benign.

Clinical Pale Brown

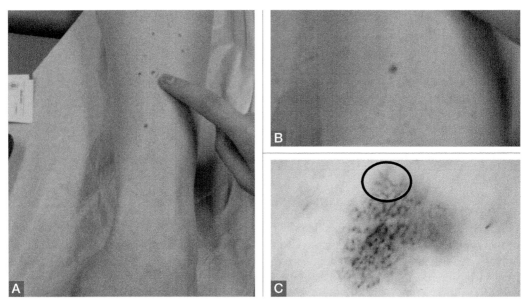

FIGURE 8.21 Clinically flat lesions that are pale brown, with a brown dermoscopic pattern. Review these clinical and dermoscopic examples of an early malignant melanoma in situ. **A,B:** Clinical examples. **C:** The dermoscopic example shows focal pseudopods and radial streaming circled in black, as well as overall asymmetry, especially at the periphery of the lesion. Remember it is the overall asymmetry of these lesions that distinguishes malignant from benign.

Figure 8.22 shows a clinically flat, pale brown lesion (Figure 8.22A, B) that is dermoscopically brown (Figure 8.22C). Dermoscopically, we see asymmetry of homogeneous nonspecific patterns and irregular pigmentation. This is an early superficial MM. Diagnosis: Early superficial spreading melanoma.

Bottom line: Malignancy, biopsy!

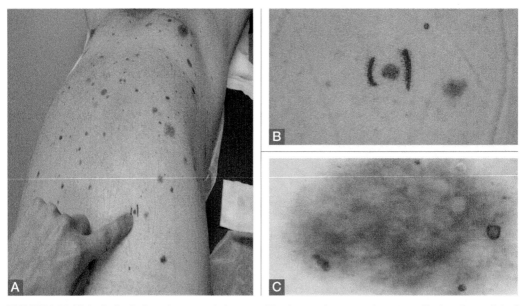

FIGURE 8.22 Clinically flat lesions that are pale brown, with a brown dermoscopic pattern. Review these clinical and dermoscopic examples of an early malignant melanoma in situ. **A,B:** Clinical examples. **C:** The dermoscopic example shows an asymmetric homogeneous nonspecific pattern. Remember it is the overall asymmetry of these lesions that distinguishes malignant from benign.

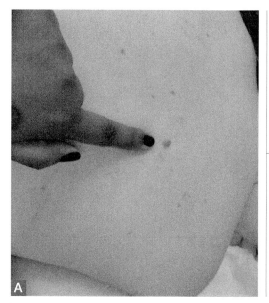
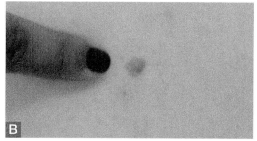
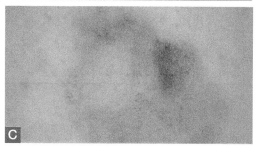

FIGURE 8.23 Clinically flat lesions that are pale brown, with a brown dermoscopic pattern. Review these clinical and dermoscopic examples of an early malignant melanoma in situ. **A,B:** Clinical examples. **C:** The dermoscopic example shows an asymmetric homogeneous nonspecific pattern, as well as asymmetric reticular and dot/globular pattern. Remember it is the overall asymmetry of these lesions that distinguishes malignant from benign.

Figure 8.23 shows a clinically flat, pale brown lesion (Figure 8.23A, B) that is dermoscopically brown (Figure 8.23C). Dermoscopically, we see asymmetry of all three melanocytic patterns: asymmetric homogeneous, reticular, and dot/globular. The asymmetry is what distinguishes this lesion from benign. This is an early superficial MM. Diagnosis: Early superficial spreading melanoma.

Bottom line: Malignancy, biopsy!

Lentigo Maligna

Pearls

- Flat/Pale Brown/Brown
  - This diagnosis is based on the clinical history. Most of the time you see these, they will be isolated pale patches on the face, but occasionally, they can occur elsewhere on the body.
  - These will look like lentigines but with nonspecific, asymmetric homogeneous patterns. However, in this category of pale brown, the patterns are often very difficult and dermoscopy is less helpful than in other categories.
  - We will revisit these lesions in the clinically dark brown lesion chapter where we can often see more specific patterns.
- **Step 4 Patterns: Remember your patterns from Chapter 1!**
  - Asymmetric, nonspecific, homogeneous
- **Bottom line: Malignant, biopsy!**

Examples

Figures 8.24 and 8.25 demonstrate clinically flat, pale brown lesions (A, B) that are dermoscopically brown (C). Dermoscopically, these lesions show vague, nonspecific findings. These are two examples of isolated patches found on the face. These are examples of early lentigo maligna melanoma in situ. Diagnosis: Lentigo maligna.

Bottom line: Malignant, biopsy!

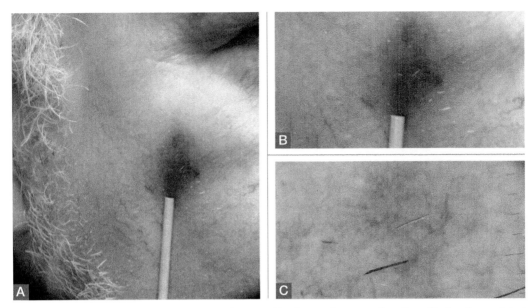

FIGURE 8.24 Clinically flat lesions that are pale brown, with a brown dermoscopic pattern. Review these clinical and dermoscopic examples of an early lentigo maligna melanoma in situ of the face. **A,B:** Clinical examples. **C:** The dermoscopic example shows an asymmetric nonspecific homogeneous pattern. Remember it is the overall asymmetry of these lesions that distinguishes malignant from benign.

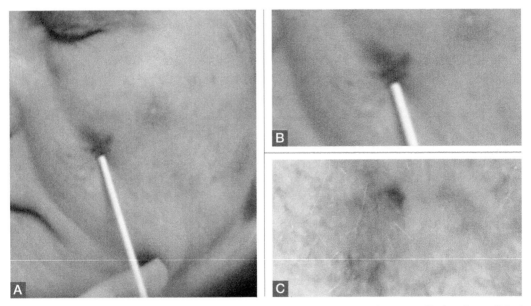

FIGURE 8.25 Clinically flat lesions that are pale brown, with a brown dermoscopic pattern. Review these clinical and dermoscopic examples of an early lentigo maligna melanoma in situ of the face. **A,B:** Clinical examples. **C:** The dermoscopic example shows an asymmetric nonspecific homogeneous pattern. Remember it is the overall asymmetry of these lesions that distinguishes malignant from benign.

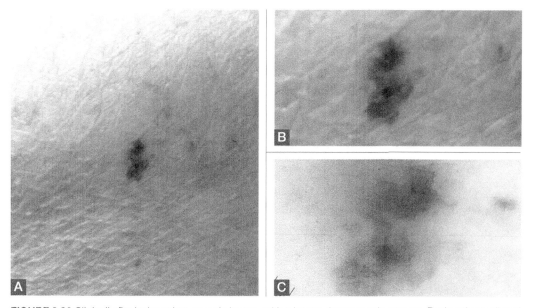

FIGURE 8.26 Clinically flat lesions that are pale brown, with a brown dermoscopic pattern. Review these clinical and dermoscopic examples of an early lentigo maligna melanoma in situ of the body. **A,B:** Clinical examples. **C:** The dermoscopic example shows an asymmetric nonspecific homogeneous pattern. Remember it is the overall asymmetry of these lesions that distinguishes malignant from benign.

Figures 8.26 to 8.31 demonstrate clinically flat, pale brown lesions (A, B) that are dermoscopically brown (C). Dermoscopically, these lesions show vague, nonspecific findings. These are examples of isolated patches found elsewhere on the body, a more atypical clinical scenario when it comes to early lentigo maligna in situ. Diagnosis: Lentigo maligna.

Bottom line: Malignant, biopsy!

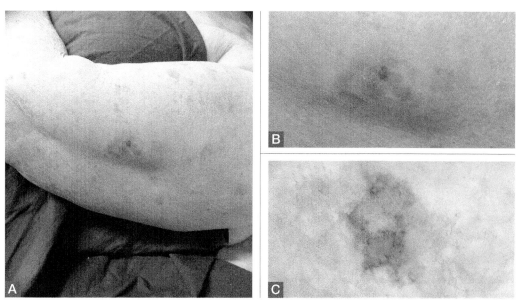

FIGURE 8.27 Clinically flat lesions that are pale brown, with a brown dermoscopic pattern. Review these clinical and dermoscopic examples of an early lentigo maligna melanoma in situ of the body. **A,B:** Clinical examples. **C:** The dermoscopic example shows an asymmetric nonspecific homogeneous pattern. Remember it is the overall asymmetry of these lesions that distinguishes malignant from benign.

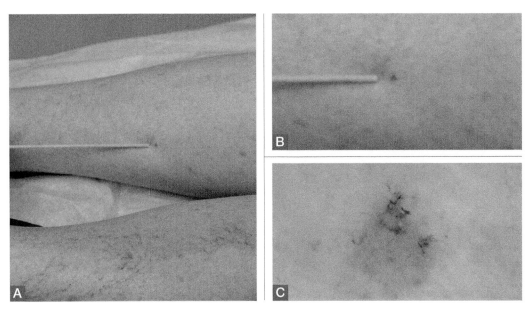

FIGURE 8.28 Clinically flat lesions that are pale brown, with a brown dermoscopic pattern. Review these clinical and dermoscopic examples of an early lentigo maligna melanoma in situ of the body. **A,B:** Clinical examples. **C:** The dermoscopic example shows an asymmetric nonspecific homogeneous pattern. Remember it is the overall asymmetry of these lesions that distinguishes malignant from benign.

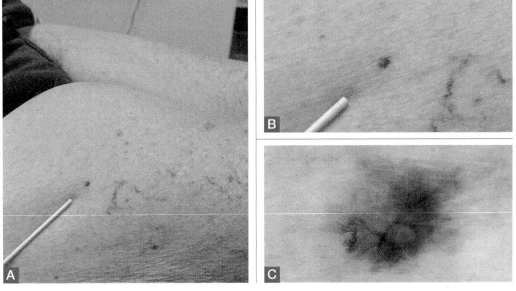

FIGURE 8.29 Clinically flat lesions that are pale brown, with a brown dermoscopic pattern. Review these clinical and dermoscopic examples of an early lentigo maligna melanoma in situ of the body. **A,B:** Clinical examples. **C:** The dermoscopic example shows an asymmetric nonspecific homogeneous pattern. Remember it is the overall asymmetry of these lesions that distinguishes malignant from benign.

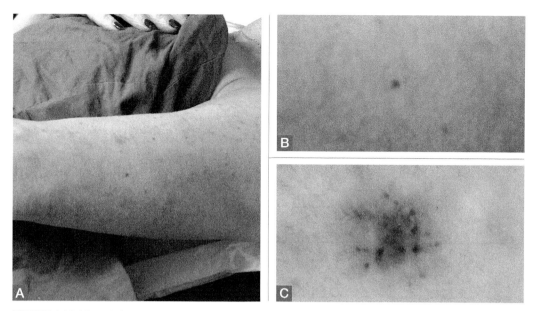

FIGURE 8.30 Clinically flat lesions that are pale brown, with a brown dermoscopic pattern. Review these clinical and dermoscopic examples of an early lentigo maligna melanoma in situ of the body. **A,B:** Clinical examples. **C:** The dermoscopic example shows an asymmetric nonspecific homogeneous pattern. Remember it is the overall asymmetry of these lesions that distinguishes malignant from benign.

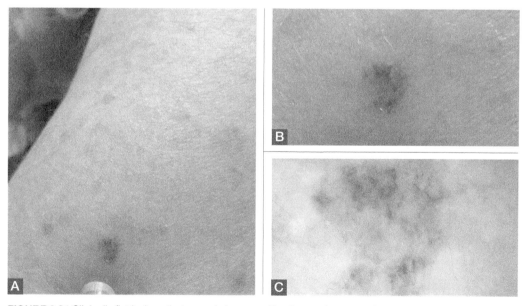

FIGURE 8.31 Clinically flat lesions that are pale brown, with a brown dermoscopic pattern. Review these clinical and dermoscopic examples of an early lentigo maligna melanoma in situ of the body. **A,B:** Clinical examples. **C:** The dermoscopic example shows an asymmetric nonspecific homogeneous pattern. Remember it is the overall asymmetry of these lesions that distinguishes malignant from benign.

Clinical Pale Brown

Squamous Cell Carcinoma In Situ: Pigmented Bowen's

Pearls

- Flat/Pale Brown/Brown
  - Pigmented Bowen's in the pale brown category often have a nonspecific homogeneous pattern similar to that of lentigo maligna.
  - You can see a dot/globular pattern that is often linear.
  - Lesions will sometimes have a reddish hue.
- **Bottom line: Malignancy, biopsy!**

Examples

Figure 8.32 is a clinically flat, pale brown, and brown dermoscopic example showing the nonspecific, asymmetric homogeneous background with small brown globules/dots in a linear pattern. The asymmetry makes this lesion likely malignant. The diagnosis is pigmented Bowen's (SCC in situ).

Bottom line: Malignant, biopsy!

Figures 8.33 to 8.35 demonstrate clinically flat, pale brown lesions (A, B) that are dermoscopically brown (C). Dermoscopically, these lesions show vague, nonspecific, asymmetric pigment pattern with speckled brown globules. The asymmetry of the pattern makes these malignant. This is an example of a pigmented Bowen's on the face. Diagnosis: Lentigo maligna.

Bottom line: Malignant, biopsy!

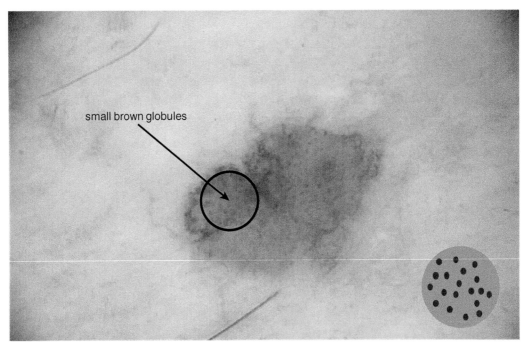

small brown globules

FIGURE 8.32 Clinically flat lesions that are pale brown, with a brown dermoscopic pattern. The diagnosis is pigmented Bowen's/early pigmented SCC in situ of the body. These views show a dermoscopic brown globular pattern.

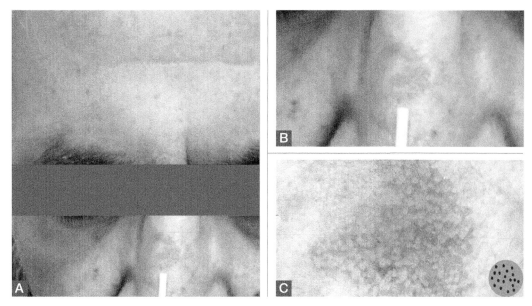

FIGURE 8.33 Clinically flat lesions that are pale brown, with a brown dermoscopic pattern. Review these clinical and dermoscopic examples of an early pigmented squamous cell skin cancer in situ of the face. **A,B:** Clinical examples. **C:** The dermoscopic example shows a speckled brown globular pattern. Remember it is the overall asymmetry of these lesions that distinguishes malignant from benign.

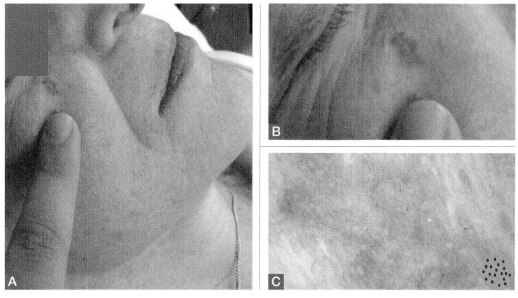

FIGURE 8.34 Clinically flat lesions that are pale brown, with a brown dermoscopic pattern. Review these clinical and dermoscopic examples of an early lentigo maligna melanoma in situ of the body. **A,B:** Clinical examples. **C:** The dermoscopic example shows an asymmetric nonspecific homogeneous pattern. Remember it is the overall asymmetry of these lesions that distinguishes malignant from benign.

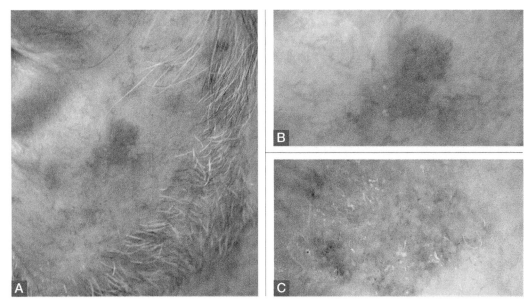

FIGURE 8.35 Clinically flat lesions that are pale brown, with a brown dermoscopic pattern. Review these clinical and dermoscopic examples of an early lentigo maligna melanoma in situ of the body. **A,B:** Clinical examples. **C:** The dermoscopic example shows an asymmetric nonspecific homogeneous pattern. Remember it is the overall asymmetry of these lesions that distinguishes malignant from benign.

Chapter 9 Flat/Pale Brown/Multicolored

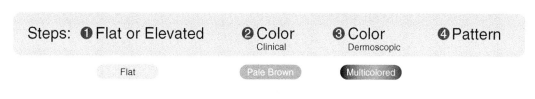

Steps: ❶ Flat or Elevated   ❷ Color *Clinical*   ❸ Color *Dermoscopic*   ❹ Pattern

Flat   Pale Brown   Multicolored

Clinical

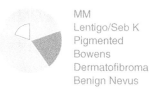

MM
Lentigo/Seb K
Pigmented
Bowens
Dermatofibroma
Benign Nevus

Dermoscopic

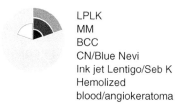

LPLK
MM
BCC
CN/Blue Nevi
Ink jet Lentigo/Seb K
Hemolized
blood/angiokeratoma

Malignant   Benign

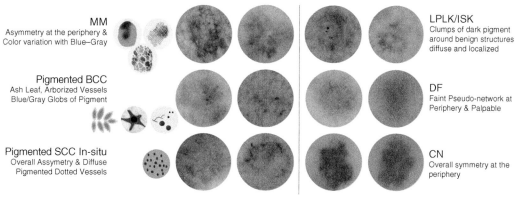

MM
Asymmetry at the periphery &
Color variation with Blue–Gray

Pigmented BCC
Ash Leaf, Arborized Vessels
Blue/Gray Globs of Pigment

Pigmented SCC In-situ
Overall Assymetry & Diffuse
Pigmented Dotted Vessels

LPLK/ISK
Clumps of dark pigment
around benign structures
diffuse and localized

DF
Faint Pseudo-network at
Periphery & Palpable

CN
Overall symmetry at the
periphery

FIGURE 9.1 Color wheel: flat/pale brown/multicolored.

Step 1: Is the lesion flat or raised? **Flat**

Step 2: What color is the lesion on clinical assessment? **Pale Brown**

Step 3: What is the dermoscopic color? **Multicolored**

Step 4: Is further elucidation needed to decide whether to biopsy or not? **Yes**

Is this a malignant or benign pattern?

Take a look at the color wheel in Figure 9.1.

These lesions really expand our differential, but the majority of the time, pale brown, flat lesions are generally benign.

Our malignancies include malignant melanoma, pigmented basal cell carcinoma (BCC), and pigmented squamous cell carcinomas (SCCs).

Our benign lesions include lichen planus–like keratosis or ISK, dermatofibroma, and congenital/junctional nevi.

Benign Lesions

Pearls

- Flat/Pale Brown/Multicolored
  - Clinically, these will have been present since childhood.
  - If these are a result of iatrogenic causes such as UV light or rubbing/irritation, this can result in multiple colors. You may see shades of brown and sometimes black.
  - They will resemble other lesions in the area. Patients will have their own "signature" lesion.
- **Step 4 Pattern Highlights: Review your patterns from** Chapter 1!
  - Symmetrical reticular pattern with darker dots
  - Overall, symmetry, especially at the periphery
- **Bottom line: Benign, biopsy unnecessary.**

Junctional/Combined Congenital Nevi

Examples

Figures 9.2 to 9.5 show a clinically flat, pale brown lesion (A, B) that is dermoscopically multicolored (brown + other = gray, pink, and/or yellow). Dermoscopically, we can see a symmetric reticular network pattern with dark dots of gray within the network. Often, these lesions will look similar to other nevi in the area—each patient may have his or her own "signature lesions!" Diagnosis: Junctional/combined congenital nevi.

Bottom line: benign, biopsy unnecessary.

Figures 9.4A–D and 9.5A, B are examples of a patient's "signature lesions." The patient's lesions in Figure 9.4A–D all have a similar coloring and pattern with the dark dots of gray in the center of the network. The lesions from the patient in Figure 9.5A, B have a very different appearance but are similar to one another. The darker brown/gray pigment is scattered in a horseshoe-like distribution at the periphery of the lesions. Diagnosis: Junctional/combined congenital nevi.

Bottom line: Benign, biopsy unnecessary

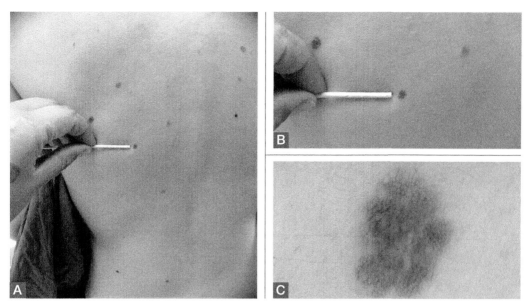

FIGURE 9.2 Clinically flat lesions that are pale brown, with a multicolored (brown + other = gray, pink, and/or yellow) dermoscopic pattern. Review these clinical and dermoscopic examples of a junctional nevi/congenital nevus. **A,B:** Clinical examples. **C:** The dermoscopic example shows a symmetric reticular network pattern with dark dots on the network. These lesions often resemble other nevi—signature nevi.

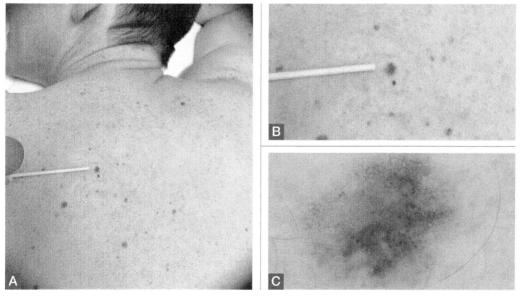

FIGURE 9.3 Clinically flat lesions that are pale brown, with a multicolored (brown + other = gray, pink, and/or yellow) dermoscopic pattern. Review these clinical and dermoscopic examples of a junctional nevi/congenital nevus. **A,B:** Clinical examples. **C:** The dermoscopic example shows a symmetric reticular network pattern with dark dots on the network. These lesions often resemble other nevi—signature nevi.

Clinical Pale Brown

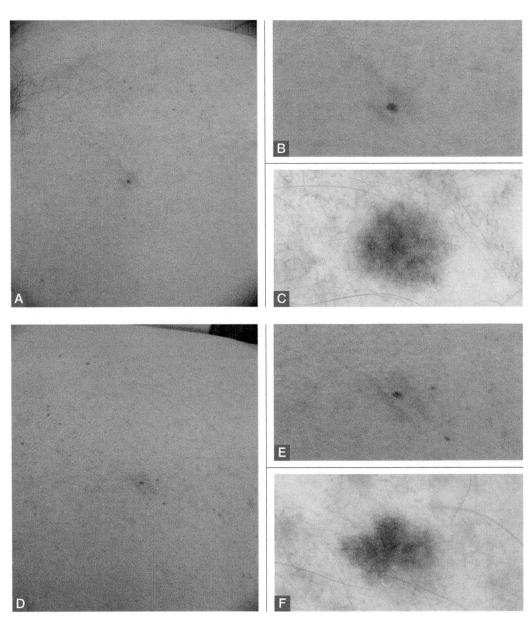

FIGURE 9.4 A–D: Multiple congenital nevi that resemble each other. These are examples of a patient's "signature lesions," that is, lesions that resemble each other. **A–C:** Clinically flat lesions that are pale brown, with a multicolored (brown + other = gray, pink, and/or yellow) dermoscopic pattern. Review these clinical and dermoscopic examples of a junctional nevi/congenital nevus. **A,B:** Clinical examples. **C:** The dermoscopic example shows a symmetric reticular network pattern with dark dots on the network. This lesion often resembles other nevi—signature nevi. **D–F:** Clinically flat lesions that are pale brown, with a multicolored (brown + other = gray, pink, and/or yellow) dermoscopic pattern. Review these clinical and dermoscopic examples of a junctional nevi/congenital nevus. **D,E:** Clinical examples. **F:** The dermoscopic example shows a symmetric reticular network pattern with dark dots on the network. This lesion often resembles other nevi—signature nevi.

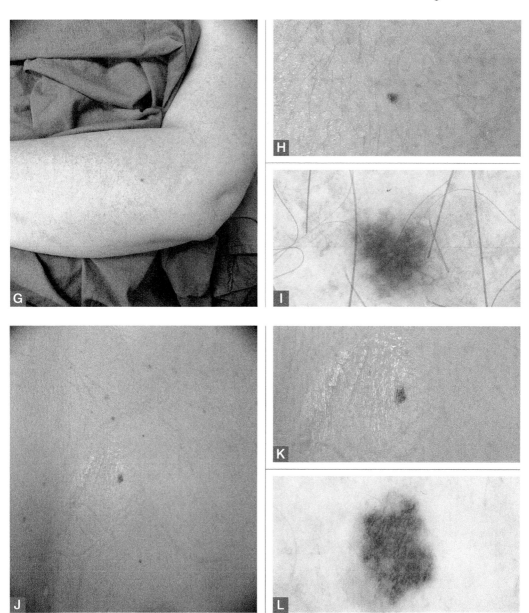

FIGURE 9.4 (*Continued*) **G–I:** Clinically flat lesions that are pale brown, with a multicolored (brown + other = gray, pink, and/or yellow) dermoscopic pattern. Review these clinical and dermoscopic examples of a junctional nevi/congenital nevus. **G,H:** Clinical examples. **I:** The dermoscopic example shows a symmetric reticular network pattern with dark dots on the network. This lesion often resembles other nevi—signature nevi. **J–L:** Clinically flat lesions that are pale brown, with a multicolored (brown + other = gray, pink, and/or yellow) dermoscopic pattern. Review these clinical and dermoscopic examples of a junctional nevi/congenital nevus. **J,K:** Clinical examples. **L:** The dermoscopic example shows a symmetric reticular network pattern with dark dots on the network. This lesion often resembles other nevi—signature nevi.

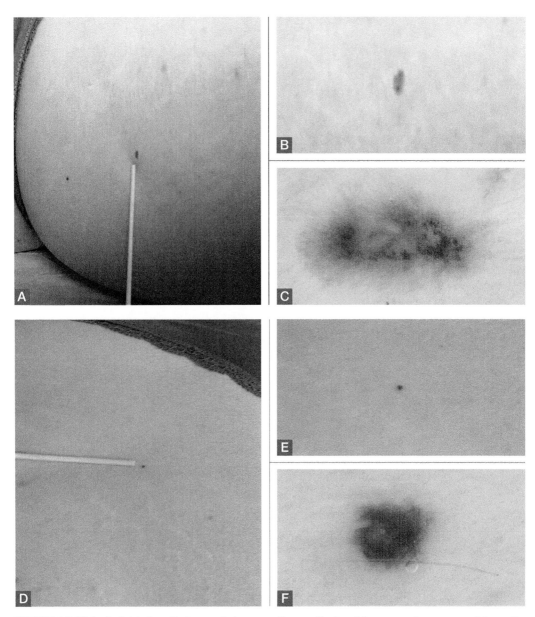

FIGURE 9.5 Clinically flat lesions that are pale brown, with a multicolored (brown + other = gray, pink, and/or yellow) dermoscopic pattern. Review these clinical and dermoscopic examples of a junctional nevi/congenital nevus. **A,B:** Clinical examples. **C:** The dermoscopic example shows a symmetric reticular network pattern with dark dots on the network. This lesion often resembles other nevi—signature nevi. **D–F:** Clinically flat lesions that are pale brown, with a multicolored (brown + other = gray, pink, and/or yellow) dermoscopic pattern. Review these clinical and dermoscopic examples of a junctional nevi/congenital nevus. **D,E:** Clinical examples. **F:** The dermoscopic example shows a symmetric reticular network pattern with dark dots on the network. This lesion often resembles other nevi—signature nevi.

Lichen Planus–Like Keratosis or Benign Lichenoid

Pearls

- Flat/Pale Brown/Multicolored
- There are two possibilities for the origin of these lesions:
  - A solar lentigo undergoing regression or an inflammatory reaction
  - A seborrheic keratosis undergoing regression or an inflammatory reaction
- When trying to distinguish between melanomas, it is useful to note the following:
  - LPLKs have more substance on palpation than superficial spreading MMs.
  - Pale brown, clinically flat lesions are usually benign.
  - LPLKs will typically show up on skin types 2 and 3.
  - LPLKs will generally resemble other lesions on the patient.
- **Step 4 Pattern Highlights: Review your patterns from** Chapter 1!
  - The inflammation leads to a nonspecific vascular pattern.
  - Often, you will see clumps of dark pigment around benign structures:
    - Diffusely on a background of hypomelanosis
    - Localized in small clusters
  - Look for clues of benign features: ridges, sharp borders, moth-eaten borders, fingerprint patterns, milia-like cysts, and comedo-like openings.
- These are often the most difficult lesions to differentiate from malignant melanoma and nonmelanoma skin cancers, so we will biopsy these lesions *often*!

Examples

Figure 9.6 is a clinically flat, pale brown lesion (Figure 9.6A, B) with a dermoscopically multicolored (brown + other = gray, pink, or yellow) pattern (Figure 9.6C). We can see diffuse granularity within the lesion dermoscopically, which can be difficult to distinguish from melanoma,

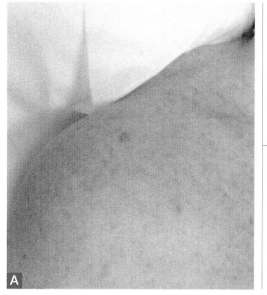
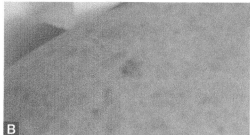
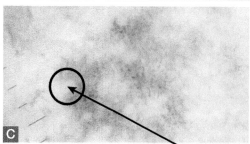

Moth-eaten border

FIGURE 9.6 Clinically flat lesions that are pale brown, with a multicolored (brown + other = gray, pink, and/ or yellow) dermoscopic pattern. Review these clinical and dermoscopic examples of benign lichen planus–like keratosis. **A,B:** Clinical examples. **C:** The dermoscopic example shows the diffuse granularity that can be difficult to distinguish from melanoma. Note the moth-eaten border, seen in benign lentigo.

Clinical Pale Brown

but note the moth-eaten border that is characteristic of a benign lentigo undergoing regression. Diagnosis: Lichen planus–like keratosis or benign lichenoid.

Bottom line: Use caution; biopsy is recommended.

Figure 9.7 is a clinically flat, pale brown lesions (Figure 9.7A, B) with a dermoscopically multicolored (brown + other = gray, pink, or yellow) pattern (Figure 9.7C). We can see diffuse granularity and nonspecific inflammation within the lesion dermoscopically, which can be difficult to distinguish from melanoma, but note the moth-eaten border that is characteristic of a benign or irritated seborrheic keratosis. Diagnosis: Lichen planus–like keratosis or benign lichenoid.

Bottom line: Use caution; biopsy is recommended.

Figure 9.8 is a clinically flat, pale brown lesion (Figure 9.8A, B) with a dermoscopically multicolored (brown + other = gray, pink, or yellow) pattern (Figure 9.8C). We can see localized granularity within the lesion dermoscopically, again making it difficult to distinguish from melanoma, but note the clear ridges and moth-eaten border that are characteristic of a benign lentigo or irritated seborrheic keratosis. Diagnosis: Lichen planus–like keratosis or benign lichenoid.

Bottom line: Use caution; biopsy is recommended.

Figure 9.9 is a clinically flat, pale brown lesion (Figure 9.9A, B) with a dermoscopically multicolored (brown + other = gray, pink, or yellow) pattern (Figure 9.9C). We can see some localized granularity and nonspecific inflammation within the lesion dermoscopically, which can be difficult to distinguish from melanoma, but note the moth-eaten border that is characteristic of a benign lentigo undergoing regression. Diagnosis: Lichen planus–like keratosis or benign lichenoid.

Bottom line: Use caution; biopsy is recommended.

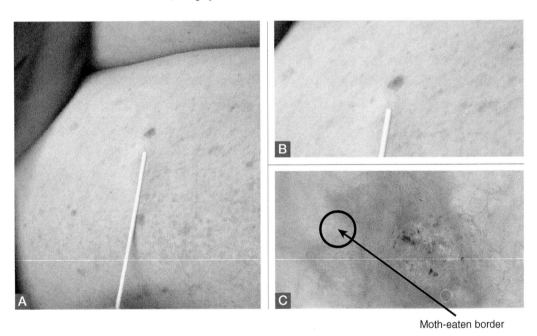

Moth-eaten border

FIGURE 9.7 Clinically flat lesions that are pale brown, with a multicolored (brown + other = gray, pink, and/or yellow) dermoscopic pattern. Review these clinical and dermoscopic examples of benign lichen planus–like keratosis/irritated seborrheic keratosis. **A,B:** Clinical examples. **C:** The dermoscopic example shows the diffuse granularity that can be difficult to distinguish from melanoma. Note the moth-eaten border seen in benign lentigo and irritated seborrheic keratoses.

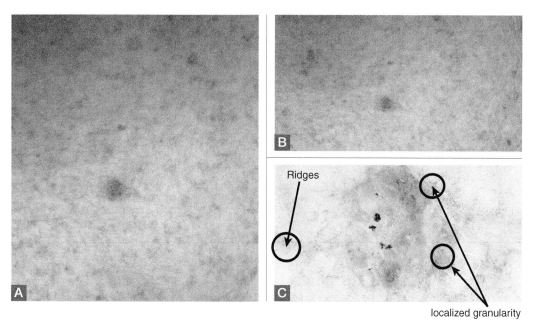

FIGURE 9.8 Clinically flat lesions that are pale brown, with a multicolored (brown + other = gray, pink, and/or yellow) dermoscopic pattern. Review these clinical and dermoscopic examples of benign lichen planus–like keratosis/irritated seborrheic keratosis. **A,B:** Clinical examples. **C:** The dermoscopic example shows the diffuse granularity that can be difficult to distinguish from melanoma. Note the moth-eaten border seen in benign lentigo and irritated seborrheic keratoses. Also note that the ridges are consistent with benign seborrheic keratosis.

Figure 9.10 is a clinically flat, pale brown lesion (Figure 9.10A, B) with a dermoscopically multicolored (brown + other = gray, pink, or yellow) pattern (Figure 9.10C). We can see diffuse and localized clumps of granularity within the lesion dermoscopically, which can be difficult

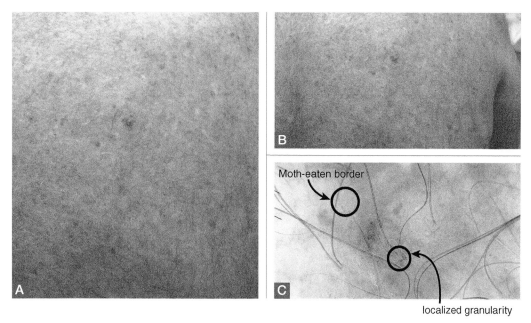

FIGURE 9.9 Clinically flat lesions that are pale brown, with a multicolored (brown + other = gray, pink, and/or yellow) dermoscopic pattern. Review these clinical and dermoscopic examples of benign lichen planus–like keratosis/irritated seborrheic keratosis. **A,B:** Clinical examples. **C:** The dermoscopic example shows the diffuse granularity that can be difficult to distinguish from melanoma. Note the moth-eaten border seen in benign lentigo and irritated seborrheic keratoses. Also note that the ridges are consistent with benign seborrheic keratosis.

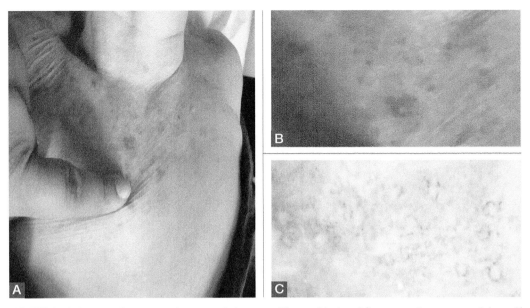

FIGURE 9.10 Clinically flat lesions that are pale brown, with a multicolored (brown + other = gray, pink, and/or yellow) dermoscopic pattern. Review these clinical and dermoscopic examples of benign lichen planus–like keratosis and actinic keratosis (pre-nonmelanoma skin cancer). **A,B:** Clinical examples. **C:** The dermoscopic example shows the diffuse granularity that can be difficult to distinguish from melanoma and which can also have a precancer component of nonmelanoma skin cancer. This lesion should be biopsied. Note there are also no signs of a benign lesion.

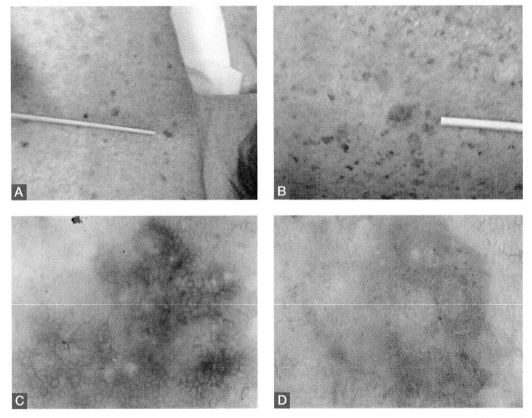

FIGURE 9.11 Clinically flat lesions that are pale brown with a multicolored (brown + other = gray, pink, and/or yellow) dermoscopic pattern. **A:** A clinical example of malignant melanoma. **B:** A clinical example of benign lichen planus–like keratosis. Note that **(A)** is smooth and flat, while there are components of **(B)** that are elevated and rough. **C,D:** The corresponding dermoscopic examples of **(A)**, malignant melanoma, and **(B)**, benign lichen planus–like keratosis. Both have diffuse granularity, making it difficult to differentiate benign from malignant. Note that **(A)** is smooth and flat, while there are components of **(B)** that are elevated and rough.

to distinguish from melanoma. There are no clear signs of a benign lesion. Diagnosis: Lichen planus–like keratosis or benign lichenoid.

Bottom line: Biopsy should be performed.

Let's look at a few comparisons of LPLKs and MMs side by side to compare.

Figure 9.11A, B shows clinically flat, pale brown lesions (Figure 9.11A, B) that have a dermoscopically multicolored (brown + other = gray, pink, or yellow) pattern (Figure 9.11C). Image A is a malignant melanoma, and clinically, it is very smooth.

Image B is a benign lichen planus–like keratosis. It is clinically rough, with more substance to palpate. Dermoscopically, the two lesions are very difficult to differentiate from one another. They both demonstrate areas of diffuse granularity.

Biopsy is necessary to determine the diagnosis.

Figure 9.12A, B shows clinically flat, pale brown lesions (Figure 9.12A, B) that have a dermoscopically multicolored (brown + other = gray, pink, or yellow) pattern (Figure 9.12C). Image A is a malignant melanoma, and clinically, it is very smooth.

Image B is a benign lichen planus–like keratosis. It is clinically rough, with more substance to palpate. Dermoscopically, the two lesions are very difficult to differentiate from one another. They both demonstrate areas of diffuse granularity.

Biopsy is necessary to determine the diagnosis.

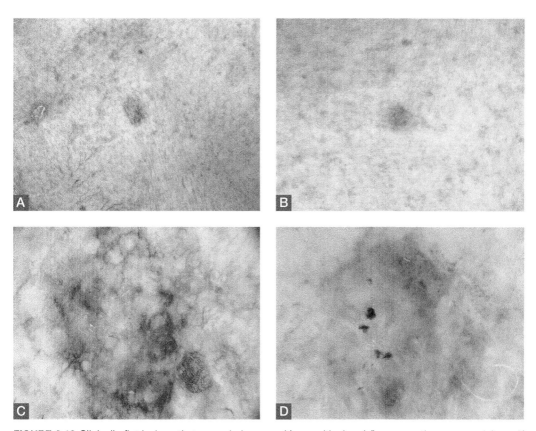

FIGURE 9.12 Clinically flat lesions that are pale brown, with a multicolored (brown + other = gray, pink, and/or yellow) dermoscopic pattern. **A:** A clinical example of malignant melanoma. **B:** A clinical example of benign lichen planus–like keratosis. Note that **(A)** is smooth and flat, while there are components of **(B)** that are elevated and rough. **C,D:** The corresponding dermoscopic examples of **(A)**, malignant melanoma, and **(B)**, benign lichen planus–like keratosis. Both have diffuse granularity, making it difficult to differentiate benign from malignant. Note that **(A)** is smooth and flat, while there are components of **(B)** that are elevated and rough.

Early Dermatofibroma

Pearls

- Flat/Pale Brown/Multicolored
  - These "flat" dermatofibromas are typically found at an early stage.
- Flat, but firmly palpable
  - Characteristically smooth and well circumscribed
- **Step 4 Patterns:** Remember your patterns from Chapter 1!
  - Faint pseudo network-like/lace-like network pattern
  - Faint pigmented network
  - Central white/depigmentation scar-like patch
- **Bottom line: Benign; biopsy not necessary.**

Examples

Figure 9.13A, B is a clinically flat, pale brown lesion (Figure 9.13A, B) with a dermoscopically multicolored (brown + other = gray, pink, or yellow) pattern (Figure 9.13C). Dermoscopically, we see a fine network-like pattern at the periphery and a central white/pink scar-like area. Note the faint dotted vessels that can be seen at the center of the lesion (Figure 9.14B). Clinically, this lesion is palpable. Diagnosis: Early dermatofibroma.

    Bottom line: Benign, biopsy not necessary.

Figure 9.14 is a clinically flat, pale brown lesion (Figure 9.14A, B) with a dermoscopically multicolored (brown + other = gray, pink, or yellow) pattern (Figure 9.14C). Dermoscopically, we see a fine network-like pattern at the periphery and a central white/pink scar-like area. Clinically, this lesion is palpable. Diagnosis: Early dermatofibroma.

    Bottom line: Benign, biopsy not necessary.

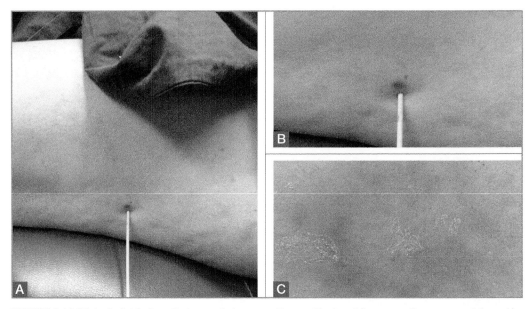

FIGURE 9.13 Clinically flat lesions that are pale brown, with a multicolored (brown + other = gray, pink, and/or yellow) dermoscopic pattern. Review these clinical and dermoscopic examples of dermatofibroma. **A,B:** Clinical examples. **C:** The dermoscopic example shows a peripheral fine network-like structure and a central white/pink scar-like area. Note the faint dotted vessels that can be seen at the center. Remember, a dermatofibroma is palpable.

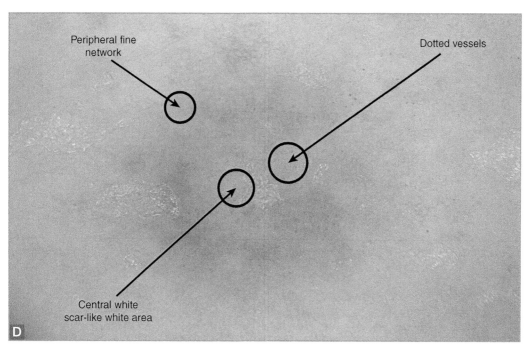

Peripheral fine network

Dotted vessels

Central white scar-like white area

FIGURE 9.13 (*Continued*) **D:** Close-up dermoscopy.

Figure 9.15 is a clinically flat, pale brown lesion (Figure 9.15A, B) with a dermoscopically multicolored (brown + other = gray, pink, or yellow) pattern (Figure 9.15C). Dermoscopically, we see a fine network-like pattern at the periphery and a central white/pink scar-like area. Clinically, this lesion is palpable. Diagnosis: Early dermatofibroma.

Bottom line: Benign, biopsy not necessary.

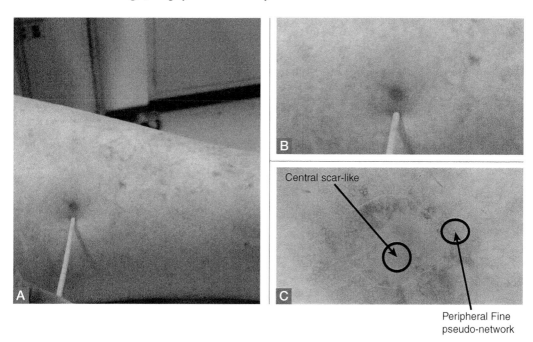

Central scar-like

Peripheral Fine pseudo-network

FIGURE 9.14 Clinically flat lesions that are pale brown with a multicolored (brown + other = gray, pink, and/or yellow) dermoscopic pattern. Review these clinical and dermoscopic examples of dermatofibroma. **A,B:** Clinical examples. **C:** The dermoscopic example shows a peripheral fine network-like structure and a central white/pink scar-like area. Remember, a dermatofibroma is palpable.

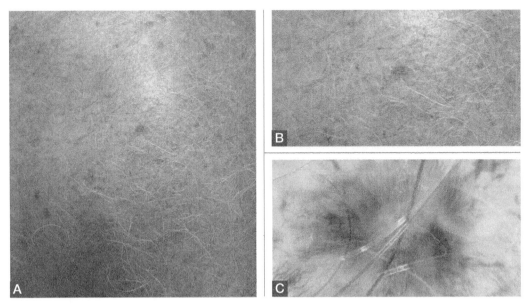

FIGURE 9.15 Clinically flat lesions that are pale brown, with a multicolored (brown + other = gray, pink, and/or yellow) dermoscopic pattern. Review these clinical and dermoscopic examples of dermatofibroma. **A,B:** Clinical examples. **C:** The dermoscopic example shows a peripheral fine network-like structure and a central white/pink scar-like area. Remember, a dermatofibroma is palpable.

Malignant Lesions

For this section, we will consider all three of our malignant possibilities together.

Malignant Melanoma, Basal Cell Carcinoma, and Squamous Cell Carcinoma

---

Pearls

- **Step 4 Patterns:** We will be using our patterns, but remember it is not necessary to distinguish one malignancy from another! They will all need to be biopsied. Check back with Chapter 1 to review your malignant patterns, but some of the things you will be looking for include
  - Disorganization of the melanocytic patterns and blue-gray granularity for our malignant melanomas.
  - BCC structures such as ash leaf patterns, arborized vessels, blue-gray globs of pigment, and ulceration.
  - Pigmented SCC in situ includes overall asymmetry and diffuse pigmented and dotted vessels.
- **Bottom line: Biopsy!**

Examples

Figure 9.16 is a clinically flat, pale brown lesion (Figure 9.16A, B) with a dermoscopically multicolored (brown + other = gray, yellow, or pink) pattern (Figure 9.16C). This is an example of an early pigmented SCC in situ. We can see diffuse pigmented, dotted vessels, but it is the overall asymmetry of this lesion, especially at the border, that distinguished this from a benign lesion. **Diagnosis:** Early pigmented SCC in-situ.

   Bottom line: Malignancy, biopsy!

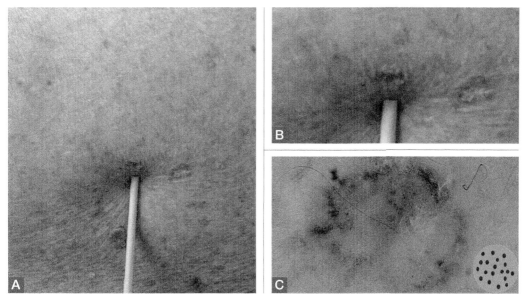

FIGURE 9.16 Clinically flat lesions that are pale brown, with a multicolored (brown + other = gray, pink, and/or yellow) dermoscopic pattern. Review these clinical and dermoscopic examples of an early pigmented squamous cell skin cancer in situ. **A,B:** Clinical examples. **C:** The dermoscopic example shows diffuse pigmented dotted vessels. Remember, it is the overall asymmetry of these lesions that distinguishes malignant from benign.

Figure 9.17 is a clinically flat, pale brown lesion (Figure 9.17A, B) with a dermoscopically multicolored (brown + other = gray, yellow, or pink) pattern (Figure 9.17C). This is an example of an early pigmented BCC. We can see globular-like structures that somewhat resemble a spoke wheel. Additionally, we can also see an ash leaf structure at the periphery with some ulceration. However, it is the overall asymmetry that distinguishes this from a benign lesion. **Diagnosis:** Early pigmented BCC.

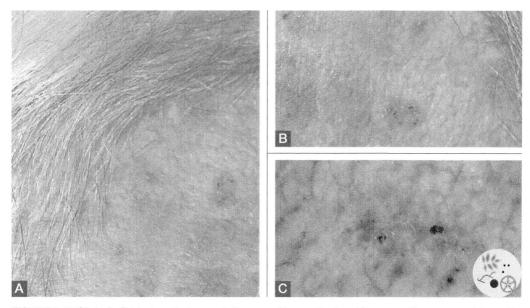

FIGURE 9.17 Clinically flat lesions that are pale brown, with a multicolored (brown + other = gray, pink, and/or yellow) dermoscopic pattern. Review these clinical and dermoscopic examples of an early pigmented basal cell skin cancer. **A,B:** Clinical examples. **C:** The dermoscopic example shows globular-like structures resembling a spoke wheel. You can also see an ash leaf pattern at the periphery and some ulceration. Remember it is the overall asymmetry of these lesions that distinguishes malignant from benign.

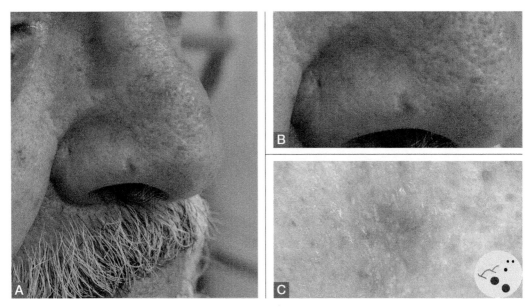

FIGURE 9.18 Clinically flat lesions that are pale brown, with a multicolored (brown + other = gray, pink, and/or yellow) dermoscopic pattern. Review these clinical and dermoscopic examples of an early pigmented basal cell skin cancer. **A,B:** Clinical examples. **C:** The dermoscopic example shows globular-like structures and arborized vessels.

Bottom line: Malignancy, biopsy!

Figure 9.18 is a clinically flat, pale brown lesion (Figure 9.18A, B) with a dermoscopically multicolored (brown + other = gray, yellow, or pink) pattern (Figure 9.18C). This is an example of an early pigmented BCC. We can see globular-like, as well as a few arborizing, sharp vessels. However, it is the overall asymmetry that distinguishes this from a benign lesion. **Diagnosis:** Early pigmented BCC.

Bottom line: Malignancy, biopsy!

Figure 9.19 is a clinically flat, pale brown lesion (Figure 9.19A, B) with a dermoscopically multicolored (brown + other = gray, yellow, or pink) pattern (Figure 9.19C). This is an example

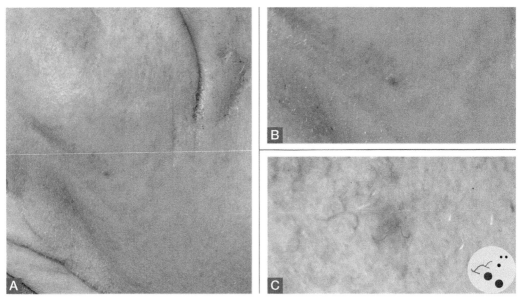

FIGURE 9.19 Clinically flat lesions that are pale brown, with a multicolored (brown + other = gray, pink, and/or yellow) dermoscopic pattern. Review these clinical and dermoscopic examples of an early pigmented basal cell skin cancer. **A,B:** Clinical examples. **C:** The dermoscopic example shows globular-like structures and arborized vessels.

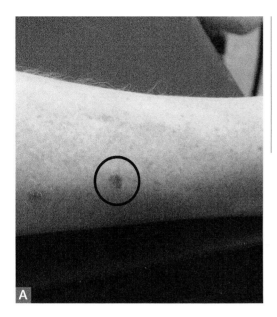

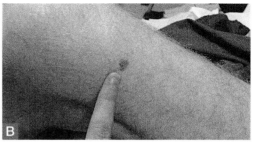

FIGURE 9.20 Clinically flat lesions that are pale brown with a multicolored (brown + other = gray, pink, and/ or yellow) dermoscopic pattern. **A:** A clinical example of basal cell carcinoma. **B:** Malignant melanoma. Note that both lesions need a biopsy and are malignant.

of an early pigmented BCC. We can see globular-like structures, as well as a few arborizing, sharp vessels. However, it is the overall asymmetry that distinguishes this from a benign lesion. **Diagnosis:** Early pigmented BCC.

   Bottom line: Malignancy, biopsy!

   Figure 9.20A, B is two clinically flat, pale brown lesions (Figure 9.20A, B) with corresponding dermoscopically multicolored (brown + other = gray, yellow, or pink) patterns (Figure 9.21A, B).

   Figure 9.21A shows an example of an early pigmented BCC. We can see globular-like structures that somewhat resemble a spoke wheel, white crystalline structures, and an area with a brown/blue ovoid nest. However, it is the overall asymmetry that distinguishes this from a benign lesion. Diagnosis: Early pigmented BCC.

   Bottom line: Malignancy, biopsy!

   Figure 9.21B shows an example of a malignant melanoma in situ. We can appreciate asymmetry at the periphery but also blue-gray granularity at the center of the lesion. This lesion could be confused for an LPLK going through regression, as we discussed earlier in this chapter, but there are no clear signs of this being a benign lesion. Diagnosis: Malignant melanoma in situ.

   Bottom line: Malignancy, biopsy!

KEY POINTS

The lesson learned from the lesions shown in Part A and Part B is that they are both clinically dark brown and flat (the basal cell being ever so slightly raised), they are both dermoscopically multicolored with malignant features, and they both require biopsy. Again, we see that is not so important that we distinguish between basal cell and melanoma but rather that we recognize the need for removal.

Clinical Pale Brown

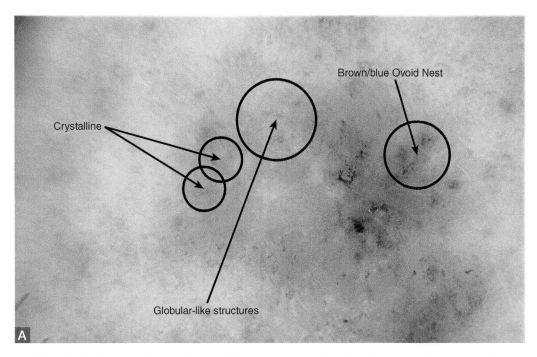

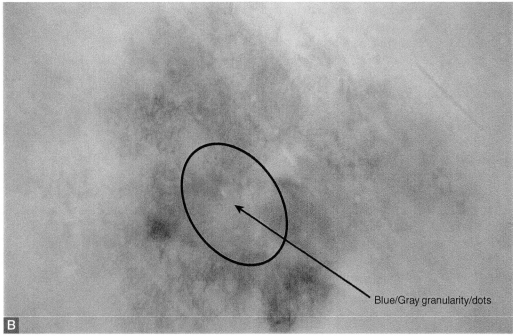

FIGURE 9.21 A: The corresponding dermoscopic examples of (A), superficial basal cell carcinoma with globular-like structures, brown/blue ovoid nests, and crystalline scar-like structures. B: The corresponding dermoscopic examples of (B), malignant melanoma in situ with localized fine blue-gray granularity, indicating a malignant feature of regression in this smooth flat lesion.

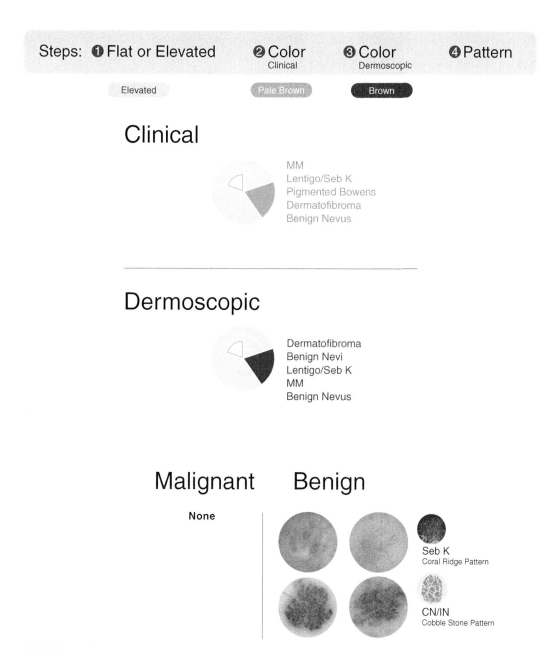

FIGURE 10.1 Color wheel: elevated/pale brown/brown.

Step 1: Is the lesion flat or raised? **Elevated**

Step 2: What color is the lesion on clinical assessment? **Pale Brown**

Step 3: What is the dermoscopic color? **Brown**

Step 4: Is further elucidation needed to decide whether to biopsy or not? **No**

Take a look at the color wheel in Figure 10.1.

What's missing on the differential? Malignant lesions!

Elevated/pale brown/brown are your best friends, your bread and butter, your walk in the park. If you evaluate a lesion and determine it is a clinically elevated, pale brown, and dermoscopically brown lesion, you are done. You will not need to biopsy these lesions.

Our differential includes only benign entities, congenital and intradermal nevi, as well as seborrheic keratosis. There are no malignancies on our list.

This being said, there are always exceptions to rules, and there may come a day that you in fact will find a malignancy in this category. However, in the overwhelming majority of cases, malignancy need not be of concern.

Let's look at some examples in order to show why we don't need to biopsy these lesions and can move on in the examination of our patients. Pattern evaluation will not be necessary for these lesions.

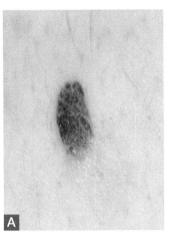
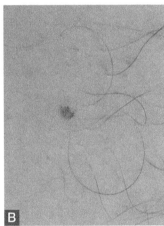
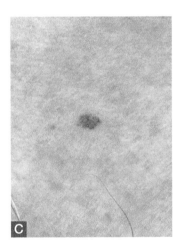

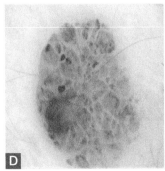
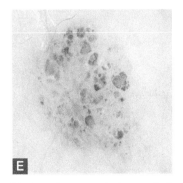
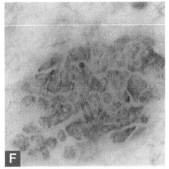

FIGURE 10.2 A–C: Clinically elevated lesions that are pale brown. **A–C** show a brown dermoscopic pattern. These are examples of three congenital nevi. **D–F:** The dermoscopic pattern of the corresponding figures **D–F** shows a dot/globular pattern.

Examples

Figure 10.2A–C shows three clinically elevated, pale brown lesions (A–C). Figure 10.2D–F shows their dermoscopic counterparts. We see brown dermoscopically. You can also immediately notice the globular dot pattern, but the pattern is not necessary in this case. These are congenital nevi. Diagnosis: Congenital nevi.

Bottom line: Benign, biopsy not necessary.

Figures 10.3 to 10.6 show more examples of clinically elevated, pale brown (A, B) lesions that are dermoscopically brown (C). Remember that congenital nevi will look similar to other

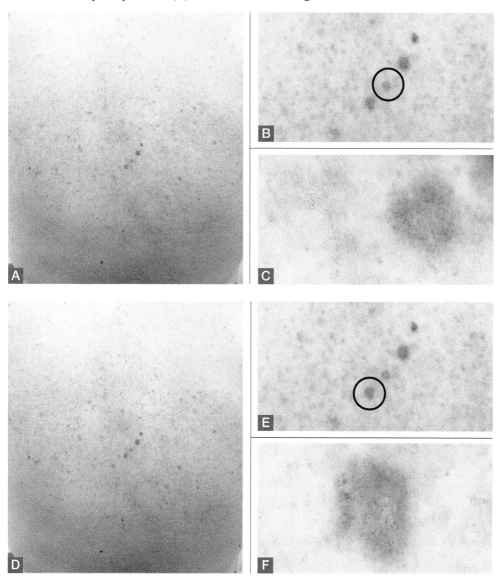

FIGURE 10.3 **A–C:** These clinically elevated lesions are pale brown, with a brown dermoscopic pattern. Review these clinical and dermoscopic examples of a congenital nevus. **A,B:** Clinical examples. **C:** The dermoscopic example shows the dot/globular pattern. Note that it can be difficult to distinguish flat from elevated lesions based on an image. It is usually easier to make this distinction during live clinical exam. Either way, unless a lesion is grossly elevated, the color wheel will still guide you to the right outcome to biopsy or not. **D–F:** These clinically elevated lesions are pale brown, with a brown dermoscopic pattern. Review these clinical and dermoscopic examples of a congenital nevus. **D,E:** Clinical examples. **F:** The dermoscopic example shows the dot/globular pattern. Note that it can be difficult to distinguish flat from elevated lesions based on an image. It is usually easier to make this distinction during live clinical exam. Either way, unless a lesion is grossly elevated, the color wheel will still guide you to the right outcome to biopsy or not. This is the same patient from Figure 10.3. Remember that congenital nevi resemble other nevi on the patient.

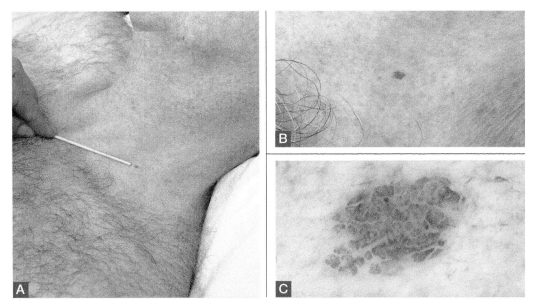

FIGURE 10.4 These clinically elevated lesions are pale brown, with a brown dermoscopic pattern. Review these clinical and dermoscopic examples of a congenital nevus. **A,B:** Clinical examples. **C:** The dermoscopic example shows a dot/globular pattern.

nevi surrounding them. The pattern is unnecessary to evaluate, but you can appreciate our benign melanocytic patterns, including diffuse reticular, globular, and homogenous patterns. Diagnosis:

Bottom line: benign biopsy not necessary.

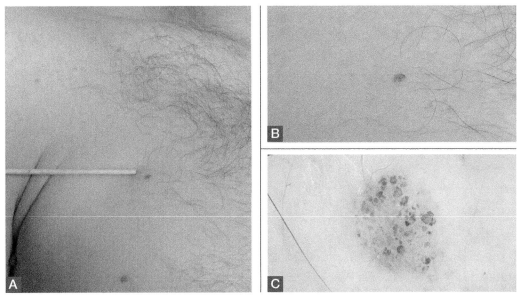

FIGURE 10.5 These clinically elevated lesions are pale brown, with a brown dermoscopic pattern. Review these clinical and dermoscopic examples of a congenital nevus. **A,B:** Clinical examples. **C:** The dermoscopic example shows a dot/globular pattern.

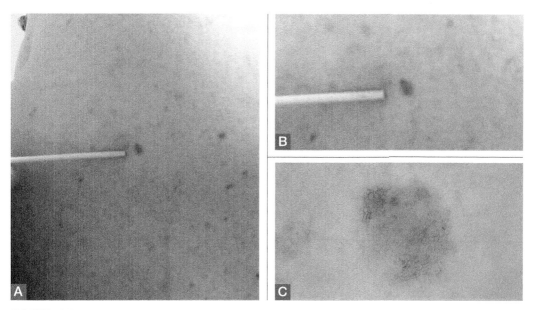

FIGURE 10.6 These clinically elevated lesions are pale brown, with a brown dermoscopic pattern. Review these clinical and dermoscopic examples of a compound congenital nevus. **A,B:** Clinical examples. **C:** The dermoscopic example shows a central dot/globular pattern, as well as a reticular pattern symmetrically at the periphery.

Figures 10.7 to 10.11 demonstrate the pattern of fissures and ridges that you were introduced to in Chapter 1; these are patterns characteristic of seborrheic keratosis. Specifically, the seborrheic keratosis that you will see is elevated, pale brown, and brown lesions. Diagnosis: Seborrheic keratosis.

Bottom line: Benign, biopsy not necessary.

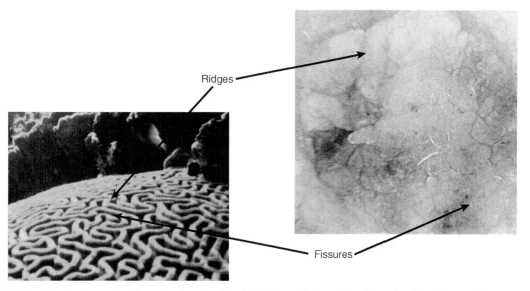

FIGURE 10.7 This coral pattern of seborrhea keratosis demonstrates ridges (elevations) and fissures (depressions). (Coral Image: Jerry Reid, US Fish & Wildlife Service via Wikimedia Commons)

Clinical Pale Brown

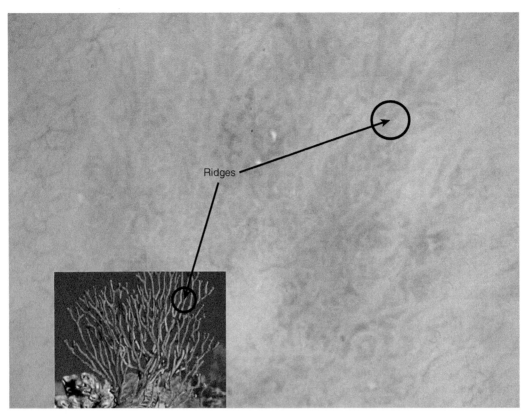

FIGURE 10.8 An example of the coral pattern of seborrheic keratosis demonstrating ridges.

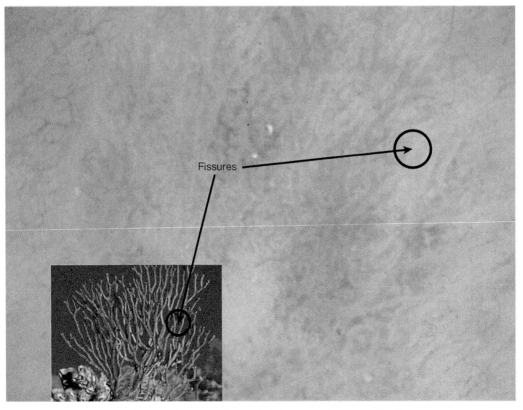

FIGURE 10.9 An example of the coral pattern of seborrheic keratosis demonstrating fissures.

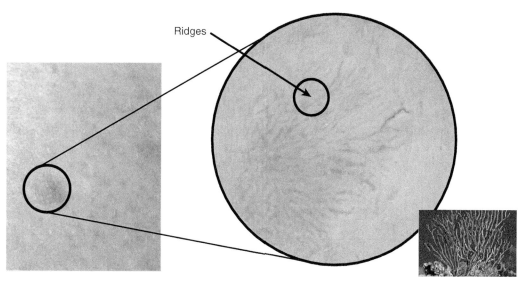

FIGURE 10.10 An example of the coral pattern of seborrheic keratosis demonstrating ridges.

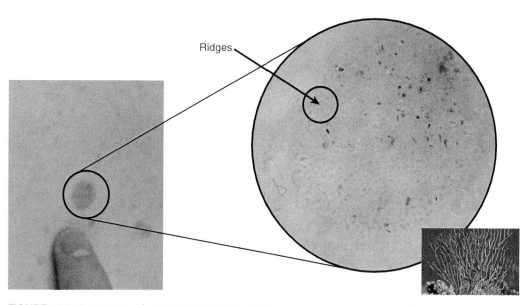

FIGURE 10.11 An example of the coral pattern of seborrheic keratosis demonstrating ridges.

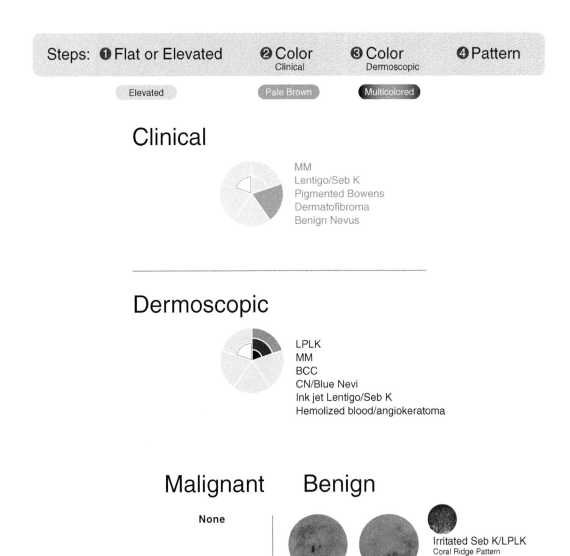

Steps: ❶ Flat or Elevated ❷ Color
Clinical
❸ Color
Dermoscopic
❹ Pattern

Elevated | Pale Brown | Multicolored

Clinical

MM
Lentigo/Seb K
Pigmented Bowens
Dermatofibroma
Benign Nevus

Dermoscopic

LPLK
MM
BCC
CN/Blue Nevi
Ink jet Lentigo/Seb K
Hemolized blood/angiokeratoma

Malignant ## Benign

None

Irritated Seb K/LPLK
Coral Ridge Pattern
Non-specific Inflammation

CN/IN
Cobble Stone Pattern
Wobble Sign

FIGURE 11.1 Color wheel: elevated/pale brown/multicolored.

Step 1: Is the lesion flat or raised? **Elevated**

Step 2: What color is the lesion on clinical assessment? **Pale Brown**

Step 3: What is the dermoscopic color? **Multicolored**

Step 4: Is further elucidation needed to decide whether to biopsy or not? **Sometimes**

Take a look at the color wheel in Figure 11.1.

What's missing on the differential? Malignant lesions!

If you evaluate a lesion and determine that it is a clinically elevated, pale brown and dermoscopically multicolored lesion, you are likely home free. You will not need to biopsy these lesions, with one important exception.

Our differential includes only benign entities, congenital and intradermal nevi, as well as irritated seborrheic keratosis or lichen planus–like keratosis. There are no malignancies on our list. Occasionally, actinic keratosis may grow within an irritated seborrheic keratosis or LPLK, and this would need to be biopsied. Unfortunately, there is no reliable way to determine malignant growth inside a benign seborrheic keratosis, so if the lesion is clinically inflamed or irritated, it should be biopsied.

Let's look at some examples in order to show when we don't need to biopsy these lesions and can move on in the examination of our patients. Pattern evaluation will not be necessary for these lesions. When dealing with inflamed lesions, we need to take a slightly different approach. When the inflammation is great, it obscures the benign features of the lesion, and biopsy is often necessary to rule out malignancy. If the inflammation is minimal and benign features—ridges, milia-like cysts—are more prominent, observation, instead of biopsy, is warranted.

Examples

Figure 11.2 shows a clinically elevated, pale brown lesion (Figure 11.2A, B) with a dermoscopically multicolored (brown + other = gray, pink, or yellow) pattern. This is an example of a congenital nevus, and pattern assessment is not necessary. However, if you remember from

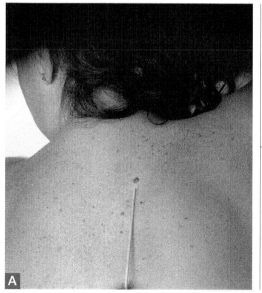
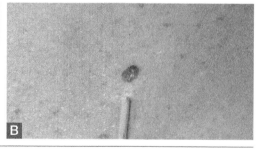
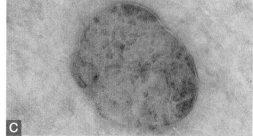

FIGURE 11.2 Clinically elevated lesions that are pale brown, with a multicolored (brown + other = gray, pink, and/or yellow) dermoscopic pattern. Review these clinical and dermoscopic examples of a congenital nevus. **A,B:** Clinical examples. **C:** The dermoscopic example shows a dot/globular pattern. You can see comma-like vessels and dark dots on the network. Additionally, this lesion wobbles when a contact scope is applied to it.

Chapter 1, we may see comma-like vessels and a globular dot pattern. Additionally, this lesion wobbles when in contact with the dermatoscope (Figure 11.3A, B). Diagnosis: Congenital nevus.

Bottom line: Biopsy unnecessary!

Figure 11.4 shows a clinically elevated, pale brown lesion (Figure 11.3A, B) with a dermoscopically multicolored (brown + other = gray, pink, or yellow) pattern. This is an example of a congenital nevus, and pattern assessment is not necessary. Again, we can remember that we

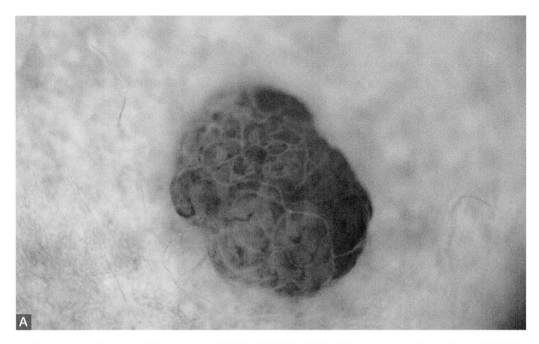

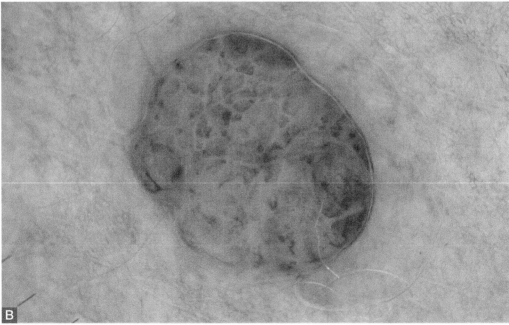

FIGURE 11.3 A: Congenital nevus wobbles when moved back and forth. **B:** Congenital nevus wobbles when moved back and forth.

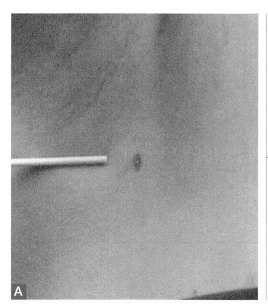
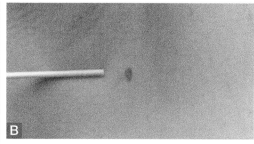
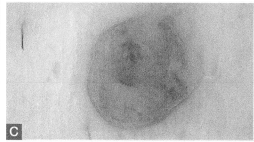

FIGURE 11.4 Clinically elevated lesions that are pale brown, with a multicolored (brown + other = gray, pink, and/or yellow) dermoscopic pattern. Review these clinical and dermoscopic examples of a congenital nevus. **A,B:** Clinical examples. **C:** The dermoscopic example shows a dot/globular pattern. You can see comma-like vessels and dark dots on the network. Additionally, this lesion wobbles when a contact scope is applied to it.

may see comma-like vessels and a globular dot pattern. Additionally, this lesion also wobbles when in contact with the dermatoscope. Diagnosis: Congenital nevus.

Bottom line: Biopsy unnecessary!

Figure 11.5 shows a clinically elevated, pale brown lesion (Figure 11.4A, B) with a dermo-scopically multicolored (brown + other = gray, pink, or yellow) pattern. This is an example of a benign lichen planus–like keratosis or irritated seborrheic keratosis. There is peripheral pink inflammation seen with a crust and dermoscopic ridges. Occasionally, actinic keratosis can grow within these lesions and will need to be biopsied. Diagnosis: Benign lichen planus–like keratosis or irritated seborrheic keratosis.

Bottom line: biopsy to rule out potential actinic keratosis.

Figure 11.6 shows a clinically elevated, pale brown lesion (Figure 11.5A, B) with a dermo-scopically multicolored (brown + other = gray, pink, or yellow) pattern. This is an example of a benign lichen planus–like keratosis or irritated seborrheic keratosis. There is peripheral pink inflammation seen with a crust and dermoscopic ridges. Occasionally, actinic keratosis can grow within these lesions and will need to be biopsied. Diagnosis: Benign lichen planus–like keratosis or irritated seborrheic keratosis.

Bottom line: Biopsy to rule out potential actinic keratosis.

Figure 11.7 shows a clinically elevated, pale brown lesion (Figure 11.6A, B) with a dermo-scopically multicolored (brown + other = gray, pink, or yellow) pattern. This is an example of a benign lichen planus–like keratosis or irritated seborrheic keratosis. There is peripheral pink inflammation seen with a crust and dermoscopic ridges. Occasionally, actinic keratosis can grow within these lesions and will need to be biopsied. Diagnosis: Benign lichen planus–like keratosis or irritated seborrheic keratosis.

Bottom line: Biopsy to rule out potential actinic keratosis.

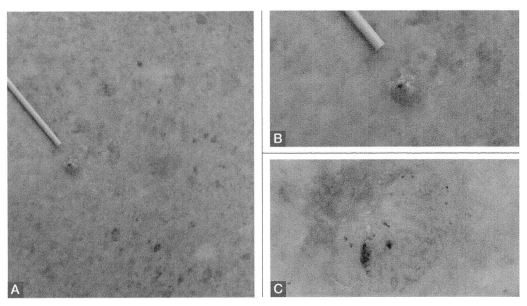

FIGURE 11.5 Clinically elevated lesions that are pale brown, with a multicolored (brown + other = gray, pink, and/or yellow) dermoscopic pattern. Review these clinical and dermoscopic examples of benign lichen planus–like keratosis/irritated seborrheic keratosis. **A,B:** Clinical examples. **C:** The dermoscopic example shows peripheral pink inflammation, crust, and ridges. Sometimes, these lesions can harbor actinic keratoses and are also irritating to the patient. Usually, they are biopsied.

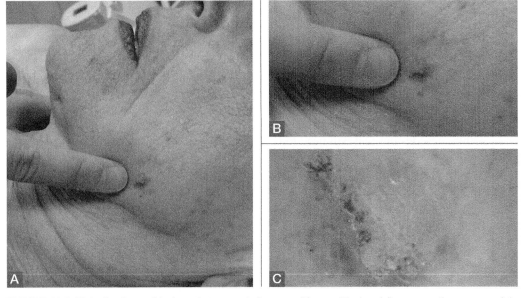

FIGURE 11.6 Clinically elevated lesions that are pale brown, with a multicolored (brown + other = gray, pink, and/or yellow) dermoscopic pattern. Review these clinical and dermoscopic examples of benign lichen planus–like keratosis/irritated seborrheic keratosis. **A,B:** Clinical examples. **C:** The dermoscopic example shows peripheral pink inflammation, crust, and ridges. Sometimes, these lesions can harbor actinic keratoses and are also irritating to the patient. Usually, they are biopsied. Note that there is some blue-gray regression, which is also seen in flat superficial spreading melanoma.

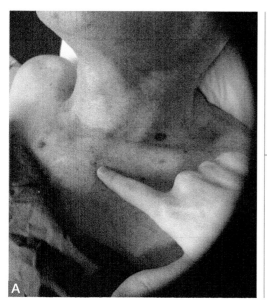
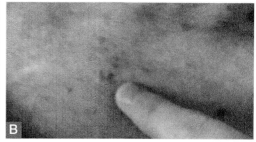
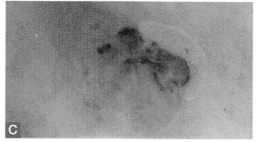

FIGURE 11.7 Clinically elevated lesions that are pale brown, with a multicolored (brown + other = gray, pink, and/or yellow) dermoscopic pattern. Review these clinical and dermoscopic examples of benign lichen planus–like keratosis/irritated seborrheic keratosis. **A,B:** Clinical examples. **C:** The dermoscopic example shows peripheral pink inflammation, crust, and ridges. Sometimes, these lesions can harbor actinic keratoses and are also irritating to the patient. Usually, they are biopsied.

Clinical Pale Brown

Chapter 12 Flat/Brown-Black/Brown

Steps: **❶ Flat or Elevated**   **❷ Color** Clinical   **❸ Color** Dermoscopic   **❹ Pattern**

Flat   Brown/Black   Brown

Clinical

MM
Ink-jet Lentigo/Seb K
Pigmented Bowens
Dermatofibroma
Benign Nevus

Dermoscopic

Dermatofibroma
Benign Nevi
Lentigo/Seb K
MM
Benign Nevus

Malignant   Benign

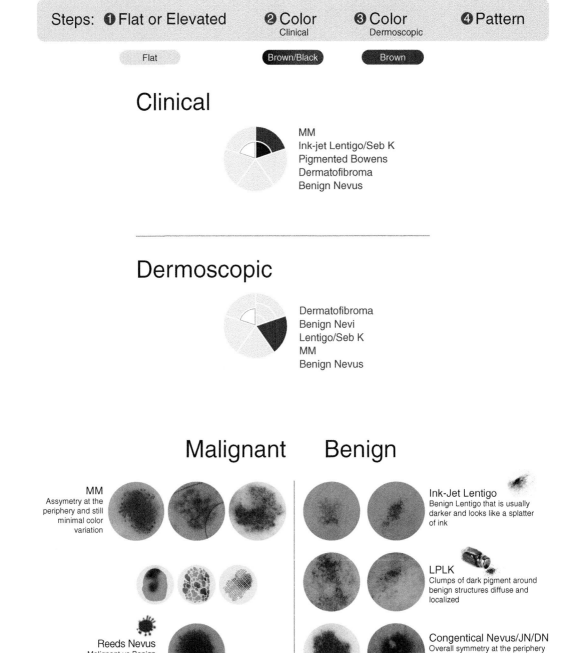

MM
Assymetry at the periphery and still minimal color variation

Reeds Nevus
Malignant vs Benign Starburst Pattern

Ink-Jet Lentigo
Benign Lentigo that is usually darker and looks like a splatter of ink

LPLK
Clumps of dark pigment around benign structures diffuse and localized

Congentical Nevus/JN/DN
Overall symmetry at the periphery

FIGURE 12.1 Color wheel: flat/brown-black/brown.

Step 1: Is the lesion flat or raised? **Flat**

Step 2: What color is the lesion on clinical assessment? **Brown/Black**

Step 3: What is the dermoscopic color? **Brown**

Step 4: Is further elucidation needed to decide whether to biopsy or not? **Yes**

Is this a malignant or benign pattern?

Take a look at the color wheel in Figure 12.1.

We've moved into the world of Dark Brown! When we are looking at flat, clinically brown-black, dermoscopically brown lesions, we have to consider malignancies that are *early* in their development. This is good, because we want to catch them early!

Early malignant melanoma (MM) and lentigo maligna are in our differential. Reed or Spitz nevus is also in our differential; these are typically seen in younger patients. However, in older patients, they are treated as malignancy.

Our benign lesions include ink-jet lentigo, lichen planus–like keratosis (LPLK), and congenital/junctional nevus.

Benign Lesions

Ink-Jet Lentigo

Pearls

- Flat/Brown-Black/Brown
- Usually referred to in lay terms as "sun spots" or "freckles."
- These benign lesions can have any of the benign melanocytic patterns from Chapter 1!
- These, in particular, are darker than the "typical" lentigo and look like a splatter on ink.
- They can sometimes be difficult to differentiate from dark precancers such as:
  - Pigmented actinic keratosis, a precursor to squamous cell cancer
  - Atypical intraepidermal melanocytic proliferation, which can be a precursor to a superficial spreading-type melanoma or lentigo maligna
- **Step 4 Patterns:** Fingerprint pattern, reticular network pattern, diffuse globular, diffuse light brown structureless area, and moth-eaten or sharply demarcated borders
- **Bottom line: Benign, biopsy not necessary, but biopsy if difficult to differentiate with any doubt.**

Examples

Figures 12.2 to 12.4 are clinically flat, brown-black lesions (A, B) that are dermoscopically brown (C). Dermoscopically, they look like a splatter of ink with moth-eaten borders. They can be difficult to differentiate from dark pigmented actinic keratosis because of the diffuse granularity of pigment. Diagnosis: Ink-jet lentigo.

Bottom line: Benign, but biopsy if uncertain.

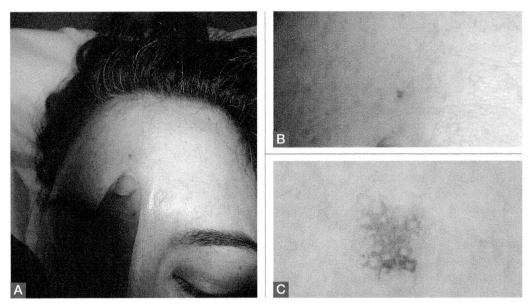

FIGURE 12.2 These clinically flat lesions are dark brown, with a brown dermoscopic pattern. Review these clinical and dermoscopic examples of an ink-jet lentigo (sun spot). **A,B:** Clinical examples. **C:** The dermoscopic examples shows a splatter of ink pattern. Sometimes it can be difficult to differentiate these lesions from dark precancers, like pigmented actinic keratosis, which is a precursor to squamous cell skin cancer.

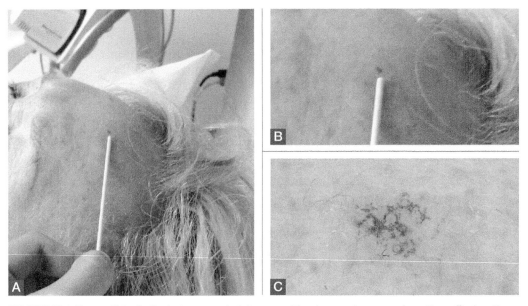

FIGURE 12.3 These clinically flat lesions are dark brown, with a brown dermoscopic pattern. Review these clinical and dermoscopic examples of an ink-jet lentigo (sun spot). **A,B:** Clinical examples. **C:** The dermoscopic example shows a splatter of ink pattern. Sometimes, it can be difficult to differentiate these lesions from dark precancers, like pigmented actinic keratosis, which is a precursor to squamous cell skin cancer.

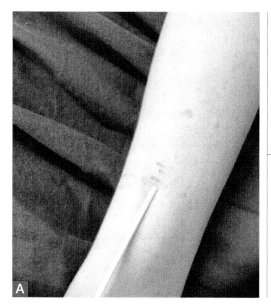
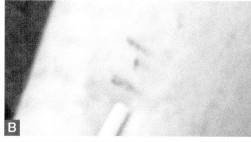
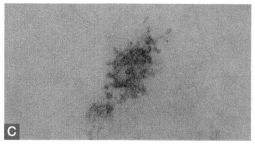

FIGURE 12.4 These clinically flat lesions are dark brown, with a brown dermoscopic pattern. Review these clinical and dermoscopic examples of an ink-jet lentigo (sun spot). **A,B:** Clinical examples. **C:** The dermoscopic example shows a splatter of ink pattern. Sometimes, it can be difficult to differentiate these lesions from dark precancers, like pigmented actinic keratosis, which is a precursor to squamous cell skin cancer.

Lichen Planus–like Keratosis or Benign Lichenoid

Pearls

- Flat/Brown-Black/Brown
  - There are two possibilities for the origin of these lesions:
    - A solar lentigo undergoing regression or an inflammatory reaction
    - A seborrheic keratosis undergoing regression or inflammatory reaction
  - When trying to distinguish melanoma, it is useful to note the following:
    - LPLKs have more substance/crust on palpation than superficial spreading MMs.
    - LPLKs will typically show up on skin types 2 and 3.
    - LPLKs will generally resemble other lesions on the patient.
- **Step 4 Pattern Highlights: Review your patterns from Chapter 1!**
  - The inflammation leads to a nonspecific vascular pattern.
  - Often, you will see clumps of dark pigment around benign structures:
    - Diffusely on a background of hypomelanosis
    - Localized in small clusters
  - Look for clues of benign features: ridges, sharp borders, moth-eaten borders, fingerprint patterns, milia-like cysts, and comedo-like openings.
- These are often the most difficult lesions to differentiate from malignant melanoma and nonmelanoma skin cancers, so **we will biopsy** these lesions *often*!

Examples

Figure 12.5 is a clinically flat, brown-black lesion (Figure 12.5A, B), with a dermoscopically brown pattern (Figure 12.5C). This is an example of a LPLK. We can see clumps of pigment, like the sprinkling of pepper, with a moth-eaten border. Without these benign features, this lesion would be difficult to differentiate from dark precancers. Remember that flat melanomas will be smooth and not demonstrate the surface changes that we can feel with these lesions. Diagnosis: Lichen planus–like keratosis or benign lichenoid.

Bottom line: Use caution, biopsy often recommended.

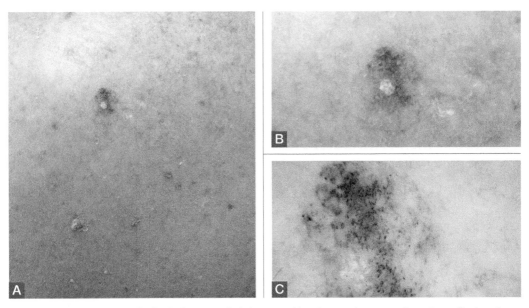

FIGURE 12.5 These clinically flat lesions are dark brown, with a brown dermoscopic pattern. Review these clinical and dermoscopic examples of lichen planus–like keratosis. **A,B:** Clinical examples. **C:** The dermoscopic example shows clumps of pigment, like a sprinkling of pepper with a moth-eaten border or other features consistent with a benign lentigo or seborrheic keratosis undergoing regression. When the features of a benign lesion are absent, these lesions are difficult to differentiate from dark precancers, like pigmented actinic keratosis, which is a precursor to squamous cell skin cancer. Remember melanomas with these features are flat and do not have all the surface changes of LPLK.

Figure 12.6 is a clinically flat, brown-black lesion (Figure 12.6A, B), with a dermoscopically brown pattern (Figure 12.6C). This is another example of an LPLK. We can see clumps of diffuse pigment, like the sprinkling of pepper. Without these benign features, this lesion would be

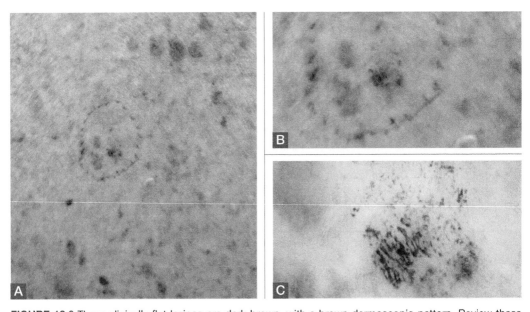

FIGURE 12.6 These clinically flat lesions are dark brown, with a brown dermoscopic pattern. Review these clinical and dermoscopic examples of lichen planus–like keratosis. **A,B:** Clinical examples. **C:** The dermoscopic example shows clumps of pigmented/diffuse granularity like a sprinkling of pepper. When the features of a benign lesion are absent, these lesions are difficult to differentiate from dark precancers, like pigmented actinic keratosis, which is a precursor to squamous cell skin cancer. Remember, melanomas with these features are flat and do not have all the surface changes of LPLK.

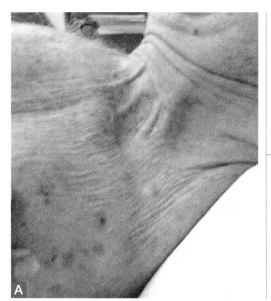
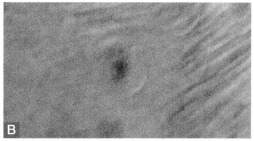
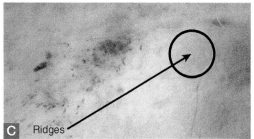

FIGURE 12.7 These clinically flat lesions are dark brown, with a brown dermoscopic pattern. Review these clinical and dermoscopic examples of lichen planus–like keratosis. **A,B:** Clinical examples. **C:** The dermoscopic example shows clumps of pigmented/diffuse granularity, like a sprinkling of pepper. When the features of a benign lesion are absent, these lesions are difficult to differentiate from dark precancers, like pigmented actinic keratosis, which is a precursor to squamous cell skin cancer. Remember, melanomas with these features are flat and do not have all the surface changes of LPLK.

difficult to differentiate from dark precancers. Remember that flat melanomas will be smooth and not demonstrate the surface changes that we can feel with these lesions. Diagnosis: Lichen planus–like keratosis or benign lichenoid.

Bottom line: Use caution, biopsy often recommended.

Figure 12.7 is a clinically flat, brown-black lesion (Figure 12.7A, B), with a dermoscopically brown pattern (Figure 12.7C). This is an example of an LPLK. We can see clumps of pigment, like the sprinkling of pepper. We are also able to see a few ridges, which are characteristic of a benign lesion. Without these benign features, this lesion would be difficult to differentiate from dark precancers. Remember that flat melanomas will be smooth and not demonstrate the surface changes that we can feel with these lesions. Diagnosis: Lichen planus–like keratosis or benign lichenoid.

Bottom line: Use caution, biopsy is recommended.

Junctional Nevi

Pearls

- Flat/Brown-Black/Brown
  - Clinically, these will have been present since childhood.
  - If these are a result of iatrogenic causes such as UV light or rubbing/irritation, this can result in multiple colors. You may see shades of brown and sometimes black.
  - They will resemble other lesions in the area; patients will have their own "signature" lesion.
- **Step 4 Pattern Highlights: Review the patterns described in Chapter 1!**
  - Symmetrical reticular pattern with darker dots
  - Perifollicular hypopigmentation
  - Overall symmetry especially at the periphery
- **Bottom line: Benign, Biopsy not necessary**

Clinical Brown-Black

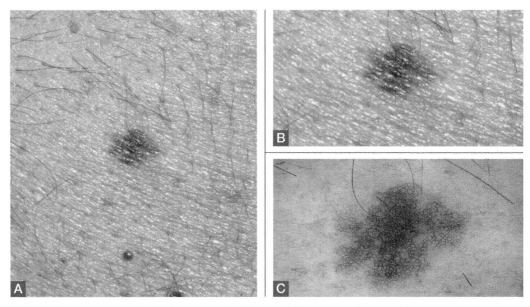

FIGURE 12.8 These clinically flat lesions are dark brown, with a brown dermoscopic pattern. Review these clinical and dermoscopic examples of a junctional nevus. **A,B:** Clinical examples. **C:** The dermoscopic example shows a dark brown reticular network with perifollicular hypopigmentation (light color around a hair follicle). There is overall symmetry.

Examples

Figures 12.8 to 12.13 show clinically flat, brown-black lesions (A, B) that are dermoscopically brown (C). These lesions are characteristic of junctional nevi and show a symmetric reticular network pattern, with perifollicular hypopigmentation. Diagnosis: Junctional nevi.

Bottom line: Benign, biopsy unnecessary

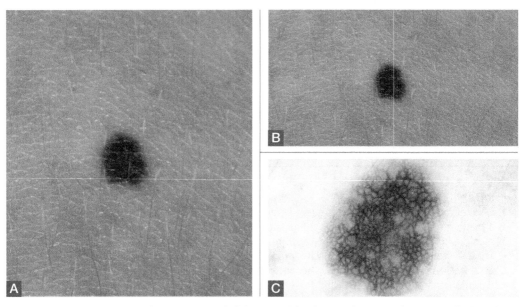

FIGURE 12.9 These clinically flat lesions are dark brown, with a brown dermoscopic pattern. Review these clinical and dermoscopic examples of a junctional nevus. **A,B:** Clinical examples. **C:** The dermoscopic example shows a dark brown reticular network with perifollicular hypopigmentation (light color around a hair follicle). There is overall symmetry.

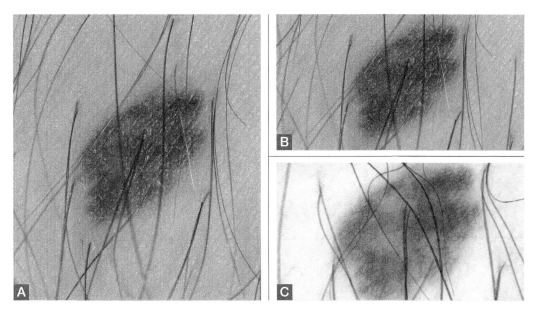

FIGURE 12.10 These clinically flat lesions are dark brown, with a brown dermoscopic pattern. Review these clinical and dermoscopic examples of junctional nevus. **A,B:** Clinical examples. **C:** The dermoscopic example shows a dark brown reticular network with perifollicular hypopigmentation (light color around a hair follicle). There is overall symmetry.

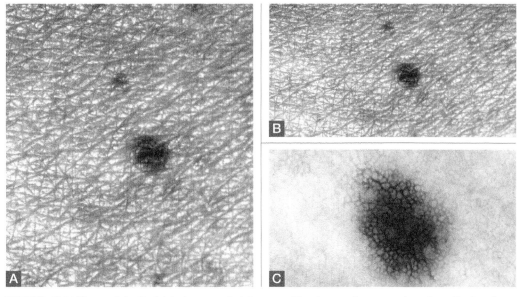

FIGURE 12.11 These clinically flat lesions are dark brown, with a brown dermoscopic pattern. Review these clinical and dermoscopic examples of junctional nevus. **A,B:** Clinical examples. **C:** The dermoscopic example shows a dark brown reticular network.

Clinical Brown-Black

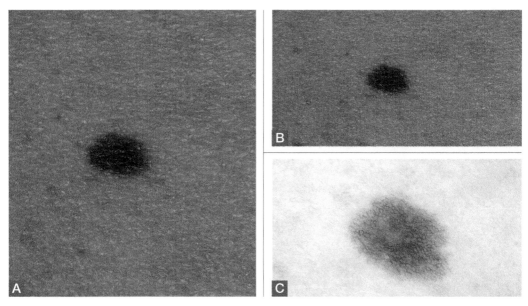

FIGURE 12.12 These clinically flat lesions are dark brown, with a brown dermoscopic pattern. Review these clinical and dermoscopic examples of junctional nevus. **A,B:** Clinical examples. **C:** The dermoscopic example shows a dark brown reticular network.

Figures 12.14 and 12.15 show clinically flat, brown-black lesions (A, B) that are dermoscopically brown (C). These lesions are characteristic of congenital nevi and show a symmetric reticular network pattern with dark dots on the network centrally. Diagnosis: Congenital nevi.

Bottom line: Benign, biopsy unnecessary

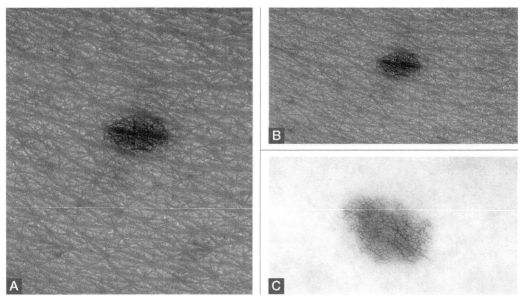

FIGURE 12.13 These clinically flat lesions are dark brown, with a brown dermoscopic pattern. Review these clinical and dermoscopic examples of junctional nevus. **A,B:** Clinical examples. **C:** The dermoscopic example shows a dark brown reticular network.

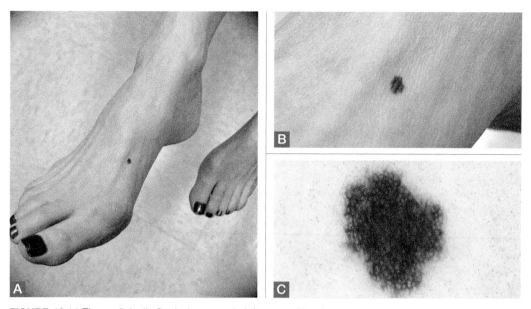

FIGURE 12.14 These clinically flat lesions are dark brown, with a brown dermoscopic pattern. Review these clinical and dermoscopic examples of congenital nevus. **A,B:** Clinical examples. **C:** The dermoscopic examples show a dark brown reticular network, with dark dots centrally located on the network.

Figure 12.16 shows a clinically flat, brown-black lesion (Figure 12.16A, B) that is dermoscopically brown (Figure 12.16C). This lesion is characteristic of a dysplastic (atypical) nevus. The reticular network is almost completely filled in, but still visible on the periphery. Diagnosis: Dysplastic (atypical) nevus.

Bottom line: Biopsy or short-term monitoring; biopsy when any change appears. An atypical nevus is a perfect segue into malignancies!

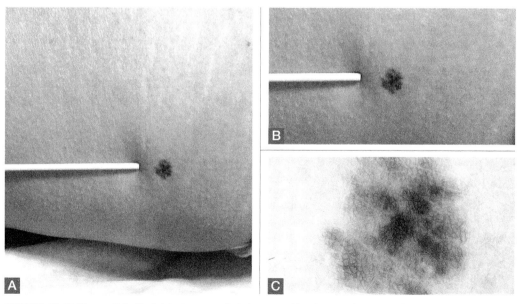

FIGURE 12.15 These clinically flat lesions are dark brown, with a brown dermoscopic pattern. Review these clinical and dermoscopic examples of congenital nevus. **A,B:** Clinical examples. **C:** The dermoscopic example shows a dark brown reticular network, with areas of darker pigment centrally located.

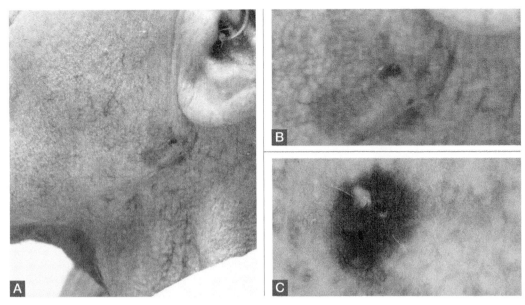

FIGURE 12.16 These clinically flat lesions are dark brown, with a brown dermoscopic pattern. Review these clinical and dermoscopic examples of a dysplastic (atypical) nevus. **A,B:** Clinical examples. **C:** The dermoscopic example shows a dark brown reticular network, with areas of darker pigment centrally located. When these lesions are atypical, they need to be biopsied or require short-term mole monitoring.

Malignant Lesions

Early Superficial Spreading Melanoma

Pearls

- Flat/Brown-Black/Brown
  - This is the **most common** presentation of MM that you will encounter.
- **Step 4 patterns: Review your patterns from Chapter 1!**
  - Irregular pigmentation
  - Asymmetry of homogenous, globular, and reticular patterns
  - Streaks, radial streaming, and pseudopods at the periphery
- **Bottom line: Malignant, biopsy!**

Examples

Figure 12.17 shows a clinically flat, brown-black lesion (Figure 12.17A, B) that is dermoscopically brown (Figure 12.17C). Dermoscopically, we see an asymmetric distribution of pigmentation, especially at the periphery. Diagnosis: This is an early superficial MM.

 Bottom line: Malignancy, biopsy!

 Figure 12.18 shows a clinically flat, brown-black lesion (Figure 12.18A, B) that is dermoscopically brown (Figure 12.18C). Dermoscopically, we see an asymmetric homogenous pattern with a peripherally asymmetric distribution of pigmentation. Diagnosis: This is an early superficial MM.

 Bottom line: Malignancy, biopsy!

 Figure 12.19 shows a clinically flat, brown-black lesion (Figure 12.19A, B) that is dermoscopically brown (Figure 12.19C). Dermoscopically, we see an asymmetric dot/globular pattern; pay close attention to the periphery. Diagnosis: This is an early superficial MM.

 Bottom line: Malignancy, biopsy!

 Reeds Nevus or Pigmented Spitz Nevus

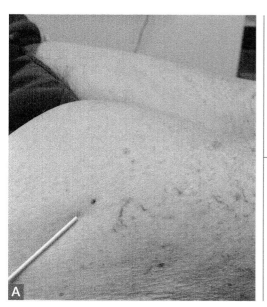
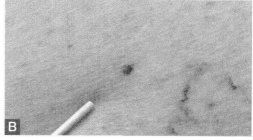
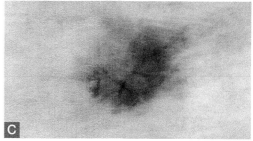

FIGURE 12.17 These clinically flat lesions are dark brown, with a brown dermoscopic pattern. Review these clinical and dermoscopic examples of a malignant melanoma in situ. **A,B:** Clinical examples. **C:** The dermoscopic example shows dark brown pigmentation with asymmetry. The diagnosis is lentigo maligna of the body melanoma in situ.

Pearls

- Flat/Brown-Black/Brown
  - Usually small dark lesions on younger patients
- **Step 4 patterns: Remember your patterns from Chapter 1!**
  - Star-burst pattern: pseudopods or streaming that is uniform around the periphery.
- **Bottom line: Treat as malignant, especially in adults, Biopsy!**

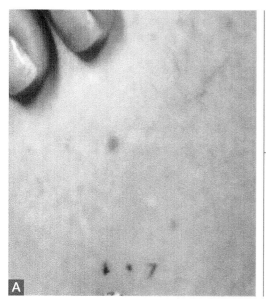
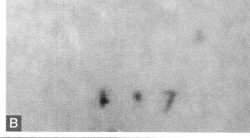
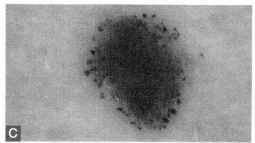

FIGURE 12.18 These clinically flat lesions are dark brown, with a brown dermoscopic pattern. Review these clinical and dermoscopic examples of a malignant melanoma in situ. **A,B:** Clinical examples. **C:** The dermoscopic example shows a dark brown asymmetric homogenous pattern, with peripheral asymmetric dots. The diagnosis is melanoma in situ.

Clinical Brown-Black

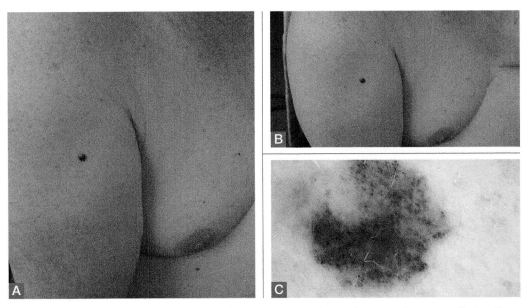

FIGURE 12.19 These clinically flat lesions are dark brown, with a brown dermoscopic pattern. Review these clinical and dermoscopic examples of a malignant melanoma in situ. **A,B:** Clinical examples. **C:** The dermoscopic example shows a dark brown asymmetric dot/globular pattern. The diagnosis is melanoma in situ.

Example

Figure 12.20 shows a clinically flat, brown-black lesion (Figure 12.20A, B) that is dermoscopically brown (Figure 12.20C). We can see a small, dark brown lesion with a uniform star-burst pattern around the periphery. In adults, treat as a malignancy. Diagnosis: Reeds nevus or pigmented spitz nevus.

Bottom line: Malignancy, biopsy!

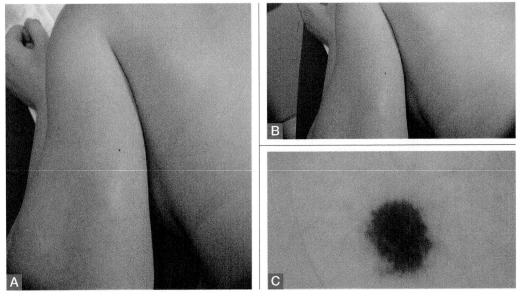

FIGURE 12.20 These clinically flat lesions are dark brown, with a brown dermoscopic pattern. Review these clinical and dermoscopic examples of a pigmented Spitz nevus (Reed nevus), which in adults is treated like a malignancy. **A,B:** Clinical examples. **C:** The dermoscopic example shows a dark brown starburst pattern. The diagnosis is Reed nevus.

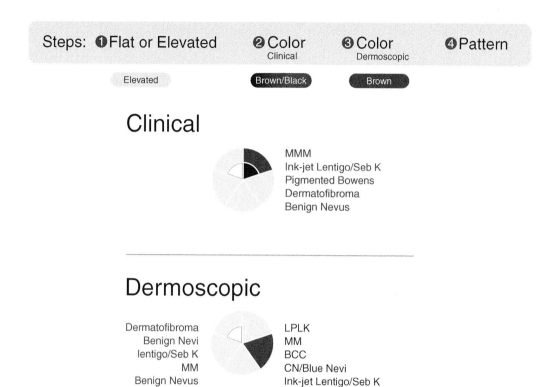

Steps: ❶Flat or Elevated ❷Color Clinical ❸Color Dermoscopic ❹Pattern

Elevated   Brown/Black   Brown

Clinical

MMM
Ink-jet Lentigo/Seb K
Pigmented Bowens
Dermatofibroma
Benign Nevus

Dermoscopic

Dermatofibroma
Benign Nevi
lentigo/Seb K
MM
Benign Nevus

LPLK
MM
BCC
CN/Blue Nevi
Ink-jet Lentigo/Seb K
Hemolized blood/angiokeratoma

Malignant   Benign

None

CN
Cobblestone pattern

Seb K
Sharp Borders, Ridges,
Milia-like Cysts &
Comedo-like Openings

Combined CN
Reticular & Cobblestone
& Dot/Globular

FIGURE 13.1 Color wheel: elevated/brown-black/brown.

Step 1: Is the lesion flat or raised? **Elevated**

Step 2: What color is the lesion on clinical assessment? **Brown-Black**

Step 3: What is the dermoscopic color? **Brown**

Step 4: Is further elucidation needed to decide whether to biopsy or not? **Sometimes**

Take a look at the color wheel in Figure 13.1.
What's missing on the differential? Malignant lesions!

If you evaluate a lesion and determine that it is a clinically elevated, brown-black, and dermoscopically brown lesion, you are dealing with a benign lesion. You will not need to biopsy these lesions.

Our differential includes only benign entities, congenital and combined nevi, as well as seborrheic keratosis.

There are no malignancies on our list. By definition, malignancies that are elevated have already progressed to an advanced stage and will be clinically suspicious. If any of these elevated lesions have more atypical features, and truly do not resemble their neighbors, a biopsy should be done. However, this category would be an exception to the rule.

Congenital or Combined Nevi

Pearls

- Elevated/Brown-Black/Brown
  - Will have been present since birth
  - May wobble with contact
- **Step 4 Pattern:** Remember to review your Chapter 1, Patterns.
  - You can see all of the benign melanocytic patterns: homogenous, globular/cobblestone, or reticular.
  - Shades of brown should not be considered multicolored! The darkest shade seen in the lesion will classify which color wheel category to choose.
  - Sometimes you can see a few visible comma vessels and milia-like cysts.
- **Bottom line: Benign, biopsy not necessary.**

Examples

Figure 13.2 shows a clinically elevated, brown-black lesion (Figure 13.2A, B), with a dermoscopically brown pattern (Figure 13.2C). This is a classic example of a congenital nevus with a symmetric, diffuse globular pattern. Diagnosis: Congenital nevus.

Bottom line: Benign, biopsy unnecessary.

Figure 13.3 shows a clinically elevated, brown-black lesion (Figure 13.3A, B), with a dermoscopically brown pattern (Figure 13.3C). This is a classic example of a congenital nevus with a symmetric, diffuse globular pattern. This lesion will wobble with contact. Diagnosis: Congenital nevus.

Bottom line: Benign, biopsy unnecessary.

Figure 13.4 shows a clinically elevated, brown lesion (Figure 13.4A, B), with a dermoscopically brown pattern (Figure 13.4C). This is a classic example of a compound nevus. You can appreciate comma-like vessels and faint pigmentation. The lesion also wobbles. Often, there is an associated reticular network with compound lesions, but you cannot see this more superficial pattern in this example. Diagnosis: Compound nevus.

Bottom line: Benign, biopsy unnecessary.

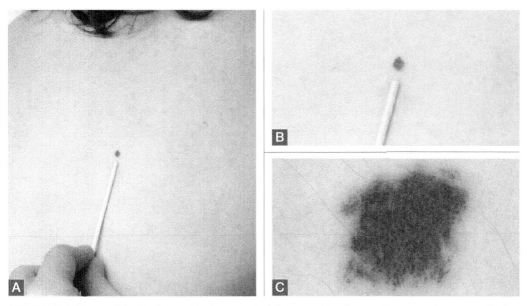

FIGURE 13.2 These clinically elevated lesions are dark brown, with a brown dermoscopic pattern. Review these clinical and dermoscopic examples of a melanocytic nevus. **A,B:** Clinical examples. **C:** The dermoscopic example shows a dot/globular pattern.

Figure 13.5 shows an example of a two-toned lesion; it is best to choose the darkest clinical color for the color wheel. We can see a clinically elevated, brown-black lesion (Figure 13.5A, B) with a dermoscopically brown pattern (Figure 13.5C). This is a classic example of a congenital nevus. You can appreciate a globular dot pattern. There is also an eccentric peripheral reticular pigmentation, but the lack of other malignant features in light of this lesion being clinically elevated and dark brown makes malignancy unlikely. Often, there is an associated reticular

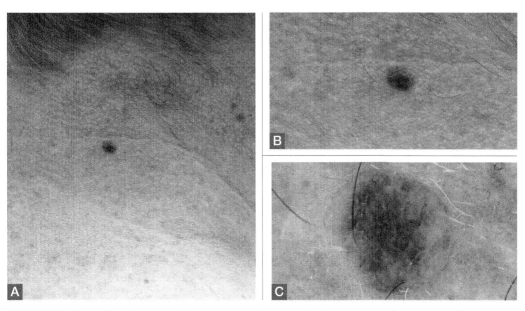

FIGURE 13.3 These clinically elevated lesions are pale brown, with a brown dermoscopic pattern. Review these clinical and dermoscopic examples of a congenital nevus. **A,B:** Clinical examples. **C:** The dermoscopic example shows a dot/globular pattern. This lesion should wobble with contact dermoscopy.

Clinical Brown-Black

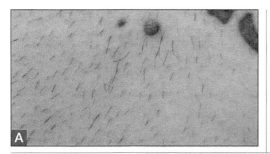
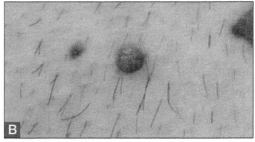
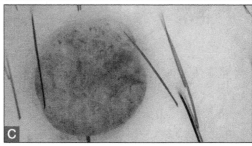

FIGURE 13.4 These clinically elevated lesions are pale brown, with a brown dermoscopic pattern. Review these clinical and dermoscopic examples of a compound nevus with melanocytic features. **A,B:** Clinical examples. **C:** The dermoscopic example shows a pattern similar to an intradermal nevus, with comma-like vessels and faint pigmentation; the lesion wobbles with a contact dermatoscope. Often, there is an associated reticular network with compound/combined lesions, but one cannot appreciate the more superficial reticular pattern in this lesion. Remember that the color wheel is used to distinguish benign lesions from malignant ones. These patterns are all benign.

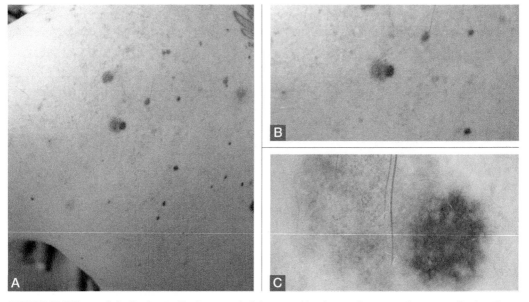

FIGURE 13.5 These clinically elevated lesions are dark brown, with a brown dermoscopic pattern. Review these clinical and dermoscopic examples of a congenital nevus with melanocytic features. **A,B:** Clinical examples. **C:** The dermoscopic example shows a dot/globular pattern. Note that this lesion also appears to have eccentric peripheral reticular pigmentation, but the lack of additional colors and other malignant features such as a negative network or streaks at the periphery makes this lesion less likely to be malignant. Remember that different shades of brown are not considered to be multicolored, but it is usually best to go with the clinical color wheel with the darkest tone, that is, dark brown clinical. However, you must also remember that if a lesion is elevated or palpable, it is not a candidate for short-term mole monitoring.

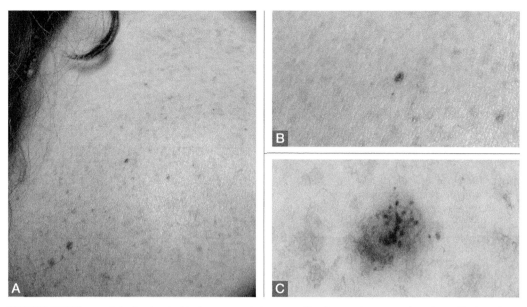

FIGURE 13.6 These clinically elevated lesions are pale brown, with a brown dermoscopic pattern. Review these clinical and dermoscopic examples of a compound melanocytic nevus. **A,B:** Clinical examples. **C:** The dermoscopic example shows a dot/globular pattern, as well as some reticular network pattern. Note that the dots are located asymmetrically at the periphery. If this dermoscopic pattern does not resemble its neighbors, this lesion is a candidate for short-term mole monitoring or biopsy.

network with compound lesions, but you cannot see this more superficial pattern in this example. Diagnosis: Congenital nevus.

Bottom line: Benign, biopsy unnecessary.

Figures 13.6 and 13.7 show a clinically elevated, brown lesion (A, B), with a dermoscopically brown pattern (C). Note that if you determine that this lesion is pinker in color, as opposed

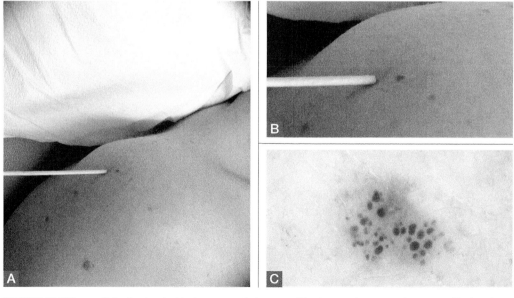

FIGURE 13.7 These clinically elevated lesions are pale brown, with a brown dermoscopic pattern. Review these clinical and dermoscopic examples of a compound melanocytic nevus. **A,B:** Clinical examples. **C:** The dermoscopic example shows a dot/globular pattern, as well as some reticular network pattern. Note that the dots are located symmetrically throughout the lesion in contrast to Figure 13.6.

to dark brown, you will still arrive at the same outcome. This is an example of a compound nevus. You can appreciate a globular pattern, as well as a reticular network. Notice in Figure 13.6 that the globules are located asymmetrically at the periphery. If this lesion does not resemble its neighbors, it should be biopsied. Diagnosis: Compound nevus.

Bottom line: Benign, biopsy unnecessary.

Seborrheic Keratoses

Pearls

- Elevated/Brown-Black/Brown
- **Step 4 Pattern:** Remember to look for your Chapter 1, Patterns
  - Any of the seborrheic patterns can be found, but especially:
    - Sharply demarcated borders, milia-like cysts, comedo-like openings (crypts)
- **Bottom line: Benign, biopsy not necessary.**

Examples

Figures 13.8 to 13.15 show examples of clinically elevated, brown (A, B) lesions that are brown dermoscopically (C). These are clear examples of the comedo-like openings, milia-like cysts, and sharp borders that are characteristic of seborrheic keratosis. Diagnosis: Seborrheic keratosis.

Bottom line: Benign, biopsy unnecessary.

Figure 13.16 shows a clinically elevated, two-toned lesion. Remember that it is best to pick the darkest clinical color from the color wheel. Thus, we have a clinically elevated, dark brown-black lesion (Figure 13.16A, B) that is dermoscopically brown (Figure 13.16C). This lesion is a good example of the starry sky appearance that SK can take on. You can also appreciate the coral-like ridge pattern. Diagnosis: Seborrheic keratosis.

Bottom line: Benign, biopsy unnecessary.

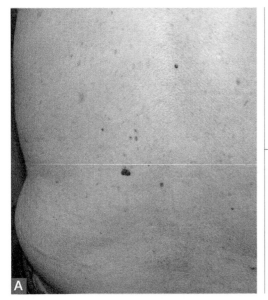
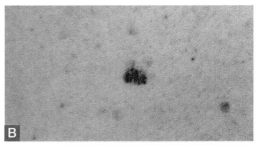
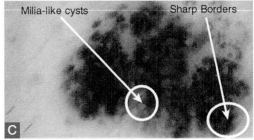

Milia-like cysts — Sharp Borders

FIGURE 13.8 These clinically elevated lesions are pale brown, with a brown dermoscopic pattern. Review these clinical and dermoscopic examples of a seborrheic keratosis. **A,B:** Clinical examples. **C:** The dermoscopic example shows comedo-like openings and sharp borders.

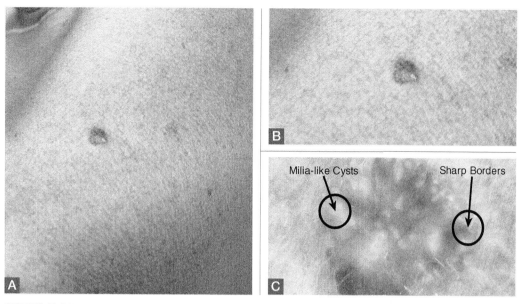

FIGURE 13.9 These clinically elevated lesions are pale brown, with a brown dermoscopic pattern. Review these clinical and dermoscopic examples of a seborrheic keratosis. **A,B:** Clinical examples. **C:** The dermoscopic example shows comedo-like openings and sharp borders.

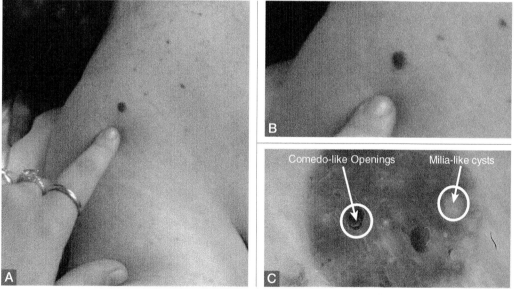

FIGURE 13.10 These clinically elevated lesions are pale brown, with a brown dermoscopic pattern. Review these clinical and dermoscopic examples of a seborrheic keratosis. **A,B:** Clinical examples. **C:** The dermoscopic example shows comedo-like openings, milia-like cysts, and sharp borders.

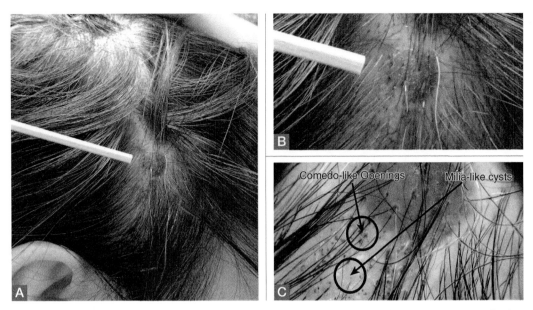

FIGURE 13.11 These clinically elevated lesions are pale brown, with a brown dermoscopic pattern. Review these clinical and dermoscopic examples of a seborrheic keratosis. **A,B:** Clinical examples. **C:** The dermoscopic example shows comedo-like openings, milia-like cysts, and sharp borders.

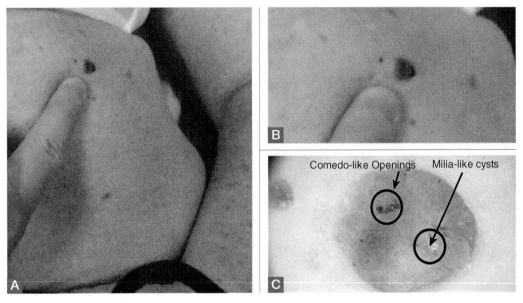

FIGURE 13.12 These clinically elevated lesions are pale brown, with a brown dermoscopic pattern. Review these clinical and dermoscopic examples of a seborrheic keratosis. **A,B:** Clinical examples. **C:** The dermoscopic example shows comedo-like openings, milia-like cysts, and sharp borders.

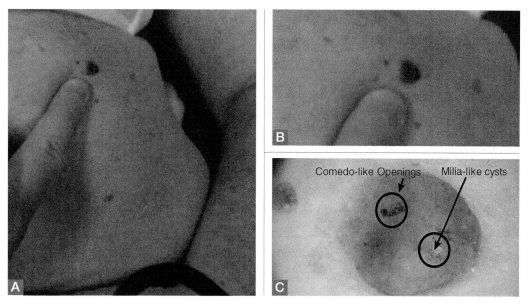

FIGURE 13.13 These clinically elevated lesions are pale brown, with a brown dermoscopic pattern. Review these clinical and dermoscopic examples of a seborrheic keratosis. **A,B:** Clinical examples. **C:** The dermoscopic example shows comedo-like openings, milia-like cysts, and sharp borders.

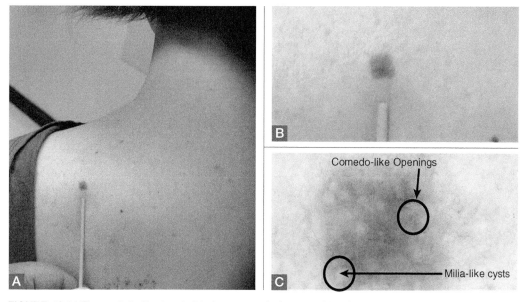

FIGURE 13.14 These clinically elevated lesions are pale brown, with a brown dermoscopic pattern. Review these clinical and dermoscopic examples of a seborrheic keratosis. **A,B:** Clinical examples. **C:** The dermoscopic example shows comedo-like openings, milia-like cysts, and sharp borders.

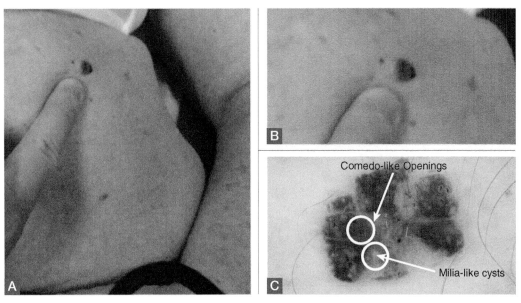

FIGURE 13.15 These clinically elevated lesions are pale brown, with a brown dermoscopic pattern. Review these clinical and dermoscopic examples of a seborrheic keratosis. **A,B:** Clinical examples. **C:** The dermoscopic example shows comedo-like openings, milia-like cysts, and sharp borders.

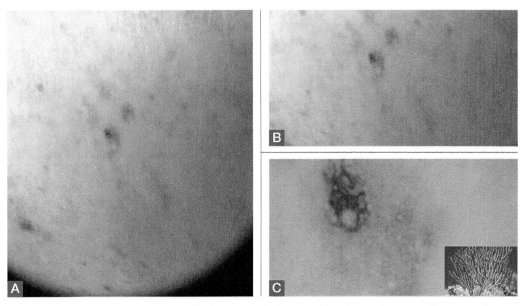

FIGURE 13.16 These clinically elevated lesions are pale brown, with a brown dermoscopic pattern. Review these clinical and dermoscopic examples of a seborrheic keratosis. **A,B:** Clinical examples. **C:** The dermoscopic example shows a coral-like ridge pattern and milia-like cysts. Note that seborrheic keratoses often have two tones of brown. It is usually best to choose the color wheel pattern with the darkest tone.

Chapter 14 Flat/Brown-Black/Multicolored

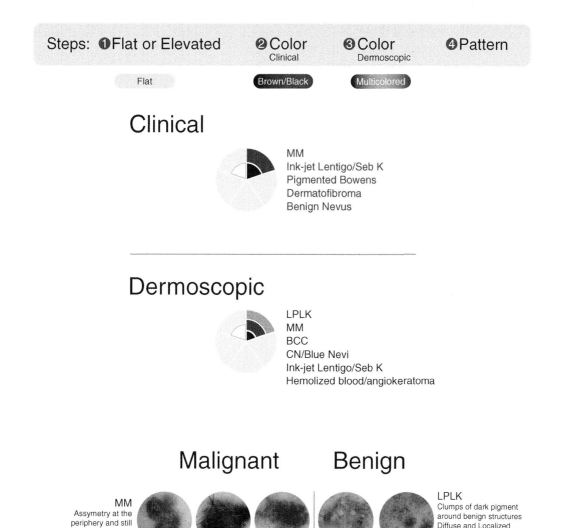

Steps: ❶Flat or Elevated ❷Color Clinical ❸Color Dermoscopic ❹Pattern

Flat   Brown/Black   Multicolored

Clinical

MM
Ink-jet Lentigo/Seb K
Pigmented Bowens
Dermatofibroma
Benign Nevus

Dermoscopic

LPLK
MM
BCC
CN/Blue Nevi
Ink-jet Lentigo/Seb K
Hemolized blood/angiokeratoma

Malignant   Benign

MM
Assymetry at the
periphery and still
minimal color variation

LPLK
Clumps of dark pigment
around benign structures
Diffuse and Localized
Often portions are elevated

Blue Nevus
Homogenous Blue
Face around
follicular openings

Early Pigmented BCC
Ash Leaf, Arborized Vessels
Blue/Gray Globs of Pigment

Melanocytic Nevus
Overall symmetry
at the periphery

FIGURE 14.1 Color wheel: flat/brown-black/multicolored.

> **Step 1:** Is the lesion flat or raised? **Flat**
>
> **Step 2:** What color is the lesion on clinical assessment? **Brown-Black**
>
> **Step 3:** What is the dermoscopic color? **Multicolored**
>
> **Step 4:** Is further elucidation needed to decide whether to biopsy or not? **Yes**
>
> Is this a malignant or benign pattern?

Take a look at the color wheel in Figure 14.1.

We've moved into the world of Dark Brown! When we are looking at flat, clinically brown-black, dermoscopically multicolored lesions we are looking at a differential similar to Flat, Brown/Black and Brown, but with a few differences.

Our benign lesions include lichen planus–like keratosis (LPLK) and congenital/junctional nevus.

Our malignancies include superficial malignant melanoma again, but early-pigmented basal cell also makes the list.

Importantly, the majority of dysplastic nevi fall into this category as well. We often struggle to categorize these lesions properly as benign or malignant. While they are not malignant, they should not be treated so simply as benign. Because we are in the world of "flat" lesions, we can recommend short-term monitoring of any dysplastic nevi. However, keep in mind that if the lesion shows any elevation, it must be biopsied. If it is in fact malignant, its elevation would mean that it is already at a more advanced stage and needs immediate removal.

Benign Lesions

Lichen Planus–like Keratosis or Benign Lichenoid

Pearls

- Flat/Brown-Black/Multicolored
  - There are two possibilities for the origin of these lesions:
    - A solar lentigo undergoing regression or an inflammatory reaction
    - A seborrheic keratosis undergoing regression or inflammatory reaction
  - When trying to distinguish between melanoma it is useful to note the following:
    - LPLKs have more substance/crust on palpation than do superficial spreading MMs.
    - LPLKs will typically show up on skin types 2 and 3.
    - LPLKs will generally resemble other lesions on the patient.
- **Step 4 Pattern Highlights: Review the patterns described in Chapter 1!**
  - The inflammation leads to a nonspecific vascular pattern.
  - Often, you will see clumps of dark pigment around benign structures:
    - Diffusely on a background of hypomelanosis
    - Localized in small clusters
  - Look for clues of benign features: ridges, sharp borders, moth-eaten borders, fingerprint patterns, milia-like cysts, and comedo-like openings.
- These are often the most difficult lesions to differentiate from malignant melanoma and nonmelanoma skin cancers, so **we will biopsy** these lesions **often**!

Examples

Figure 14.2 shows a clinically flat, brown-black lesion (Figure 14.2A, B), with a dermoscopically multicolored (brown + other = gray, pink, or yellow) pattern (Figure 14.2C). This is an example of an LPLK. We can see a broken reticular pattern and moth-eaten borders, with isolated clumps of gray granularity, which can be difficult to differentiate from melanoma. Remember that flat melanomas will be smooth and not demonstrate the surface changes that we can feel with these lesions, but these can be very difficult to differentiate. This lesion could be classified as either flat or elevated. Diagnosis: Lichen planus–like keratosis.

Bottom line: Biopsy not necessary, but use caution.

Figure 14.3 shows a clinically flat, brown-black lesion (Figure 14.3A, B), with a dermoscopically multicolored (brown + other = gray, pink, or yellow) pattern (Figure 14.3C). This is an example of an LPLK. We can see a broken reticular pattern and moth-eaten borders, with isolated clumps of gray granularity, which can be difficult to differentiate from melanoma, but you can also appreciate the ridges seen in benign seborrheic keratosis. Remember that flat melanomas will be smooth and not demonstrate the surface changes that we can feel with these lesions. This lesion could be classified as either flat or elevated. Diagnosis: Lichen planus–like keratosis.

Bottom line: Biopsy not necessary, but use caution.

Figure 14.4 shows a clinically flat, brown-black lesion (Figure 14.4A, B), with a dermoscopically multicolored (brown + other = gray, pink, or yellow) pattern (Figure 14.4C). This is an example of an LPLK. We can see a broken reticular pattern and moth-eaten borders, with isolated clumps of gray granularity, which can be difficult to differentiate from melanoma; however, you can also appreciate the ridges and a moth-eaten border seen in benign lentigo. Remember that flat melanomas will be smooth and not demonstrate the surface changes that we can feel with these lesions. This lesion could be classified as either flat or elevated. Diagnosis: Lichen planus–like keratosis.

Bottom line: Biopsy not necessary, but use caution.

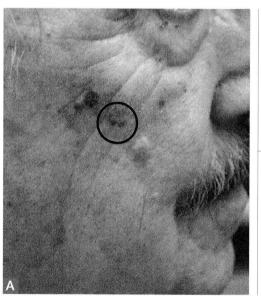
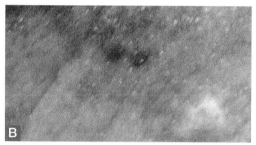
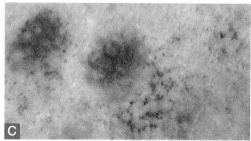

FIGURE 14.2 These clinically flat lesions are dark brown, with a multicolored (brown + other = gray, pink, and/or yellow) dermoscopic pattern. Review these clinical and dermoscopic examples of lichen planus–like keratosis (LPLK). **A,B:** Clinical examples. **C:** The dermoscopic example shows a broken reticular pattern and moth-eaten borders, with isolated gray granularity, which can be difficult to distinguish from melanoma. The evidence of the ridges seen in benign seborrheic keratosis, as well as the slight elevations within the lesion, helps make the diagnosis. These lesions can be classified as elevated or flat.

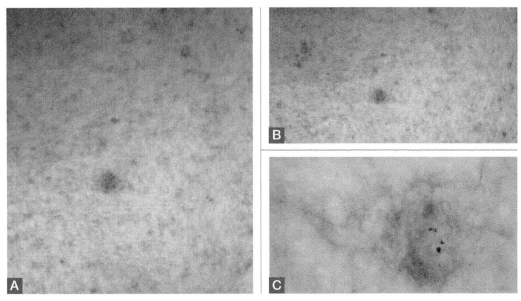

FIGURE 14.3 These clinically flat lesions are dark brown, with a multicolored (brown + other = gray, pink, and/or yellow) dermoscopic pattern. Review these clinical and dermoscopic examples of lichen planus–like keratosis (LPLK). **A,B:** Clinical examples. **C:** The dermoscopic example shows a broken reticular pattern and moth-eaten borders, with isolated gray granularity, which can be difficult to distinguish from melanoma. The evidence of the ridges seen in benign seborrheic keratosis, as well as the slight elevations within the lesion, help make the diagnosis. These lesions can be classified as elevated or flat.

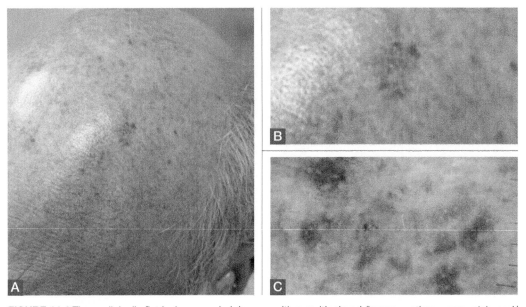

FIGURE 14.4 These clinically flat lesions are dark brown, with a multicolored (brown + other = gray, pink, and/or yellow) dermoscopic pattern. Review these clinical and dermoscopic examples of lentigo (sun spot)/LPLK. **A,B:** Clinical examples. **C:** The dermoscopic example shows a broken reticular pattern and moth-eaten borders, with isolated gray granularity. This can be difficult to distinguish from melanoma, but the evidence of the moth-eaten border seen in benign lentigo and irritated seborrheic keratosis helps make the diagnosis.

Junctional/Combined Nevi

Pearls

- Flat/Brown-Black/Multicolored
  - Clinically, these will have been present since childhood.
  - If these are a result of iatrogenic causes, such as UV light or rubbing/irritation, the result is multiple colors. You may see shades of brown and sometimes black.
  - These will resemble other lesions in the area. Patients will have their own "signature" lesion.
- **Step 4 Pattern Highlights: Review the patterns described in Chapter 1!**
  - Symmetrical reticular pattern with darker dots.
  - Perifollicular hypopigmentation.
  - Overall symmetry, especially at the periphery.
  - Skin types 3 and up will have blue-white veils in benign lesions.
- **Bottom line: Benign, biopsy not necessary.**

Examples

Figure 14.5 shows a clinically flat, brown-black lesion (Figure 14.5A, B) that is dermoscopically multicolored (brown + other = blue/gray, pink, or yellow) (Figure 14.5C). This lesion is characteristic of a congenital nevus that resembles other lesions and has a well-defined border. Dermoscopically, we see a symmetric reticular network pattern with a blue-white veil. Diagnosis: Congenital nevus.

    Bottom line: Benign, biopsy unnecessary.

Figure 14.6 shows a clinically flat, brown-black lesion (Figure 14.6A, B) that is dermoscopically multicolored (brown + other = blue/gray, pink, or yellow) (Figure 14.6C). This lesion is characteristic of a congenital nevus that resembles other lesions and has a well-defined border. Dermoscopically, we see a symmetric reticular network pattern with a blue-white veil. Diagnosis: Congenital nevus.

    Bottom line: Benign, biopsy unnecessary.

Figure 14.7 shows a clinically flat, brown-black lesion (Figure 14.7A, B) that is dermoscopically multicolored (brown + other = blue/gray, pink, or yellow) (Figure 14.7C). This lesion is

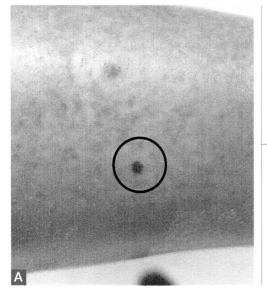
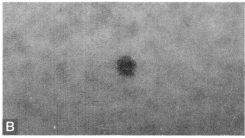
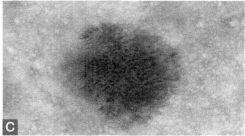

FIGURE 14.5 These clinically flat lesions are dark brown, with a multicolored (brown + other = gray, pink, and/or yellow) dermoscopic pattern. Review these clinical and dermoscopic examples of a congenital nevus. **A,B:** Clinical examples. **C:** The dermoscopic example shows a symmetric reticular network pattern, with a blue-white veil. The clinical history, as well as the patient's skin type, can help assess the benign nature of this lesion. Skin types 3 and up will have blue-white veils in benign lesions.

Clinical Brown-Black

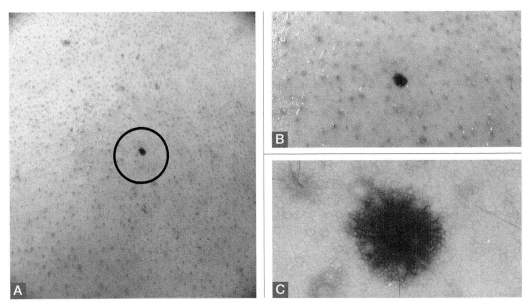

FIGURE 14.6 These clinically flat lesions are dark brown, with a multicolored (brown + other = gray, pink, and/or yellow) dermoscopic pattern. Review these clinical and dermoscopic examples of a congenital nevus. **A,B:** Clinical examples. **C:** The dermoscopic example shows a symmetric reticular network pattern with a blue-white veil. The clinical history, as well as the patient's skin type, can help assess the benign nature of this lesion. Skin types 3 and up will have blue-white veils in benign lesions.

characteristic of a congenital nevus. Dermoscopically, we see a symmetric reticular network pattern with dark dots on the network and an isolated blue-white veil. Diagnosis: Congenital nevus.

Bottom line: Benign, biopsy unnecessary.

Figure 14.8 shows a clinically flat, brown-black lesion (Figure 14.8A, B) that is dermoscopically multicolored (brown + other = blue/gray, pink, or yellow) (Figure 14.8C). This lesion is

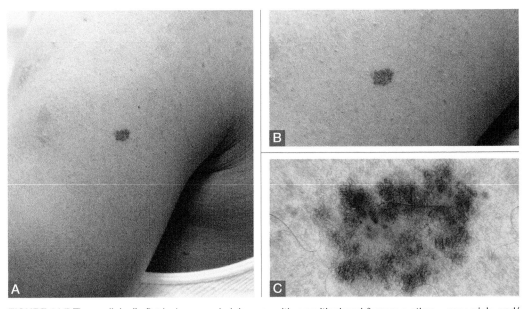

FIGURE 14.7 These clinically flat lesions are dark brown, with a multicolored (brown + other = gray, pink, and/or yellow) dermoscopic pattern. Review these clinical and dermoscopic examples of a melanocytic nevus. **A,B:** Clinical examples. **C:** The dermoscopic example shows a symmetric reticular network pattern, with dark dots on the network and an isolated blue-gray veil. The clinical history, as well as the patient's skin type, can help assess the benign nature of this lesion. Skin types 3 and up will have blue-white veils in benign lesions.

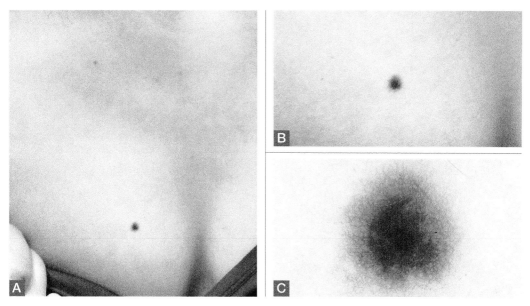

FIGURE 14.8 These clinically flat lesions are dark brown, with a multicolored (brown + other = gray, pink, and/or yellow) dermoscopic pattern. Review these clinical and dermoscopic examples of a melanocytic nevus. **A,B:** Clinical examples. **C:** The dermoscopic example shows a symmetric reticular network pattern, with dark dots on the network and an isolated blue-gray veil. Note the faint network at the periphery.

characteristic of a melanocytic nevus. Dermoscopically, we see a symmetric reticular network pattern with dark dots on the network and an isolated blue-gray veil. Diagnosis: Melanocytic nevus.

Bottom line: Benign, biopsy unnecessary.

Figure 14.9 shows a clinically flat, brown-black lesion (Figure 14.9A, B) that is dermoscopically multicolored (brown + other = blue/gray, pink, or yellow) (Figure 14.9C). This lesion is characteristic of a melanocytic compound nevus. Dermoscopically, we see a symmetric

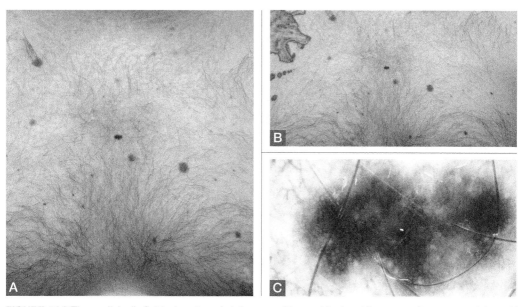

FIGURE 14.9 These clinically flat lesions tare dark brown, with a multicolored (brown + other = gray, pink, and/or yellow) dermoscopic pattern. Review these clinical and dermoscopic examples of a compound melanocytic nevus. **A,B:** Clinical examples. **C:** The dermoscopic example shows an asymmetric reticular network pattern. Often lesions that are irritated/traumatized will have multiple colors and can appear malignant. The patient's clinical history can help you differentiate by recognizing locations where the lesion gets traumatized.

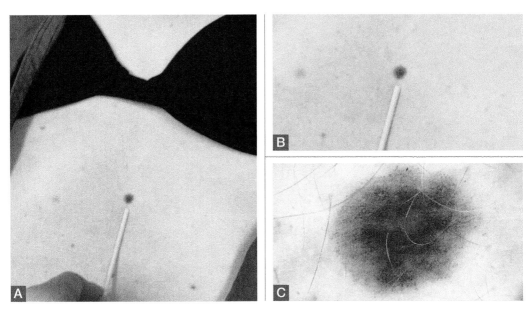

FIGURE 14.10 These clinically flat lesions are dark brown, with a multicolored (brown + other = gray, pink, and/or yellow) dermoscopic pattern. Review these clinical and dermoscopic examples of a congenital nevus. **A,B:** Clinical examples. **C:** The dermoscopic example shows a reticular network pattern, with central increased pigmentation. Note the faint network at the periphery.

reticular network pattern. Often lesions that are traumatized or irritated will have multiple colors and can appear malignant.

Your clinical history will help to determine if the lesion is being traumatized by location. Diagnosis: Melanocytic compound nevus.

Bottom line: Benign, biopsy unnecessary.

Figure 14.10 shows a clinically flat, brown-black lesion (Figure 14.10A, B) that is dermoscopically multicolored (brown + other = blue/gray, pink, or yellow) (Figure 14.10C). This lesion is characteristic of a congenital nevus. Dermoscopically, we see a symmetric reticular network pattern, with central increased pigmentation. Diagnosis: Congenital nevus.

Bottom line: Benign, biopsy unnecessary.

Blue Nevi

Pearls

- Flat/Brown-Black/Multicolored
  - Clinically, these will have been present for many years.
  - Often found on the scalp and face.
- **Step 4 Pattern Highlights: Review the patterns described in Chapter 1!**
  - Homogenous blue
  - Perifollicular hypopigmentation
- **Bottom line: Benign, biopsy not necessary.**

Examples

Figure 14.11 shows a clinically flat, brown-black lesion (Figure 14.11A, B) that is dermoscopically multicolored (brown + other = blue-gray, pink, or yellow) (Figure 14.11C). This is a classic example of a blue nevus, with a symmetric homogenous blue pattern. Diagnosis: Blue nevus.

Bottom line: Benign, biopsy unnecessary.

Figure 14.12 shows a clinically flat, brown-black lesion (Figure 14.12A, B) that is dermoscopically multicolored (brown + other = blue-gray, pink, or yellow) (Figure 14.12C). This is

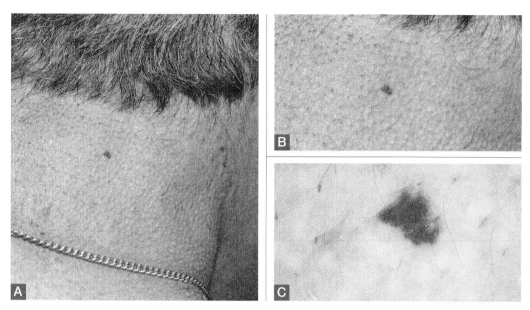

FIGURE 14.11 These clinically flat lesions are dark brown, with a multicolored (brown + other = gray, pink, and/or yellow) dermoscopic pattern. Review these clinical and dermoscopic examples of a blue nevus. **A,B:** Clinical examples. **C:** The dermoscopic example shows a symmetric homogeneous blue.

a classic example of a blue nevus. Dermoscopically, we see a symmetric homogenous blue pattern. On the face, there can be some hypopigmentation around follicular openings, which can make the lesion appear asymmetric. Look for features of basal cell carcinoma (BCC), which is the only other differential for this lesion. If you see no malignant features, such as arborizing vessels, then BCC is unlikely. Diagnosis: Blue nevus.

Bottom line: benign, biopsy unnecessary.

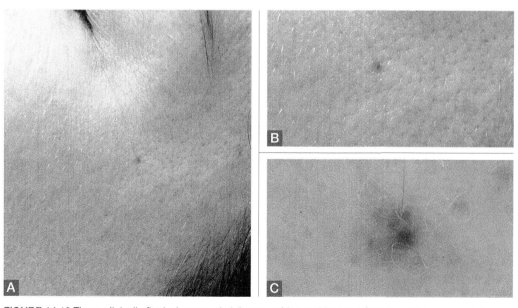

FIGURE 14.12 These clinically flat lesions are dark brown, with a multicolored (brown + other = gray, pink, and/or yellow) dermoscopic pattern. Review these clinical and dermoscopic examples of a blue nevus. **A,B:** Clinical examples. **C:** The dermoscopic example shows a symmetric homogeneous blue. On the face, there can be some hypopigmentation around follicular openings, which can make the lesion appear asymmetric. The differential for this small lesion is a small BCC, but look for other features of BCC, like an arborized vessel.

Clinical Brown-Black

Malignant Lesions

Superficial Spreading Melanoma

Pearls

- Flat/Brown-Black/Multicolored
- **Step 4 patterns: Review the patterns described in Chapter 1!**
  - Irregular pigmentation, with some minimal color variation
  - Asymmetry of homogenous, globular, and reticular patterns
  - Streaks, radial streaming, and pseudopods at the periphery
  - Blue-gray granularity/dots
  - Polymorphous and dotted vessels
  - Blue-white veil, typically seen in elevated lesions like nodular MM
- **Bottom line: Malignant, Biopsy!**

Examples

Figure 14.13 shows three clinically flat, brown-black lesions (Figure 14.13A–C) and their corresponding dermoscopic images (Figure 14.13D–F), which are multicolored (brown + other = gray/blue, pink, or yellow). Dermoscopically, we see an asymmetric distribution of pigmentation, especially at the periphery. Diagnosis: All three are melanomas.

   Bottom line: Malignancy, biopsy!

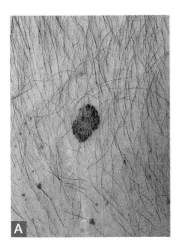 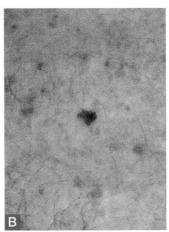 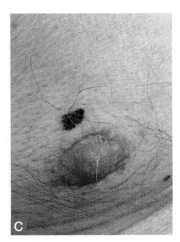

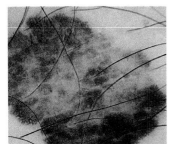 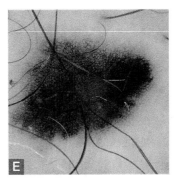 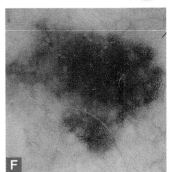

FIGURE 14.13 A–C: These clinically flat lesions are dark brown (A–C) with a multicolored (brown + other = gray, pink, and/or yellow) dermoscopic pattern. All three are melanomas. **D–F:** The dermoscopic pattern of the lesions shown in parts A-C shows a reticular disorganized pattern. All three are melanomas.

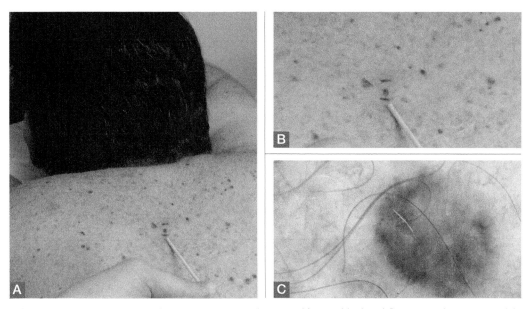

FIGURE 14.14 These clinically flat lesions are dark brown, with a multicolored (brown + other = gray, pink, and/or yellow) dermoscopic pattern. Review these clinical and dermoscopic examples of a MM. **A,B:** Clinical examples. **C:** The dermoscopic example shows an symmetric assyetric multicolored homogeneous pattern.

Figure 14.14 shows a clinically flat, brown-black (Figure 14.14A, B), dermoscopically multicolored (brown + other = gray/blue, pink, or yellow) (Figure 14.14C) lesion. We see an asymmetric distribution of pigmentation with multiple colors, especially at the periphery. Diagnosis: This is a melanoma.

Bottom line: Malignancy, biopsy!

Figure 14.15 shows a clinically flat, brown-black (Figure 14.15A, B), dermoscopically multicolored (brown + other = gray-blue, pink, or yellow) (Figure 14.15C) lesion. We see an asymmetric distribution of dot/globular pattern, as well as asymmetry of a multicolored

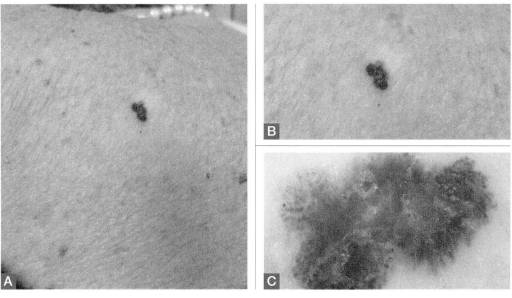

FIGURE 14.15 These clinically flat lesions are dark brown, with a multicolored (brown + other = gray, pink, and/or yellow) dermoscopic pattern. Review these clinical and dermoscopic examples of a malignant melanoma. **A,B:** Clinical examples. **C:** The dermoscopic example shows an asymmetric multicolored homogeneous pattern and an asymmetric dot/globular pattern. Note the asymmetry at the periphery of the lesion.

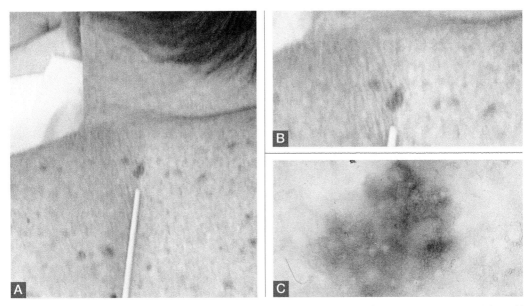

FIGURE 14.16 These clinically flat lesions are dark brown, with a multicolored (brown + other = gray, pink, and/or yellow) dermoscopic pattern. Review these clinical and dermoscopic examples of a malignant melanoma. **A,B:** Clinical examples. **C:** The dermoscopic example shows an asymmetric reticular network pattern, with gray dots and granules. This pattern shows regression.

homogenous pattern. Pay special attention to the asymmetry of the periphery. Diagnosis: This is a melanoma.

Bottom line: Malignancy, biopsy!

Figures 14.16 to 14.18 show clinically flat, brown-black (A, B), dermoscopically multicolored (brown + other = gray/blue, pink, or yellow) (C) lesions. We see asymmetric reticular patterns, with multiple colors and gray dots/granularity, especially at the periphery. This is

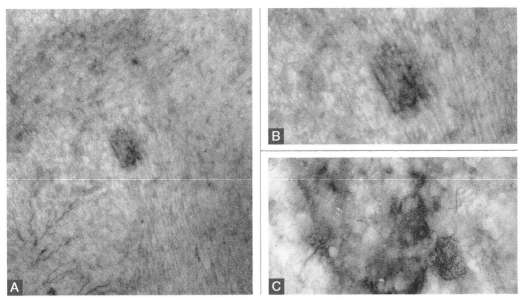

FIGURE 14.17 These clinically flat lesions are dark brown, with a multicolored (brown + other = gray, pink, and/or yellow) dermoscopic pattern. Review these clinical and dermoscopic examples of a malignant melanoma. **A,B:** Clinical examples. **C:** The dermoscopic example shows an asymmetric reticular network pattern, with gray-dot granules. This indicates a pattern of regression.

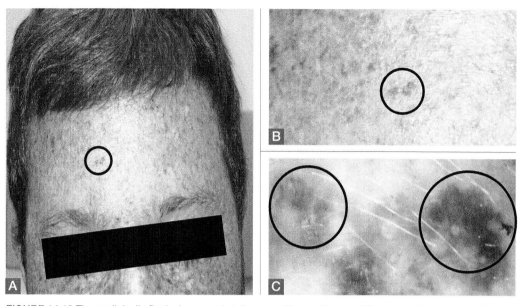

FIGURE 14.18 These clinically flat lesions are dark brown, with a multicolored (brown + other = gray, pink, and/or yellow) dermoscopic pattern. Review these clinical and dermoscopic examples of a malignant melanoma in situ. **A,B:** Clinical examples. **C:** The dermoscopic example shows an asymmetric reticular network pattern, with gray-dot granules. This indicates a pattern of regression.

the similar pattern we saw with LPLK, a pattern of regression, which is why we often biopsy LPLKs. Diagnosis: These are all melanomas.

Bottom line: Malignancy, biopsy!

Figures 14.19 and 14.20 show clinically flat, brown-black (A, B), dermoscopically multicolored (brown + other = gray/blue, pink, or yellow) (C) lesions. We see an asymmetric gray-dots/

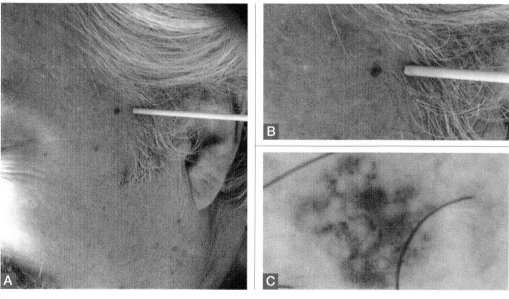

FIGURE 14.19 These clinically flat lesions are dark brown, with a multicolored (brown + other = gray, pink, and/or yellow) dermoscopic pattern. Review these clinical and dermoscopic examples of a malignant melanoma lentigo maligna type of the face. **A,B:** Clinical examples. **C:** The dermoscopic example shows gray-dot granules around follicular openings.

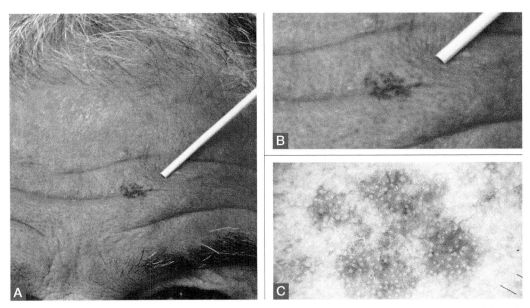

FIGURE 14.20 These clinically flat lesions are dark brown, with a multicolored (brown + other = gray, pink, and/or yellow) dermoscopic pattern. Review these clinical and dermoscopic examples of a malignant melanoma lentigo maligna melanoma in situ type of the face. **A,B:** Clinical examples. **C:** The dermoscopic example shows an annular granular pattern.

granular pattern around follicular openings. Diagnosis: These are both malignant melanomas, lentigo maligna type of the face.

Bottom line: Malignancy, biopsy!

Dysplastic Nevi

Pearls

- Flat/Brown-Black/Multicolored
  - Clinically, these may have been present since childhood.
  - The appearance of dysplasia or asymmetry of these lesions may be a result of iatrogenic causes, such as UV light or rubbing/irritation, resulting in multiple colors. If this is the case, the dysplasia or atypia would improve during short-term mole monitoring.
- **Step 4 Pattern Highlights: Review the patterns described in Chapter 1!**
  - Asymmetry of the melanocytic patterns: homogenous, globular, and reticular
- **Benign** = Observation and careful monitoring is warranted because these lesions are flat. This is in contrast to elevated lesions, in which short-term monitoring is absolutely contraindicated.

Examples

Figure 14.21 shows a clinically flat, brown-black (Figure 14.21A, B), dermoscopically multicolored (brown + other = gray, pink, or yellow) lesion (Figure 14.21C). This is an example of a dysplastic nevus. There is asymmetric homogenous, reticular, and dot/globular patterns, with asymmetry of the periphery. Diagnosis: Dysplastic nevus.

Bottom line: Caution

Figure 14.22 shows a clinically flat, brown/black (Figure 14.22A, B), dermoscopically multicolored (brown + other = gray, pink, or yellow) lesion (Figure 14.22C). This is an example of a traumatized nevus. We can see an asymmetric homogenous pattern. Diagnosis: Traumatized nevus.

Bottom line: Caution

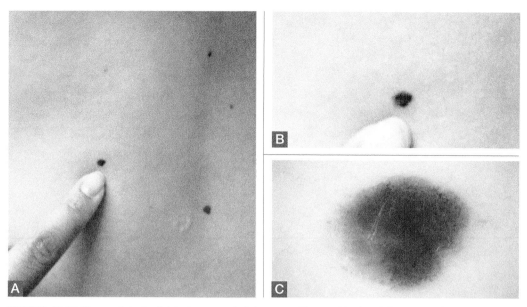

FIGURE 14.21 These clinically flat lesions are dark brown, with a multicolored (brown + other = gray, pink, and/or yellow) dermoscopic pattern. Review these clinical and dermoscopic examples of a severely dysplastic compound nevus. **A,B:** Clinical examples. **C:** The dermoscopic example shows an asymmetric homogenous, reticular, and dot/globular pattern with asymmetry at the periphery.

Figure 14.23 shows a clinically flat, brown/black (Figure 14.23A, B), dermoscopically multicolored (brown + other = gray, pink, or yellow) lesion (Figure 14.23C). This is an example of a dysplastic nevus with pigment alteration. We can see an asymmetric reticular pattern, with darkening at the periphery. Diagnosis: Dysplastic nevus with pigment alteration.

Bottom line: Caution

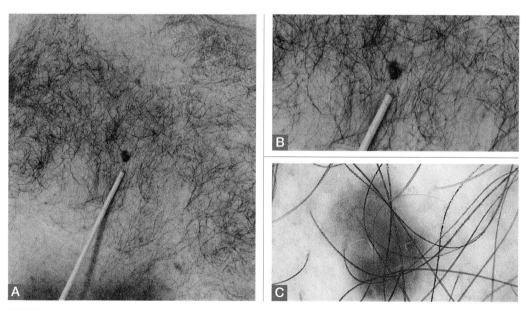

FIGURE 14.22 These clinically flat lesions are dark brown, with a multicolored (brown + other = gray, pink, and/or yellow) dermoscopic pattern. Review these clinical and dermoscopic examples of a traumatized nevus. **A,B:** Clinical examples. **C:** The dermoscopic example shows an asymmetric homogenous pattern.

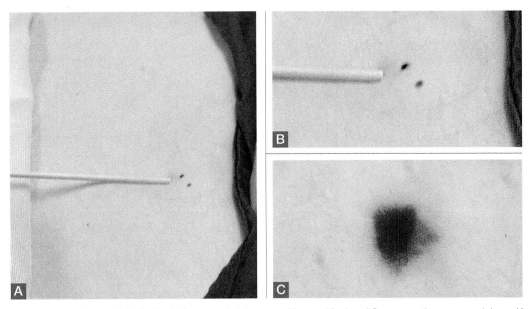

FIGURE 14.23 These clinically flat lesions are dark brown, with a multicolored (brown + other = gray, pink, and/or yellow) dermoscopic pattern. Review these clinical and dermoscopic examples of a dysplastic nevus with pigmentary alteration. **A,B:** Clinical examples. **C:** The dermoscopic example shows a reticular asymmetric pattern, with darkening at the periphery.

Figure 14.24 shows a clinically flat, brown/black (Figure 14.24A, B), dermoscopically multicolored (brown + other = gray, pink, or yellow) lesion (Figure 14.24C). This is an example of a compound nevus, dysplastic type. We can see an asymmetric reticular and dot/globular pattern, with asymmetry at the periphery. Diagnosis: Compound nevus, dysplastic type.

Bottom line: Caution

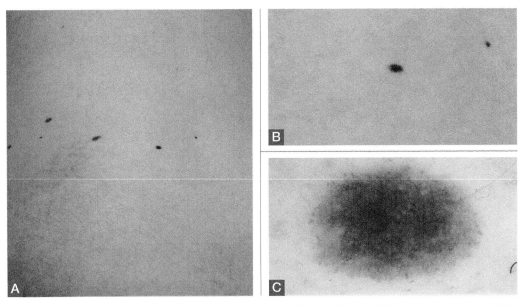

FIGURE 14.24 These clinically flat lesions are dark brown, with a multicolored (brown + other = gray, pink, and/or yellow) dermoscopic pattern. Review these clinical and dermoscopic examples of a compound nevus dysplastic type. **A,B:** Clinical examples. **C:** The dermoscopic example shows an asymmetric reticular and dot/globular pattern, with asymmetric dots at the periphery.

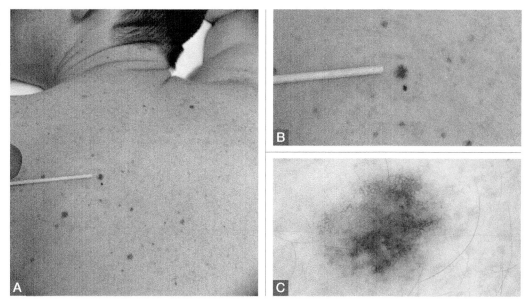

FIGURE 14.25 These clinically flat lesions are dark brown, with a multicolored (brown + other = gray, pink, and/or yellow) dermoscopic pattern. Review these clinical and dermoscopic examples of a compound nevus dysplastic type. **A,B:** Clinical examples. **C:** The dermoscopic example shows an asymmetric reticular and dot/globular pattern with asymmetric dots at the periphery.

Figure 14.25 shows a clinically flat, brown/black (Figure 14.25A, B), dermoscopically multicolored (brown + other = gray, pink, or yellow) lesion (Figure 14.25C). This is an example of a compound nevus, dysplastic type. We can see an asymmetric reticular and dot/globular pattern, with asymmetry at the periphery. Diagnosis: Compound nevus, dysplastic type.

Bottom line: Caution

Figure 14.26 shows a clinically flat, brown/black (Figure 14.26A, B), dermoscopically multicolored (brown + other = gray, pink, or yellow) lesion (Figure 14.26C). This is an example of

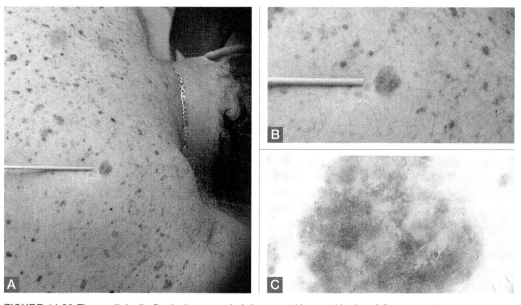

FIGURE 14.26 These clinically flat lesions are dark brown, with a multicolored (brown + other = gray, pink, and/or yellow) dermoscopic pattern. Review these clinical and dermoscopic examples of a compound nevus dysplastic type. **A,B:** Clinical examples. **C:** The dermoscopic example shows an asymmetric reticular and dot/globular pattern, with asymmetry dots at the periphery, as well as gray-dot granules.

Clinical Brown-Black

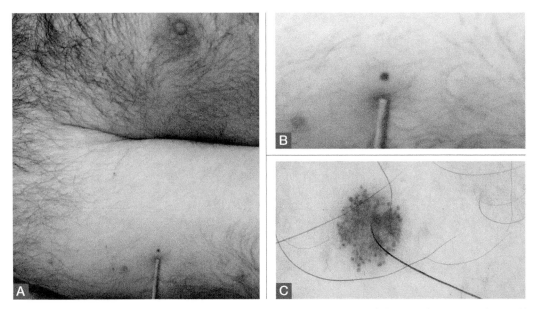

FIGURE 14.27 These clinically flat lesions are dark brown, with a multicolored (brown + other = gray, pink, and/ or yellow) dermoscopic pattern. Review these clinical and dermoscopic examples of a junctional nevus dysplastic type. **A,B:** Clinical examples. **C:** The dermoscopic example shows an asymmetric reticular and dot/globular pattern with asymmetric dots at the periphery.

a compound nevus, dysplastic type. We can see an asymmetric reticular and dot/globular pattern with asymmetry of the periphery. Additionally, we see gray dot/granules localized in the lesion. Diagnosis: Compound nevus, dysplastic type.

Bottom line: Caution

Figure 14.27 shows a clinically flat, brown/black (Figure 14.27A, B), dermoscopically multicolored (brown + other = gray, pink, or yellow) lesion (Figure 14.27C). This is an example of a junctional nevus, dysplastic type. We can see an asymmetric reticular and globular pattern with asymmetric dots at the periphery. Diagnosis: Junctional nevus, dysplastic type.

Bottom line: Caution

Figure 14.28 shows a clinically flat, brown/black (Figure 14.28A, B), dermoscopically multicolored (brown + other = gray, pink, or yellow) lesion (Figure 14.28C). This is an example of a junctional nevus, dysplastic type. We can see an asymmetric reticular and globular pattern with asymmetric dots at the periphery, as well as gray dots/granules scattered throughout. Diagnosis: Junctional nevus, dysplastic type.

Bottom line: Caution

Basal Cell Carcinoma

Pearls
- Flat/Brown-Black/Multicolored
- **Step 4 Pattern Highlights: Review the patterns described in Chapter 1!**
  - Absence of a pigment network
  - Leaf-like structures
  - Large blue-gray ovoid nests or globular-like structures
  - Arborizing telangiectasias
  - Spoke wheel areas
  - Ulceration
  - Pink-white to white shiny areas
  - Crystalline pattern
- **Bottom line: Malignant, biopsy!**

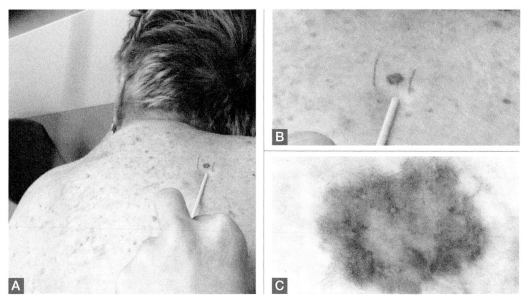

FIGURE 14.28 These clinically flat lesions are dark brown, with a multicolored (brown + other = gray, pink, and/ or yellow) dermoscopic pattern. Review these clinical and dermoscopic examples of a junctional nevus dysplastic type. **A,B:** Clinical examples. **C:** The dermoscopic example shows an asymmetric reticular and dot/globular pattern with asymmetric dots at the periphery, as well as gray-dot granules.

Examples

Figure 14.29 shows a clinically flat, brown-black (Figure 14.29A, B), dermoscopically multicolored (brown + other = gray, pink, yellow) lesion (Figure 14.29C). This is an example of an early BCC. You can appreciate the ash leaf–like structure and arborizing vessels. Diagnosis: Early basal cell carcinoma.

    Bottom line: Malignant, biopsy!

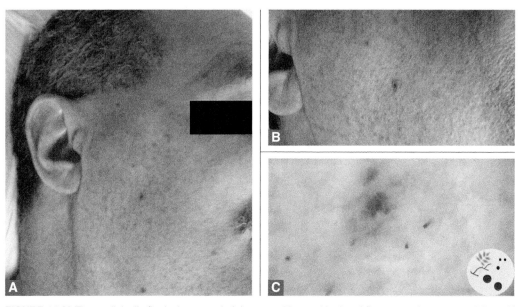

FIGURE 14.29 These clinically flat lesions are dark brown, with a multicolored (brown + other = gray, pink, and/ or yellow) dermoscopic pattern. Review these clinical and dermoscopic examples of an early pigmented basal cell skin cancer. **A,B:** Clinical examples. **C:** The dermoscopic example shows an ash leaf pattern, as well as arborized vessels.

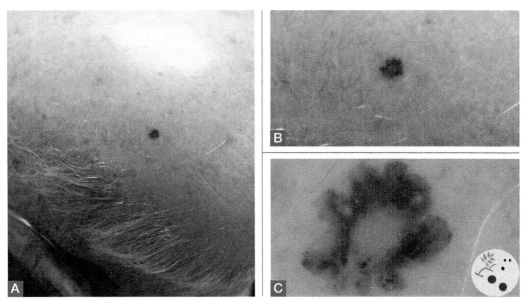

FIGURE 14.30 These clinically flat lesions are dark brown, with a multicolored (brown + other = gray, pink, and/or yellow) dermoscopic pattern. Review these clinical and dermoscopic examples of an early pigmented basal cell skin cancer. **A,B:** Clinical examples. **C:** The dermoscopic example shows an ash leaf pattern, as well as dark globular-like structures.

Figure 14.30 shows a clinically flat, brown/black (Figure 14.30A, B), dermoscopically multicolored (brown + other = gray, pink, yellow) lesion (Figure 14.30C). This is an example of an early BCC. You can appreciate the ash leaf–like structure and dark, globular-like structures. Diagnosis: Early basal cell carcinoma.

Bottom line: Malignant, biopsy!

Figure 14.31 shows a clinically flat, brown/black (Figure 14.31A, B), dermoscopically multicolored (brown + other = gray, pink, yellow) lesion (Figure 14.31C). This is an example of

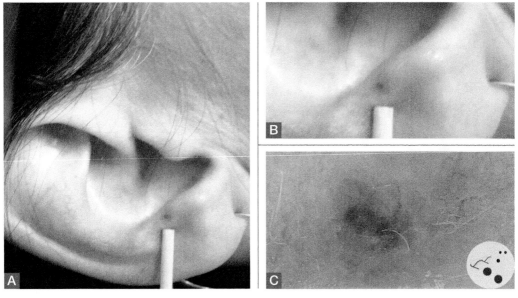

FIGURE 14.31 These clinically flat lesions are dark brown, with a multicolored (brown + other = gray, pink, and/or yellow) dermoscopic pattern. Review these clinical and dermoscopic examples of an early pigmented basal cell skin cancer. **A,B:** Clinical examples. **C:** The dermoscopic example shows a dark blue globular-like pattern, along with arborized vessels.

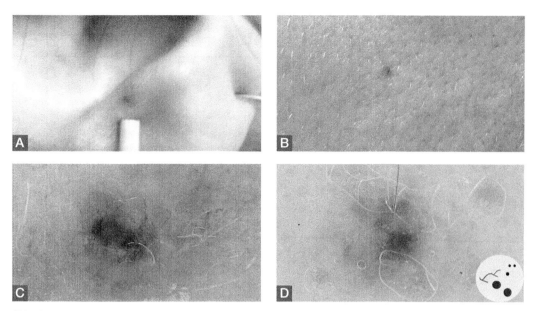

FIGURE 14.32 These clinically flat lesions are dark brown, with a multicolored (brown + other = gray, pink, and/or yellow) dermoscopic pattern. Review these clinical and dermoscopic examples of an early pigmented basal cell skin cancer. **A:** Clinical example. **B:** Clinical example. **C:** The dermoscopic example shows a dark blue, globular-like pattern, along with arborized vessels. This can be compared to a facial benign blue nevus. **D:** The dermoscopic example shows a blue homogeneous with perifollicular hypopigmentation, leading to some asymmetry within the blue homogenous pattern. Note no other features of BCC, such as arborized vessels.

an early BCC. You can appreciate the dark blue globular-like structures and arborizing vessels. Diagnosis: Early basal cell carcinoma.

Bottom line: Malignant, biopsy!

Figure 14.32 shows two clinically flat, brown/black (Figure 14.32A, B), with their corresponding dermoscopically multicolored (brown + other = gray, pink, yellow) images (Figure 14.32C, D). In A and C, you can appreciate the dark blue globular-like pattern along with arborizing vessels of a lesion on the ear. This is a BCC. This is compared to a facial lesion (Figure 14.32B), which shows a blue homogenous pattern with perifollicular hypopigmentation leading to some asymmetry (Figure 14.32D), but no other features of BCC are found. This is a benign blue nevus. Diagnosis. A and C. Basal cell carcinoma. B and D. Benign blue nevus.

Bottom line: Malignant, biopsy!

Clinical Brown-Black

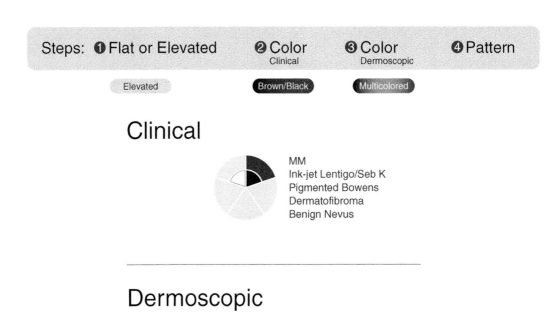

Clinical

MM
Ink-jet Lentigo/Seb K
Pigmented Bowens
Dermatofibroma
Benign Nevus

Dermoscopic

LPLK
MM
BCC
CN/Blue Nevi
Ink-jet Lentigo/Seb K
Hemolized blood/angiokeratoma

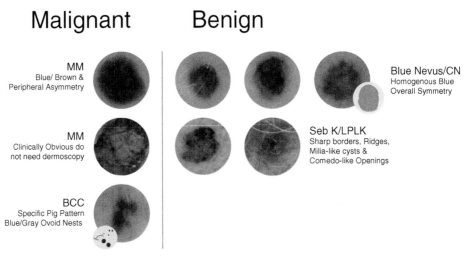

Malignant

MM
Blue/ Brown &
Peripheral Asymmetry

MM
Clinically Obvious do
not need dermoscopy

BCC
Specific Pig Pattern
Blue/Gray Ovoid Nests

Benign

Blue Nevus/CN
Homogenous Blue
Overall Symmetry

Seb K/LPLK
Sharp borders, Ridges,
Milia-like cysts &
Comedo-like Openings

FIGURE 15.1 Color wheel: elevated/brown-black/multicolored.

Step 1: Is the lesion flat or raised? **Elevated**

Step 2: What color is the lesion on clinical assessment? **Brown/Black**

Step 3: What is the dermoscopic color? **Multicolored**

Step 4: Is further elucidation needed to decide whether to biopsy or not? **Yes**

Is this a malignant or benign pattern?

Take a look at the color wheel in Figure 15.1.

When we elevate the clinically brown/black, dermoscopically multicolored lesions, we don't change the differential from the flat lesions. However, we do now include a more advanced stage of malignant melanoma. These will be clinically obvious lesions for which dermoscopy is not needed.

Our benign lesions include LPLK and seborrheic keratosis and congenital/blue nevi.

Our malignancies include malignant melanoma again, as well as clinically obvious nodular melanoma. We also will see pigmented basal cell again.

Benign Lesions

Congenital/Combined Nevi

Pearls

* Elevated/Brown-Black/Multicolored
  * These will have been present since birth.
  * May wobble with contact.
* **Step 4 Pattern:** Remember to look for your Chapter 1 Patterns
  * Any of the melanocytic patterns: homogenous, globular/cobblestone, or reticular.
  * Shades of brown are not considered multicolored!
  * Sometimes, you may see a few visible comma vessels and milia-like cysts.
* **Bottom line: Benign, biopsy not necessary.**

Examples

Figures 15.2 and 15.3 show a clinically elevated, brown/black lesions (A, B), with a dermoscopically multicolored (brown + other = gray, pink, yellow) pattern (C). These lesions are difficult to appreciate, but overall, we see a homogenous pattern with black, brown, and some blue. This lesion wobbles with contact, unless it has undergone a lot of rubbing over the years and has fibrosed to some extent. A clinical history indicates that the lesion has been present since birth and it resembles nearby lesions. Therefore, this lesion is unlikely to be malignant. Additionally, nodular melanomas are very fast growing, which would not fit this clinical picture. Diagnosis: Congenital/combined nevi.

Bottom line: Benign, biopsy unnecessary.

Figure 15.4 shows a clinically elevated, brown/black lesion (Figure 15.4A, B), with a dermoscopically multicolored (brown + other = gray, pink, yellow) pattern (Figure 15.4C). This lesion is an example of a congenital nevus. You can appreciate the dermoscopic dot/globular pattern, as well as some darker dots on the top of the network. Diagnosis: Congenital nevus.

Bottom line: benign, biopsy unnecessary.

Figure 15.5 shows a clinically elevated, brown/black lesion (Figure 15.5A, B) with a dermoscopically multicolored (brown + other = gray, pink, yellow) pattern (Figure 15.5C). This lesion is an example of a congenital nevus. You can appreciate the dermoscopic dot/globular

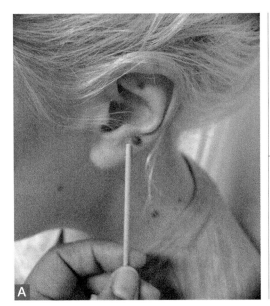
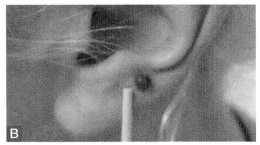
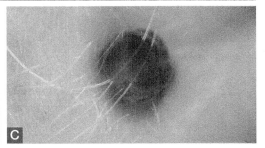

FIGURE 15.2 These clinically elevated lesions are dark brown, with a multicolored (brown + other = gray, pink, and/or yellow) dermoscopic pattern. Review these clinical and dermoscopic examples of a congenital nevus. **A,B:** Clinical examples. **C:** The dermoscopic example shows that a pattern is difficult to appreciate, but overall, it is homogeneous with black, brown, and even blue. This lesion should wobble when a contact scope is applied to it, but when lesions have been rubbed and fibrosed, it may be difficult to appreciate this feature. A clinical history will indicate that the lesion has been present since birth, resembles other lesions on the patient, and is clinically well circumscribed. The reality that nodular melanomas are very rapidly growing lesions also helps with the diagnosis of dark and multicolored congenital nevi.

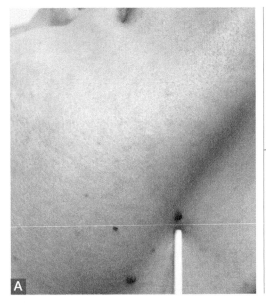
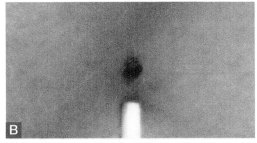
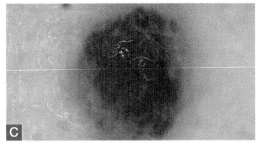

FIGURE 15.3 These clinically elevated lesions are dark brown, with a multicolored (brown + other = gray, pink, and/or yellow) dermoscopic pattern. Review these clinical and dermoscopic examples of a congenital nevus. **A,B:** Clinical examples. **C:** The dermoscopic example shows a pattern that is difficult to appreciate, but overall it is homogeneous with black, brown, and even blue. This lesion should wobble when a contact scope is applied to it, but when lesions have been rubbed and fibrosed, it may be difficult to appreciate this feature. A clinical history will indicate that the lesion has been present since birth, resembles other lesions on the patient, and is clinically well circumscribed. The reality that nodular melanomas are very rapidly growing lesions also helps with the diagnosis of dark and multicolored congenital nevi.

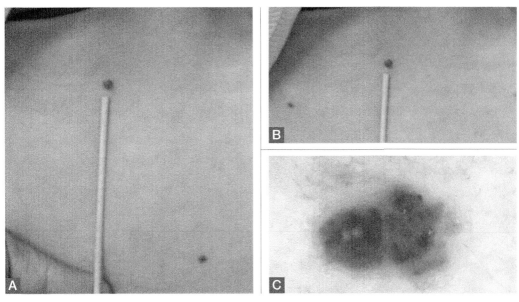

FIGURE 15.4 These clinically elevated lesions are dark brown, with a multicolored (brown + other = gray, pink, and/or yellow) dermoscopic pattern. Review these clinical and dermoscopic examples of a congenital nevus. **A,B:** Clinical examples. **C:** The dermoscopic example shows a dot/globular pattern. You can also see dark dots on the network.

and cobblestone pattern, which is specific to congenital lesions. This lesion will wobble when in contact with the scope. Diagnosis: Congenital nevus.

Bottom line: Benign, biopsy unnecessary.

Figure 15.6 shows a clinically elevated, brown/black lesion (Figure 15.6A, B) with a dermoscopically multicolored (brown + other = gray, pink, yellow) pattern (Figure 15.6C). This lesion is an example of a congenital nevus. Again, we can see the dermoscopic dot/globular pattern.

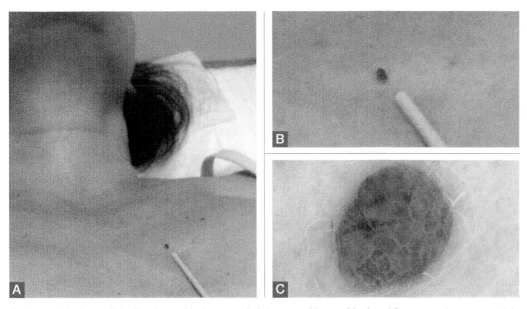

FIGURE 15.5 These clinically elevated lesions are dark brown, with a multicolored (brown + other = gray, pink, and/or yellow) dermoscopic pattern. Review these clinical and dermoscopic examples of a congenital nevus. **A,B:** Clinical examples. **C:** The dermoscopic example shows a dot/globular and cobblestone pattern that is very specific to congenital lesions. It is more difficult to see the comma-like vessels in darker lesions. Additionally, when a contact scope is applied to the lesion, it wobbles.

Clinical Brown-Black

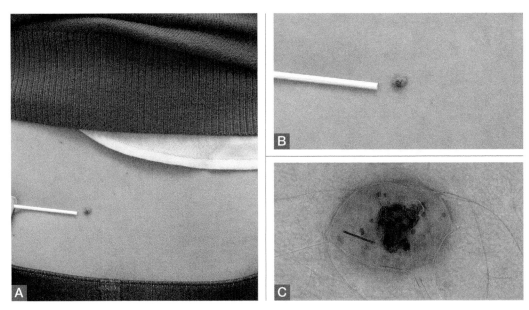

FIGURE 15.6 These clinically elevated lesions are dark brown, with a multicolored (brown + other = gray, pink, and/ or yellow) dermoscopic pattern. Review these clinical and dermoscopic examples of a congenital nevus. **A,B:** Clinical examples. **C:** The dermoscopic example shows a dot/globular pattern. Note the erosion/bleeding seen in this lesion, most likely due to outside trauma. Additionally, when a contact scope is applied to the lesion, it wobbles.

The erosion or bleeding seen in this lesion is most likely due to outside trauma. Additionally, this lesion wobbles when in contact with the scope. Diagnosis: Congenital nevus.

Bottom line: Benign, biopsy unnecessary.

Figure 15.7 shows a clinically elevated, brown/black lesion (Figure 15.7A, B), with a dermoscopically multicolored (brown + other = gray, pink, yellow) pattern (Figure 15.7C). This

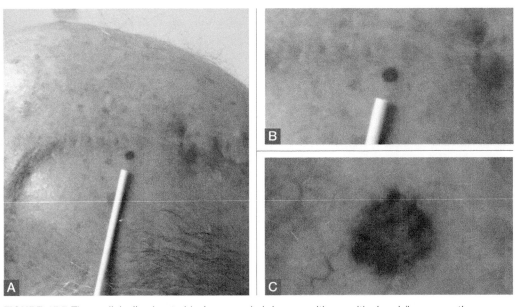

FIGURE 15.7 These clinically elevated lesions are dark brown, with a multicolored (brown + other = gray, pink, and/or yellow) dermoscopic pattern. Review these clinical and dermoscopic examples of a blue nevus. **A,B:** Clinical examples. **C:** The dermoscopic example shows a symmetric homogeneous blue that begins to have a blue-white veil appearance when elevated. This appearance makes it more difficult to distinguish from nodular melanoma. The clinical history, and lack of other malignant features often seen with the more rapidly growing and aggressive nodular melanomas, helps differentiate these lesions. New blue nevi of the scalp are often biopsied, due to reported cases of these lesions becoming locally aggressive.

is an example of an elevated blue nevus. Here, we see the homogenous blue symmetric pattern that begins to have a blue-white veil appearance because of its elevation. This makes it more difficult to differentiate from a nodular melanoma. The clinical history, and lack of other malignant features often seen with the more rapidly growing and aggressive nodular melanomas, helps to differentiate these lesions. New blue nevi that develop on the scalp, such as this one, are often biopsied due to reported cases of these lesions becoming locally aggressive. Diagnosis: Elevated blue nevus.

Bottom line: Benign, but biopsy recommend.

Seborrheic Keratosis or Lichen Planus–like Keratosis

Pearls

- Elevated/Brown-Black/Multicolored
  - For the LPLKs, there are two possibilities for their origin:
    - A solar lentigo undergoing regression or an inflammatory reaction
    - A seborrheic keratosis undergoing regression or inflammatory reaction
  - When trying to distinguish between melanomas, it is useful to note:
    - LPLKs have more substance/crust on palpation than do superficial spreading MMs.
    - LPLKs will typically show up on skin types 2 and 3.
    - LPLKs will generally resemble other lesions on the patient.
- **Step 4 Pattern Highlights: Review the patterns described in Chapter 1!**
  - The inflammation leads to a nonspecific vascular pattern.
  - Often, you will see clumps of dark pigment around benign structures:
    - Diffusely on a background of hypomelanosis
    - Localized in small clusters
  - Look for clues of benign features: ridges, sharp borders, moth-eaten borders, fingerprint patterns, milia-like cysts, and comedo-like openings.
- These are often the most difficult lesions to differentiate from malignant melanoma and nonmelanoma skin cancers, so **we will biopsy** these lesions **_often_**!

Examples

Figure 15.8 shows a clinically elevated, brown/black lesion (Figure 15.8A, B) with a dermoscopically multicolored (brown + other = gray, pink, or yellow) pattern (Figure 15.8C). You can appreciate the sharp borders, milia-like cysts, and hairpin vessels of this seborrheic keratosis. Note the dark or bluish color. Even if you cannot appreciate the multicolors of this lesion, the color wheel will help you identify this as a seborrheic keratosis! Diagnosis: Seborrheic keratosis.

Bottom line: Benign, biopsy unnecessary.

Figure 15.9 shows a clinically elevated, brown/black lesion (Figure 15.9A, B), with a dermoscopically multicolored (brown + other = gray, pink, or yellow) pattern (Figure 15.9C). You can appreciate the sharp borders and milia-like cysts of this seborrheic keratosis. Additionally, this is a good example of the cerebriform or ridge-like pattern. These darker lesions with a blue-white veil will need to be considered in the clinical context. The veil is often seen in patients with type 3 skin or higher. Diagnosis: Seborrheic keratosis.

Bottom line: Benign, biopsy unnecessary.

Figure 15.10 shows a clinically elevated, brown/black lesion (Figure 15.10A, B), with a dermoscopically multicolored (brown + other = gray, pink, or yellow) pattern (Figure 15.10C). You can appreciate the sharp borders and comedo-like openings of this seborrheic keratosis. These darker lesions with a blue-white veil will need to be considered in the clinical context. The veil is often seen in patients with type 3 skin or higher. Diagnosis: Seborrheic keratosis.

Bottom line: Benign, biopsy unnecessary.

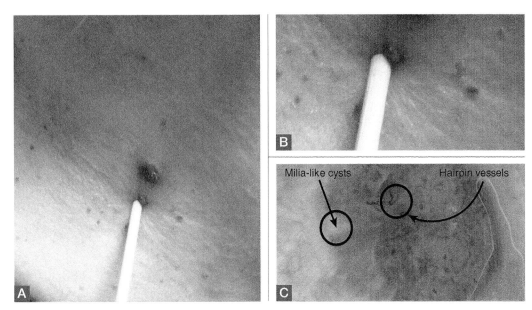

FIGURE 15.8 These clinically elevated lesions are dark brown, with a multicolored (brown + other = gray, pink, and/or yellow) dermoscopic pattern. Review these clinical and dermoscopic examples of a seborrheic keratosis. **A,B:** Clinical examples. **C:** The dermoscopic example shows milia-like cysts, hairpin vessels, and sharp borders. Note the dark/blue color. If you do not appreciate the multiple colors, do not worry; the algorithm will still help you make the diagnosis.

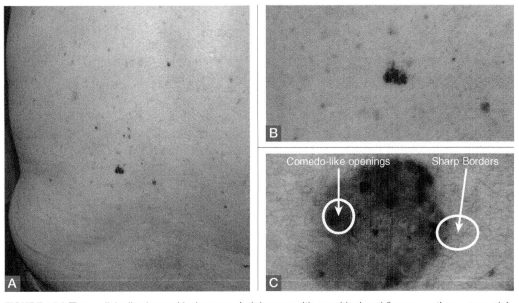

FIGURE 15.9 These clinically elevated lesions are dark brown, with a multicolored (brown + other = gray, pink, and/or yellow) dermoscopic pattern. Review these clinical and dermoscopic examples of a seborrheic keratosis. **A,B:** Clinical examples. **C:** The dermoscopic example shows comedo-like openings and sharp borders. You can also appreciate the cerebriform/ridge-like pattern. These darker lesions with a blue-white veil need to be evaluated in the patient's clinical context. These lesions are often seen in skin type 3 or greater.

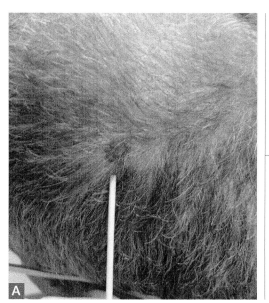
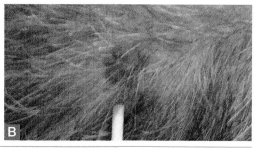
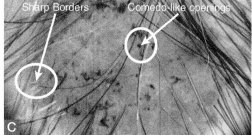

FIGURE 15.10 These clinically elevated lesions are dark brown, with a multicolored (brown + other = gray, pink, and/or yellow) dermoscopic pattern. Review these clinical and dermoscopic examples of a seborrheic keratosis. **A,B:** Clinical examples. **C:** The dermoscopic example shows comedo-like openings and sharp borders. You can also appreciate the cerebriform/ridge-like pattern. These darker lesions with a blue-white veil need to be evaluated in the patient's clinical context. These lesions are often seen in skin type 3 or greater.

Figure 15.11 shows a clinically elevated, brown/black lesion (Figure 15.11A, B), with a dermoscopically multicolored (brown + other = gray, pink, or yellow) pattern (Figure 15.11C). You can appreciate the sharp borders and comedo-like openings of this seborrheic keratosis. These darker lesions with a blue-white veil will need to be considered in the clinical context. The veil is often seen in patients with type 3 skin or higher. Diagnosis: Seborrheic keratosis.

Bottom line: Benign, biopsy unnecessary.

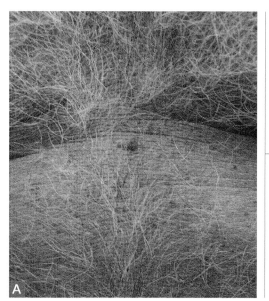
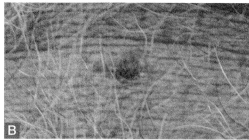
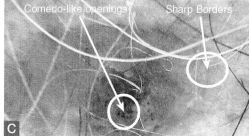

FIGURE 15.11 These clinically elevated lesions are dark brown, with a multicolored (brown + other = gray, pink, and/or yellow) dermoscopic pattern. Review these clinical and dermoscopic examples of a seborrheic keratosis. **A,B:** Clinical examples. **C:** The dermoscopic example shows comedo-like openings and sharp borders. You can also appreciate the cerebriform/ridge-like pattern. These darker lesions with a blue-white veil need to be evaluated in the patient's clinical context. These lesions are often seen in skin type 3 or greater.

Clinical Brown-Black

Figure 15.12 shows a clinically elevated, brown/black lesion (Figure 15.12A, B), with a dermoscopically multicolored (brown + other = gray, pink, or yellow) pattern (Figure 15.12C). This lesion is markedly darker, but you can still appreciate the sharp borders and comedo-like openings of this pigmented seborrheic keratosis. These darker lesions with a blue-white veil will need to be considered in the clinical context. The veil is often seen in patients with type 3 skin or higher. In lighter skin types, pigmented SKs can be tricky to distinguish from malignancy and should be biopsied. Diagnosis: Pigmented seborrheic keratosis.

Bottom line: If difficult to differentiate, biopsy.

Figures 15.13 and 15.14 are both clinically elevated, brown/black lesions (A, B), with dermoscopically multicolored (brown + other = gray, pink, or yellow) patterns (C). These are examples of lichen planus–like keratosis, likely secondary to a seborrheic keratosis. You can clearly see milia-like cysts, comedo-like opening, and sharp borders. Additionally, we can see isolated gray granularity, the sign of regression that we've seen with LPLKs in prior chapters. Remember that this is also a feature of flat superficial spreading malignant melanomas. However, in this lesion, the benign features, as well as the elevations within the lesion, help to distinguish between the two. These LPLKs can be classified as either flat or elevated, but remember that in either case, they will have more substance than the flat melanomas. Diagnosis: Lichen planus–like keratosis.

Bottom line: Benign, biopsy unnecessary.

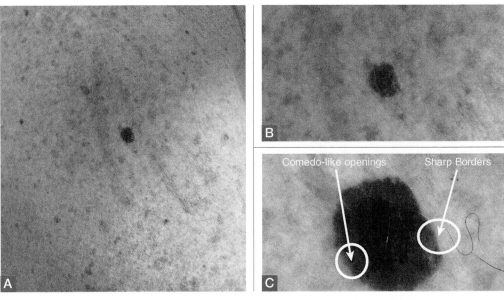

FIGURE 15.12 These clinically elevated lesions are dark brown, with a multicolored (brown + other = gray, pink, and/or yellow) dermoscopic pattern. Review these clinical and dermoscopic examples of a pigmented seborrheic keratosis. **A,B:** Clinical examples. **C:** The dermoscopic examples show comedo-like openings and sharp borders. These darker lesions with a blue-white veil need to be evaluated in the patient's clinical context. These lesions are often seen in skin type 3 or greater; however, with pigmented SKs, sometimes the skin color could be lighter. If the benign features are not obvious, these lesions can be tricky and should be biopsied.

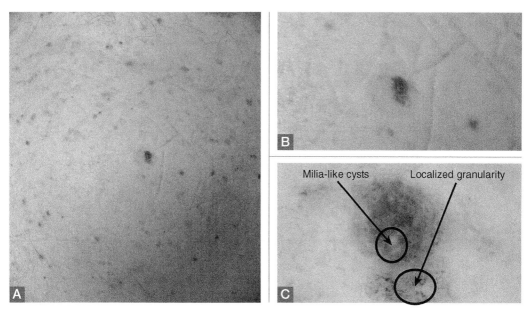

FIGURE 15.13 These clinically elevated lesions are dark brown, with a multicolored (brown + other = gray, pink, and/or yellow) dermoscopic pattern. Review these clinical and dermoscopic examples of lichen planus–like keratosis (LPLK). **A,B:** Clinical examples. **C:** The dermoscopic example shows milia-like cysts, comedo-like openings, and sharp borders. It also shows isolated gray granularity, a regression feature of flat superficial spreading type melanomas. Note the ridges seen in benign seborrheic keratosis, as well as the slight elevations within the lesion. These lesions can be classified as elevated or flat, but either way tend to have more substance than do the flat superficial spreading type melanomas.

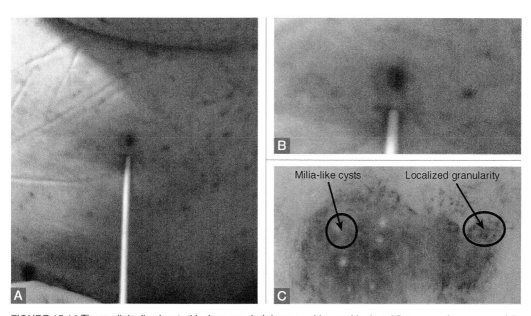

FIGURE 15.14 These clinically elevated lesions are dark brown, with a multicolored (brown + other = gray, pink, and/or yellow) dermoscopic pattern. Review these clinical and dermoscopic examples of lichen planus–like keratosis (LPLK). **A,B:** Clinical examples. **C:** The dermoscopic example shows milia-like cysts, comedo-like openings, and sharp borders. It also shows isolated areas of gray granularity, a regression feature of flat superficial spreading type melanomas. Note the ridges seen in benign seborrheic keratosis, as well as the slight elevations within the lesion. These lesions can be classified as elevated or flat, but either way tend to have more substance than the flat superficial spreading type melanomas.

Malignant Lesions

Nodular Melanoma

Pearls

- Elevated/Brown-Black/Multicolored
- **Step 4 patterns: Remember the patterns described in Chapter 1!**
  - Irregular pigmentation, with some minimal color variation
  - Asymmetry of homogenous, globular, and reticular patterns
  - Streaks, radial streaming, and pseudopods at the periphery
  - Blue-gray granularity/dots
  - Polymorphous and dotted vessels
  - Blue-white veil only in elevated lesions!
- **Bottom line: Malignant, biopsy!**

Examples

Figure 15.15 shows a clinically elevated, brown/black lesion (Figure 15.15A, B) that is dermo-scopically multicolored (brown + other = gray, pink, yellow) (Figure 15.15C). This is a 0.37-mm thick nodular melanoma. Dermoscopically, we see an asymmetric homogenous pattern with a blue-white veil. There are additional malignant features, such as the negative network and radial streaking around the periphery of the lesion. This dark papule grew within a 1-month duration. Both amelanotic and nodular pigment melanomas are aggressive and rapidly growing tumors. Diagnosis: Nodular melanoma.

Bottom line: Malignancy, biopsy!

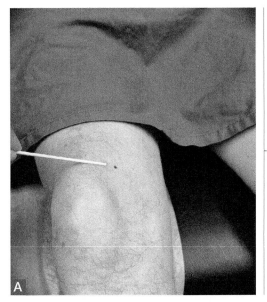
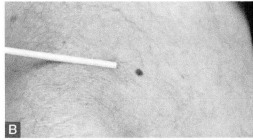
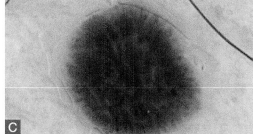

FIGURE 15.15 These clinically elevated lesions are dark brown, with a multicolored (brown + other = gray, pink, and/or yellow) dermoscopic pattern. Review these clinical and dermoscopic examples of a 0.37-mm thick malignant melanoma. **A,B:** Clinical examples. **C:** The dermoscopic example shows an asymmetric homoge-neous pattern, with the blue-white veil that is only seen in elevated lesions. The lesion also has other malignant features, such as a negative network and streaks around the periphery of the lesion. This was a dark papule of only 1 month's duration, but both amelanotic and nodular pigmented melanomas are aggressive, rapidly grow-ing tumors.

Basal Cell Carcinoma

Pearls

- Elevated/Brown-Black/Multicolored
- **Step 4 Pattern Highlights: Review the patterns described in Chapter 1!**
  - Absence of a pigment network
  - Leaf-like structures
  - Large blue-gray ovoid nests or globular-like structures
  - Arborizing telangiectasias
  - Spoke wheel areas
  - Ulceration
  - Pink-white to white shiny areas
  - Crystalline pattern
- **Bottom line: Benign, Biopsy!**

Examples

Figure 15.16 shows a clinically elevated, brown/black (Figure 15.16A, B), dermoscopically multicolored (brown + other = gray, pink, yellow) lesion (Figure 15.16C). This is an example of an early pigmented basal cell carcinoma. You can appreciate the dark blue globular structures and arborizing vessels. Diagnosis: Early pigmented basal cell carcinoma.

Bottom line: Malignant, biopsy!

Figure 15.17 shows a clinically elevated, brown/black (Figure 15.17A, B), dermoscopically multicolored (brown + other = gray, pink, yellow) lesion (Figure 15.17C). This is an example of an early pigmented basal cell carcinoma. You can appreciate the dark blue globular structure in the center with arborizing vessels. Diagnosis: Early pigmented basal cell carcinoma.

Bottom line: Malignant, biopsy!

Clinical Brown-Black

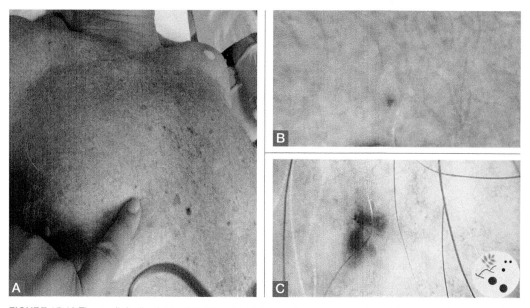

FIGURE 15.16 These clinically elevated lesions are dark brown, with a multicolored (brown + other = gray, pink, and/or yellow) dermoscopic pattern. Review these clinical and dermoscopic examples of an early pigmented basal cell skin cancer. **A,B:** Clinical examples. **C:** The dermoscopic example shows dark blue globular-like structures, along with arborized vessels.

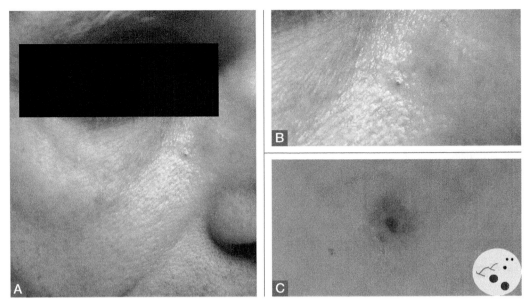

FIGURE 15.17 These clinically elevated lesions are dark brown, with a multicolored (brown + other = gray, pink, and/or yellow) dermoscopic pattern. Review these clinical and dermoscopic examples of an early pigmented basal cell skin cancer. **A,B:** Clinical examples. **C:** The dermoscopic example shows dark blue globular-like structures, along with arborized vessels.

Figure 15.18 shows a clinically elevated, brown/black (Figure 15.18A, B), dermoscopically multicolored (brown + other = gray, pink, yellow) lesion (Figure 15.18C). This is an example of an early pigmented basal cell carcinoma. You can appreciate the dark blue globular structures and arborizing vessels. Diagnosis: Early pigmented basal cell carcinoma.

Bottom line: Malignant, biopsy!

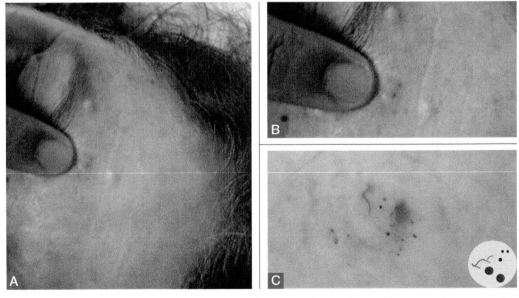

FIGURE 15.18 These clinically elevated lesions are dark brown, with a multicolored (brown + other = gray, pink, and/or yellow) dermoscopic pattern. Review these clinical and dermoscopic examples of an early pigmented basal cell skin cancer. **A,B:** Clinical examples. **C:** The dermoscopic example shows dark blue globular-like structures, along with arborized vessels.

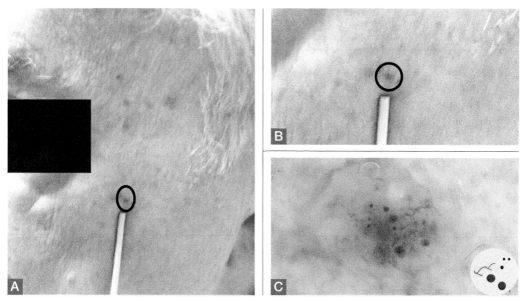

FIGURE 15.19 These clinically elevated lesions are dark brown, with a multicolored (brown + other = gray, pink, and/or yellow) dermoscopic pattern. Review these clinical and dermoscopic examples of an early pigmented basal cell skin cancer. **A,B:** Clinical examples. **C:** The dermoscopic example shows dark blue globular-like structures, along with arborized vessels. Note that basal cells can also have milia-like cysts like those seen in congenital nevi and most often associated with seborrheic keratoses.

Figure 15.19 shows a clinically elevated, brown/black (Figure 15.19A, B), dermoscopically multicolored (brown + other = gray, pink, yellow) lesion (Figure 15.19C). This is another example of an early pigmented basal cell carcinoma. You can appreciate the dark blue globular structures and arborizing vessels. Note that you may also see a milia-like cyst that we have seen in congenital nevi and most often with seborrheic keratosis. However, in the presence of the other malignant features, this lesion is without doubt malignant. Diagnosis: Early pigmented basal cell carcinoma.

Bottom line: Malignant, biopsy!

Clinical Brown-Black

Chapter 16 Flat/Elevated/Red/Red

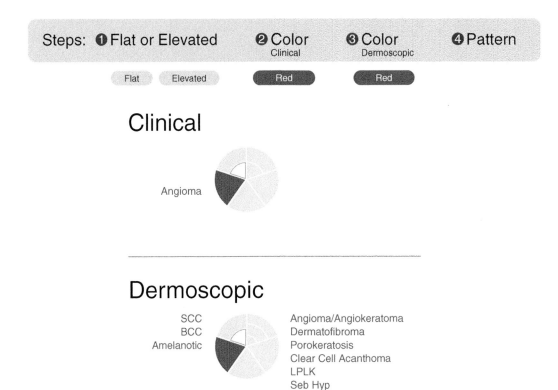

Steps: ❶ Flat or Elevated ❷ Color
Clinical
❸ Color
Dermoscopic
❹ Pattern

Flat | Elevated | Red | Red

Clinical

Angioma

Dermoscopic

SCC
BCC
Amelanotic

Angioma/Angiokeratoma
Dermatofibroma
Porokeratosis
Clear Cell Acanthoma
LPLK
Seb Hyp
Benign Nevus

Malignant | Benign

None

Angiokeratoma
Clusters of red lacunae
Can have areas of dark
hemolized blood

FIGURE 16.1 Color wheel: flat/elevated/red/red.

Step 1: Is the lesion flat or raised? **Flat or Elevated**

Step 2: What color is the lesion on clinical assessment? **Red**

Step 3: What is the dermoscopic color? **Red**

Step 4: Is further elucidation needed to decide whether to biopsy or not? **No**

Take a look at the color wheel in Figure 16.1.

We have only one diagnosis when dealing with clinically and dermoscopically purely red lesions. Regardless of their elevation, they are benign angiokeratomas, commonly called cherry angiomas.

(Cherry) Angiomas

Pearls

- Flat/Elevated/Red/Red
  - Characterized by well-demarcated round or oval structures called lacunae.
  - They are collections of blood vessels; depending on the vascularization, they will appear anywhere from bright red to blue-red or dark blue/maroon.
  - When thrombosed, they will appear as homogenous, confluent dark bluish-black pigment.

Examples

Figure 16.2 shows a closer dermoscopic example of the characteristic well-demarcated, round or oval, red to blue-red, or blue-black to maroon structures called lacunae. These structures are

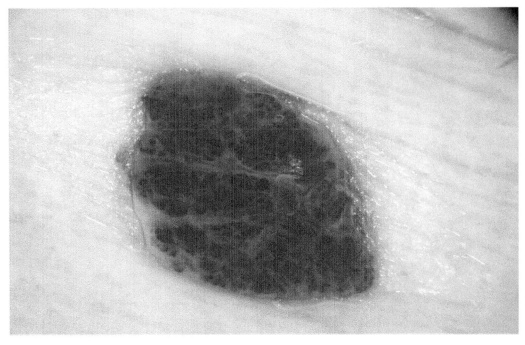

FIGURE 16.2 These clinically flat or mostly elevated lesions are red, with a vascular red lacunae dermoscopic pattern. Review these clinical and dermoscopic examples of a cherry angioma. Angiomas are characterized by well-demarcated red to blue-red or blue-black to maroon, round or oval structures (lacunae). These structures are collections of blood vessels. When thrombosed, they appear as homogeneous, confluent dark bluish-black pigment.

Clinical Other Colors—Yellow, Purple, Red

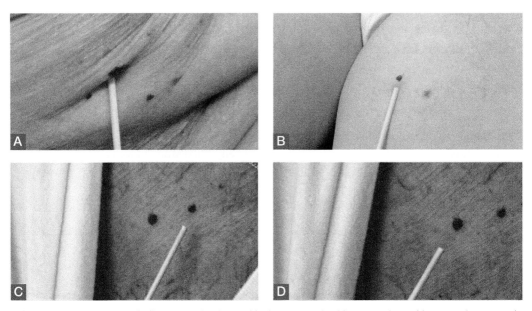

FIGURE 16.3 These clinically flat or mostly elevated lesions are red, with a vascular red lacunae dermoscopic pattern **(A–D)**. These are clinical examples of cherry angiomas.

collections of blood vessels; the state of the vessels within the lesion will determine the shade of red.

Figures 16.3 and 16.4 show clinically elevated or flat red lesions (Figure 16.3A–D), with corresponding dermoscopically red lacunar patterns (Figure 16.4A–D).

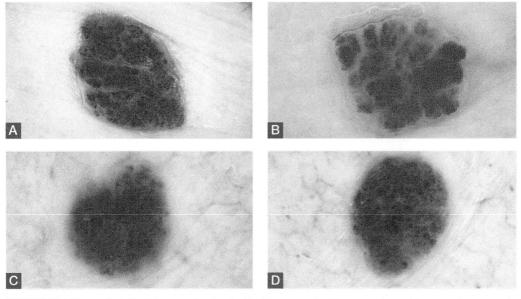

FIGURE 16.4 These clinically flat or mostly elevated lesions are red, with a vascular red lacunae dermoscopic pattern **(A–D)**. There are the corresponding dermoscopic examples of cherry angiomas from Figure 16.3.

Chapter 17 Flat/Elevated/Purple/Multicolored

Steps: ❶ Flat or Elevated ❷ Color
Clinical ❸ Color
Dermoscopic ❹ Pattern

Flat   Elevated   Purple   Multicolored

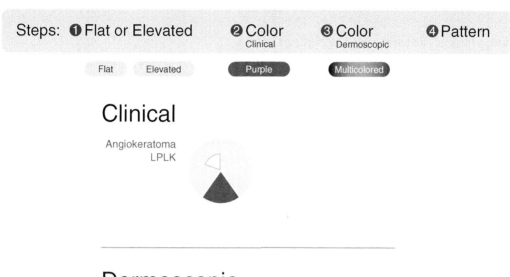

Clinical

Angiokeratoma
LPLK

Dermoscopic

LPLK
MM
BCC
CN/Blue Nevi
Ink-jet Lentigo/Seb K
Hemolized blood/angiokeratoma

Malignant | Benign

None

Angiokeratoma
Clusters of red lacunae
Can have areas of dark hemolized
blood or white veil giving it a multicolored appearance

LPLK
Can sometimes be confused with MM
The clinical violaceous color is not as
purple as with angiokeratomas

FIGURE 17.1 Color wheel: flat/elevated/purple/multicolored.

> **Step 1:** Is the lesion flat or raised? **Flat or Elevated**
>
> **Step 2:** What color is the lesion on clinical assessment? **Purple**
>
> **Step 3:** What is the dermoscopic color? **Multicolored**
>
> **Step 4:** Is further elucidation needed to decide whether to biopsy or not? **No**

Take a look at the color wheel in Figure 17.1.

When looking at clinically purple lesions, we are again dealing with **angiokeratomas**. There are patterns that have been identified as sensitive and specific for angiokeratoma that we will show briefly.

Lichen planus–like keratosis can also appear to have a violet hue clinically; however, it is not as "purple" as our angiokeratomas. We covered these lesions in Chapters 6 and 7: Flat and Elevated/Pink-Clear/Multicolored.

These lesions can be confused with melanoma, so flip back to those chapters to review those lesions.

Angiokeratoma

Pearls

- Flat/Elevated/Purple/Multicolored
  - Characterized by well-demarcated round or oval structures called lacunae
    - They are collections of blood vessels; depending on the vascularization, they will appear anywhere from bright red to blue-red or dark blue/maroon.
    - When thrombosed, they will appear as homogenous, confluent dark bluish-black pigment.
- Other patterns to help you include[1]
  - Whitish veil
  - Erythema and peripheral erythema
  - Hemorrhagic crusts

Examples

Figure 17.2 shows a dermoscopic example of some of the patterns you may see in solitary angiokeratomas, including the whitish veil, dark lacunae, and peripheral erythema.

Figures 17.3 and 17.4 show clinically elevated or flat purple lesions (Figure 17.3A–D) and their dermoscopically multicolored (bright red to blue-red or dark blue-black/maroon) counterparts (Figure 17.4A–D). You can see that the lacunae can often be different colors, but are present in each lesion. Lesions A to C demonstrate some peripheral erythema. Note the whitish veil in lesions C and D.

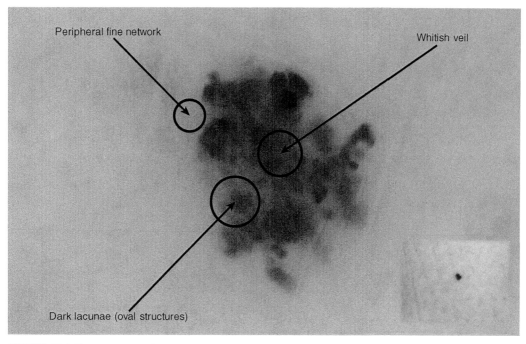

Peripheral fine network

Whitish veil

Dark lacunae (oval structures)

FIGURE 17.2 These clinically flat or mostly elevated lesions are red/purple, with a multicolored lacunae dermoscopic pattern. Review this dermoscopic example of angiokeratoma. On dermoscopy, note the dark oval structures (lacunae) and peripheral erythema and fine network, as well as the whitish veil.

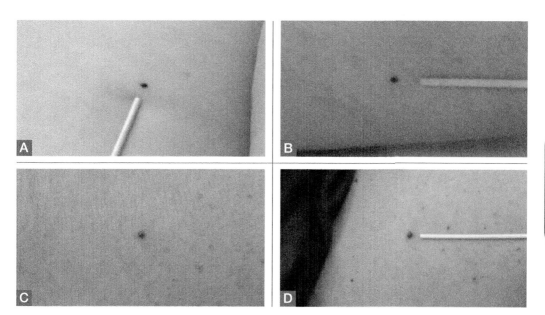

FIGURE 17.3 These clinically flat or mostly elevated lesions are red/purple, with a multicolored lacunae dermoscopic pattern (A–D). Review these clinical examples of angiokeratomas.

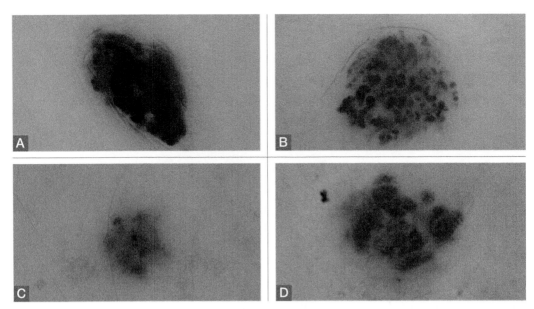

FIGURE 17.4 These clinically flat or mostly elevated lesions are red/purple, with a multicolored lacunae dermoscopic pattern **(A–D)**. These examples of angiokeratomas are from the corresponding dermoscopic examples of Figure 17.3 A–D. They have dark oval structures (lacunae), and **(A–C)** show peripheral erythema. Note that on dermoscopy, **(C)** and **(D)** have a whitish veil.

Reference

1. Zaballos P, Daufi C, Puig S, et al. Dermoscopy of solitary angiokeratomas: a morphological study. *Arch Dermatol.* 2007;143(3):318–325.

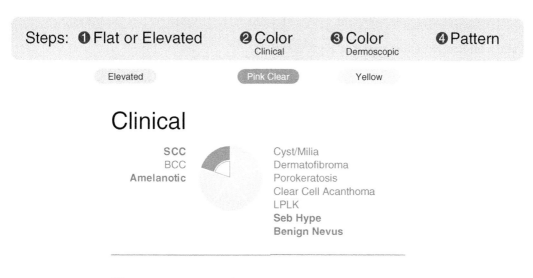

Clinical

SCC
BCC
Amelanotic

Cyst/Milia
Dermatofibroma
Porokeratosis
Clear Cell Acanthoma
LPLK
Seb Hype
Benign Nevus

Dermoscopic

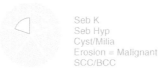

Seb K
Seb Hyp
Cyst/Milia
Erosion = Malignant
SCC/BCC

Malignant Benign

None

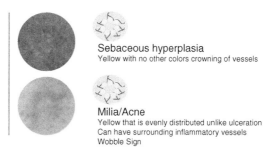

Sebaceous hyperplasia
Yellow with no other colors crowning of vessels

Milia/Acne
Yellow that is evenly distributed unlike ulceration
Can have surrounding inflammatory vessels
Wobble Sign

FIGURE 18.1 Color wheel: elevated/pink clear/yellow.

Step 1: Is the lesion flat or raised? **Elevated (Occasionally Flat)**

Step 2: What color is the lesion on clinical assessment? **Pink or Clear**

Step 3: What is the dermoscopic color? **Yellow**

Step 4: Is further elucidation needed to decide whether to biopsy or not? **Yes**

Take a look at the color wheel in Figure 18.1.

Here we will be looking at two benign lesions: **sebaceous hyperplasia** and **milia/acne**.

Both of these lesions have been **confused with basal cell carcinoma**. This chapter will help you learn how to never confuse them again!

Sebaceous Hyperplasia

Pearls

- Elevated/Pink-Clear/Yellow
  - These pink- or skin-colored papules often have a central dell or depression.
  - Remember that we first encountered these in Chapter 7 Elevated/Pink-clear/Multicolored. We will revisit them here, as they can often be yellow dermoscopically.
  - These lesions are mostly elevated, but occasionally, you'll run across a flat one.
  - Irritated sebaceous hyperplasia can clinically look like BCCs and will be important to distinguish by identifying patterns.
- **Step 4 Patterns:**
  - Yellow-white lobular structures, resembling popcorn
  - Serpentine radial vessels, resembling a crown
    ○ These radial vessels typically do not cross the midline.
  - Central indentation or dell
- **Bottom line: Benign, biopsy not necessary.**

Examples

Figure 18.2 reminds us of the patterns that we see with sebaceous hyperplasia. Clinically, these elevated, pink or clear lesions have a yellow-white lobular dermoscopic pattern. These lobular structures can look like popcorn, with serpentine radial vessels or crown vessels and central dell.

Figures 18.3 and 18.4 are examples of clinically elevated, pink or skin-colored lesions (Figure 18.3A–D) with a yellow-white dermoscopic pattern (Figure 18.4A–D). You can appreciate the yellow-white lobular popcorn pattern, with the radial serpentine vessels in all four lesions. Figures A, B, and C also have the central dell.

Figure 18.5 shows two clinically elevated, pink or skin-colored lesions (Figure 18.5A) with two different dermoscopic patterns. The differences are subtle but critically important. Figure 18.5B has a dermoscopically multicolored blue-gray globular-like structure and arborizing vessels on a pink background. Figure 18.5C has a dermoscopically yellow lobular structure with peripheral radial vessels and peripheral edema not crossing the midline. Figure 18.5B is a basal cell carcinoma, while Figure 18.5C is a sebaceous hyperplasia. Being able to distinguish between these two lesions is critically important, but if you pay attention to the steps, it is easily done (see Chapter 7).

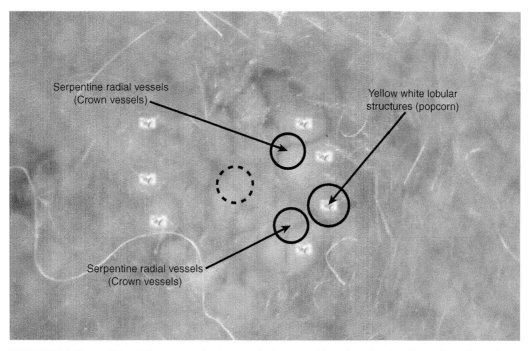

FIGURE 18.2 These clinically flat, or mostly elevated, lesions are skin-colored/pink, with a yellow-white lobular dermoscopic pattern. Review this dermoscopic example of sebaceous hyperplasia. On dermoscopy, note the white-yellow lobular structures (popcorn) and peripheral serpentine radial vessels (crown vessels), as well as the central indentation (dell).

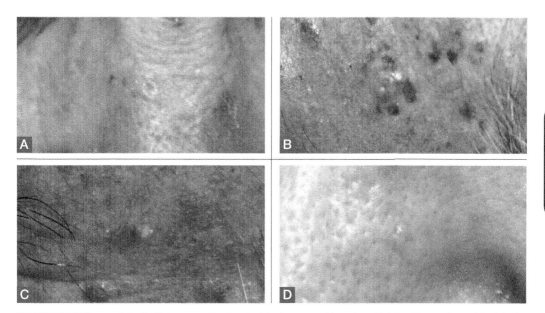

FIGURE 18.3 These clinically flat, or mostly elevated, lesions are skin-colored/pink with a yellow-white lobular dermoscopic pattern. Parts **(A–D)** show clinical examples of sebaceous hyperplasia.

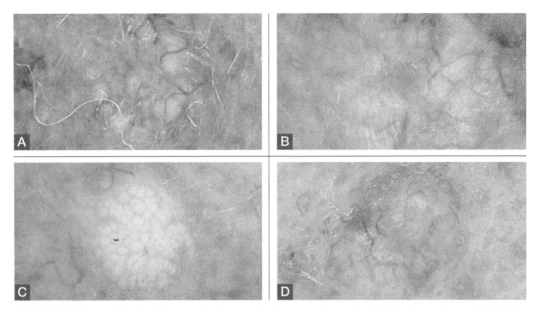

FIGURE 18.4 These clinically flat, or mostly elevated, lesions are skin-colored/pink with a yellow-white lobular dermoscopic pattern. Parts **(A–D)** show examples of sebaceous hyperplasia; these are the corresponding dermoscopic examples of Figure 18.3. Parts **(A–D)** also show white-yellow lobular structures (popcorn structures) and peripheral serpentine radial vessels (crown vessels). Note that **(A–C)** also have a central indentation (dell).

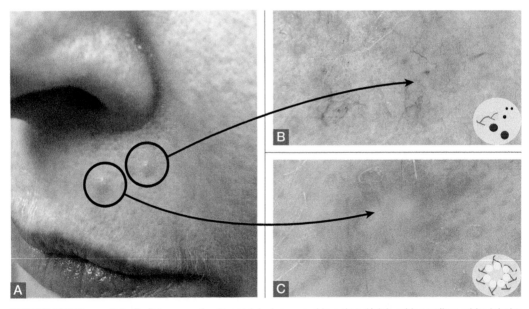

FIGURE 18.5 These clinically flat, or mostly elevated, lesions are skin-colored/pink, with a yellow-white lobular dermoscopic pattern. **A:** The clinical example and corresponding dermoscopy images show basal cell skin cancer **(B)** and sebaceous hyperplasia **(C)**. Note that the lesion shown in Part **(B)** has globular-like structures and arborized vessels on a pink background, while the lesion shown in Part **(C)** has yellow lobular-like structures, with peripheral radial erythema/vessels.

Pearls

- Elevated/Pink-Clear/Yellow
  - The patient's clinical history will be helpful. Pay attention to the age of the patient and the lesion's location!
  - While these lesions are typically seen more often in adolescents and young adults, older populations still experience acne lesions from comedones to large, tender nodules and cysts.
  - Picking can cause irritation and bleeding, making it difficult to differentiate from some presentations of early BCCs in fair-skinned, older adults.
- **Step 4 Patterns:**
  - Dermoscopic features of acne lesions can include a neutral yellow background and a central punctum.
  - If in the presence of excoriation, the yellow background can be confused for the yellow ulceration seen in basal cell carcinoma.

Milia/Acne

Example

Figure 18.6 shows a clinically elevated, pink or clear lesion, with a dermoscopically yellow pattern. You will also see the presence of some inflammation. These inflammatory vessels and yellow background from excoriation can look similar to the arborizing vessels and yellow ulceration of a BCC seen in the upper right image. However, here we see no other features of a BCC, such as blue-gray globules or dots or leaf-like structures. Diagnosis: Milia/acne.

Bottom line: Biopsy not necessary.

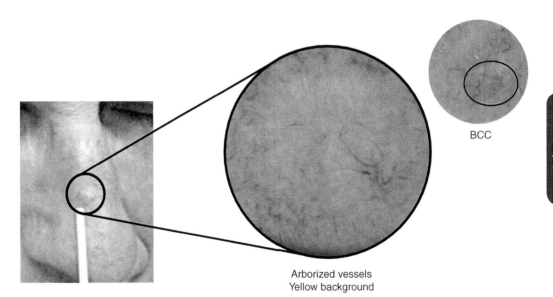

BCC

Arborized vessels
Yellow background

FIGURE 18.6 These clinically flat, or mostly elevated, lesions are skin-colored/pink, with a yellow-white lobular dermoscopic pattern. Review these clinical and dermoscopic findings of excoriated acne vulgaris lesion. **Upper right:** This example illustrates the localized yellow hue that can be seen in an ulcerated BCC.

Chapter 19 When Do You Not Use Dermoscopy?

There are a few circumstances in which dermoscopy is not necessary and where our color wheel algorithm should not be used. This is largely when it is clinically obvious that the lesion is malignant (remember the ABCDEs we discussed in Chapter 1). Typically, these tend to be more advanced lesions (but not always!) and will have multiple dermoscopic features that may not be useful in diagnosis. Furthermore, any lesions that are too thick or scaly are not indicated for dermoscopy, as you cannot appreciate features adequately.

Examples

Figure 19.1 shows an example of a clinically elevated, multicolored lesion. Any lesion that is clinically elevated and multicolored needs to be biopsied. This lesion does exhibit the associated basal cell carcinoma patterns, but sometimes lesions that are clinically obvious are dermoscopically confusing due to excessive ulceration, bleeding, or thickening of the tumor.

Figure 19.2 shows an example of a clinically elevated, multicolored lesion. Any lesion that is clinically elevated and multicolored needs to be biopsied. This lesion does exhibit the associated squamous cell carcinoma patterns, such as dotted vessels, but the dark surrounding pigmentation could be confused with melanoma. However, remember our ultimate goal is to determine whether or not to biopsy—this lesion will certainly need to be biopsied. Also, keep

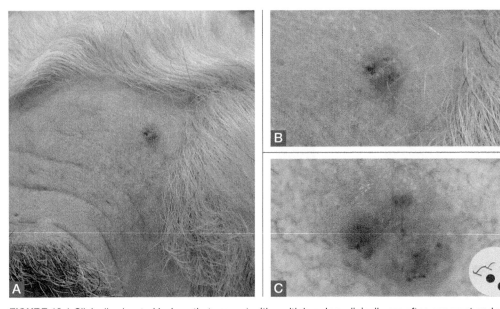

FIGURE 19.1 Clinically elevated lesions that present with multiple colors clinically are often apparent and need to be biopsied. Note that this lesion does exhibit the dermoscopic patterns associated with basal cell skin cancer such as ash leaves, arborized vessels, and blue-gray globular-like structures/ovoid nests. However, sometimes, when lesions are clinically obvious, the dermoscopic pattern can be confusing due to excessive ulceration/bleeding or thickening of the tumor/hyperkeratosis.

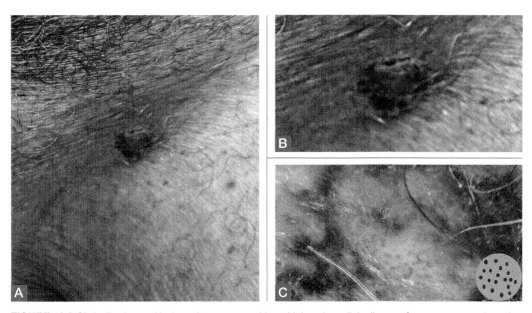

FIGURE 19.2 Clinically elevated lesions that present with multiple colors clinically are often apparent and need to be biopsied. Note that this lesion does exhibit the dermoscopic patterns associated with pigmented squamous cell skin cancer such as dotted vessels, but the dark surrounding pigmentation could be confused with melanoma. The clinical history of a lesion that has been present for a long period of time makes the lesion less consistent with melanoma. However, remember the ultimate goal of the color wheel approach is to decide whether or not to biopsy. From both a clinical and dermoscopic analysis, this lesion would need a biopsy. Clinically obvious does not always mean advanced. In this case, the lesion is still a pigmented squamous cell skin cancer in situ.

in mind that clinically obvious lesions are not synonymous with advanced lesions. This lesion is still a pigment squamous cell in situ.

Figure 19.3 shows an example of a clinically elevated, multicolored lesion. Any lesion that is clinically elevated and multicolored needs to be biopsied. This lesion does exhibit the

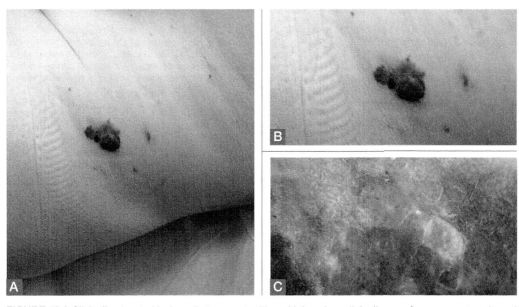

FIGURE 19.3 Clinically elevated lesions that present with multiple colors clinically are often apparent and need to be biopsied. Note that this lesion does exhibit the dermoscopic patterns associated with malignant nodular melanoma, such as polymorphous vessels, a scar-like crystalline pattern, and overall asymmetry. However, sometimes when lesions are clinically obvious, the dermoscopic pattern can be confusing due to excessive ulceration/bleeding or thickening of the tumor/hyperkeratosis.

associated malignant nodular melanoma, such as polymorphous vessels, scar-like crystalline pattern, and overall asymmetry, but sometimes lesions that are clinically obvious are dermoscopically confusing due to excessive ulceration, bleeding, or thickening of the tumor.

Figure 19.4 shows an example of a clinically elevated, multicolored lesion. Any lesion that is clinically elevated and multicolored needs to be biopsied. This lesion does exhibit the associated malignant melanoma in situ, such as polymorphous vessels, negative network pattern, and overall asymmetry especially at the periphery, but sometimes lesions that are clinically obvious are dermoscopically confusing due to excessive ulceration, bleeding, or thickening of the tumor. **Again, remember clinically obvious does not necessarily mean advanced. This is an example of a melanoma in situ**.

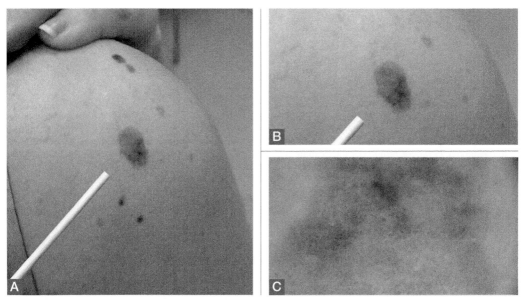

FIGURE 19.4 Clinically elevated lesions that present with multiple colors clinically are often apparent and need to be biopsied. Note that this lesion does exhibit the dermoscopic patterns associated with malignant melanoma in situ, such as polymorphous vessels, a negative network pattern, and overall asymmetry, especially at the periphery. However, sometimes when lesions are clinically obvious, the dermoscopic pattern can be confusing due to excessive ulceration/bleeding or thickening of the tumor/hyperkeratosis. Clinically obvious does not always mean advanced. This lesion is still a melanoma in situ.

Index

Note: Page numbers in *italic* denote figures

A

Acne vulgaris lesion, *271*
Amelanotic melanoma
  elevated lesions
    clinically pink-clear/dermoscopically red, 62,
      94, *95*
    clinically pink-clear/multicolored dermos-
      copy, 69
  flat/clinically pink-clear/multicolored
      dermoscopy
    dermal involvement, scar-like pattern,
      118, *119*
    diffuse glomeruloid vessels, 119, *121*
    nonspecific pigmentation, 118, *120*
Angiokeratoma, flat/elevated lesions
  lacunae dermoscopic pattern, 264, *265, 266*
  peripheral erythema, 264, *266*
Angiomas
  lacunae, 50, *51, 261,* 261–262, *262*
  peripheral erythema, 50, *51*
  whitish veil, 50, *51*

B

Basal cell carcinoma (BCC)
  characteristic patterns, 24, *25*
  elevated lesions
    clinically brown-black/multicolored
      dermoscopy, 257–259, *257–259*
    clinically pink-clear/dermoscopically red,
      98, *99, 103*
    clinically pink-clear/multicolored
      dermoscopy, 69, 142–148, *143–148*
  flat lesions
    clinically brown-black/multicolored
      dermoscopy, 242–245, *242–245*
    clinically pale brown/dermoscopically
      brown, 159, *160*
    clinically pale brown/multicolored dermoscopy,
      184, *185, 186, 188*
    clinically pink-clear/dermoscopically red,
      59, *61*
    clinically pink-clear/multicolored dermoscopy,
      65, 115–117, *116, 117*
  inflammation, 271, *271*
  telangiectasias, 80, 82, 83, *83, 84*
  vascular pattern, 80, *82*

Benign lesions
  elevated/clinically brown-black/multicolored
      dermoscopy
    congenital/combined nevi, *247–250,* 247–251
    LPLK, 251–255, *251–255*
    seborrheic keratosis, 251–255, *251–255*
  elevated/clinically pink-clear/dermoscopically red
    IN, 86–89
    clear cell acanthoma, 91, *92*
    CN, 86–89
    dermatofibroma, 89–90
    inflamed seborrheic keratosis, 91–94
  elevated/clinically pink-clear/dermoscopically
      yellow, 267–268
  elevated/clinically pink-clear/multicolored
      dermoscopy
    dermatofibroma, 126–129
    IN/CN, 132–136
    nonpigmented (pink) seborrheic keratoses,
      123–126
    sebaceous hyperplasia, 129–132
  flat/clinically brown-black/dermoscopically brown
    benign lichenoid, 205–207
    Ink-Jet Lentigo, 203–205
    junctional nevi, 207–212
    LPLK, 205–207
  flat/clinically brown-black/multicolored
      dermoscopy
    benign lichenoid, 226–228, *227, 228*
    blue nevi, 232–233, *233*
    junctional/combined nevi, 229–232, *229–232*
    LPLK, 226–228, *227, 228*
  flat/clinically pale brown/dermoscopically brown
    early dermatofibroma, 157–159
    early seborrheic keratoses, 155–157
    junctional nevi, 152, 154
    solar lentigo, 150–153
  flat/clinically pale brown/multicolored
      dermoscopy
    benign lichenoid, 177–181
    early dermatofibroma, 182–184
    junctional/combined congenital nevi, 172–176
    LPLK, 177–181
  flat/clinically pink-clear/dermoscopically red
    clear cell acanthoma, 77
    LPLK, 75–76
    porokeratosis, 59, 73–75

Benign lesions (*Continued*)
 flat/clinically pink-clear/multicolored dermoscopy
  congenital nevi, 105–106
  dermatofibroma, 106–109
  LPLK, 109–112
  nonpigmented seborrheic keratosis, 109–112
 flat/elevated/clinically purple/multicolored
  dermoscopy, 263
 flat/elevated/clinically red/dermoscopically red,
  260, 261
Benign melanocytic patterns
 globular, 5–6
 homogenous, 6–9
 reticular, 2–4
Blue-white veil, 9–10, 18, *19, 20,* 54, 229, 230, *250,*
 251, 253, 254, 256

C

Cherry angiomas, 261, *261,* 262, *262*
Clear cell acanthoma, 59, 62, 73, 77, *77,* 86, 91,
 92, 121
Color wheel
 biopsy decision-making, 58
 elevated lesions
  clinically brown-black/dermoscopically
   brown, *215,* 216
  clinically brown-black/multicolored dermoscopy, *246,* 247
  clinically pink-clear/dermoscopically red,
   62, *63*
  clinically pink clear/dermoscopically yellow,
   267, 268
  clinically pink-clear/multicolored dermoscopy,
   67, *68,* 69, *69*
 flat lesions
  clinically brown-black/multicolored
   dermoscopy, *225,* 226
  clinically pink-clear/dermoscopically red,
   59–62, *60–62*
  clinically pink-clear/multicolored dermoscopy,
   64–67, *64–67*
  elevated/clinically purple/multicolored
   dermoscopy, *263,* 264
  elevated/clinically red/dermoscopically red,
   260, 261
Compound nevus
 comma-like vessels and faint pigmentation,
  216, *218*
 elevated/clinically dark brown/dermoscopically
  black, 216, *218,* 219, *219*
 flat/clinically brown-black/multicolored
  dermoscopy, 238–241, *239–241*
 flat/clinically dark brown/multicolored
  dermoscopy, 238–241, *239–241*
 globular dot pattern, *219,* 219–220
Congenital nevi (CN)
 diffuse globular pattern, 216
 elevated lesions

 clinically brown-black/multicolored
  dermoscopy, *247–250,* 247–251
 clinically pale brown/dermoscopically
  brown, 191, *191, 192*
 clinically pale brown/multicolored
  dermoscopy, 197–199, *198, 199*
 clinically pink-clear/dermoscopically red,
  86, *89*
 clinically pink-clear/multicolored dermoscopy,
  134, 135, *135, 136*
 flat lesions
  clinically pale brown/multicolored dermoscopy,
   172, *173–176*
  clinically pink-clear/multicolored dermoscopy,
   105, 105–106, *106*
 globular pattern, 217, *218*
 symmetric, 216
Contact nonpolarized dermoscopy (CNPD), 53, *54–56*
Contact polarized dermoscopy (CPD), 53, *54–56,* 56

D

Dermatofibromas
 central vessels and erythema, 46, *48*
 central white patch, 46, *48*
 crystalline structures, 49, *49*
 elevated lesions
  clinical history, 70, *70*
  clinically pink-clear/dermoscopically red,
   89–90, *90, 91*
  clinically pink-clear/multicolored dermoscopy,
   126–129, *127–129*
 faint pseudo-network-like periphery, 46, *47*
 flat lesions
  clinically pale brown/dermoscopically
   brown, 157–159, *158, 159*
  clinically pale brown/multicolored
   dermoscopy, 182–184, *182–184*
  clinically pink-clear/multicolored dermoscopy,
   106, *107, 108,* 108–109
 globule-like/ring-like globules, 49, *49*
 network-like structures, 46, *47*
 pigmented network, 46, *48*
Dermatoscopes
 dermatofibroma, 54, *55, 56*
 junctional nevus, 56, *56*
 melanoma in situ, 54, *55*
 seborrheic keratosis
  epidermal features, 54, *54*
  nonpigmented, 54, *55*
 types
  nonpolarized, 53
  polarized, 54
Dysplastic nevi, 10, *10,* 211, *212,* 226, 238–242,
 238–243

E

Elevated lesions
 angiokeratoma, 264, *265, 266*

clinically brown-black/multicolored dermoscopy
   blue nevus, *250,* 250–251
   congenital nevus, 247–250, *248–250*
   early pigmented BCC, 257–259, *257–259*
   LPLK, 254, *255*
   malignant melanoma, 256, *256*
   seborrheic keratosis, 251–254, *252–254*
clinically dark brown/dermoscopically black
   compound nevus, 216, *218,* 219, *219*
   congenital nevus, 216, 217, *217, 218,* 219
   seborrheic keratoses, 220, *220–224*
clinically dark brown/multicolored dermoscopy
   blue nevus, *250,* 250–251
   congenital nevus, 247–250, *248–250*
   early pigmented basal cell skin cancer,
      257–259, *257–259*
   LPLK, 254, *255*
   malignant melanoma, 256, *256*
   pigmented seborrheic keratosis, 254, *254*
   seborrheic keratosis, 251–254, *252–254*
clinically pale brown/dermoscopically brown
   congenital nevi, 191, *191, 192*
   seborrheic keratosis, 193, *193–195*
clinically pale brown/multicolored dermoscopy
   congenital nevus, 197–199, *198, 199*
   irritated seborrheic keratosis, 199, *199–201*
   LPLK, 199, *199–201*
clinically pink-clear/dermoscopically red,
      62, *63*
   benign, 86–94
   malignant, 94–103
clinically pink-clear/multicolored dermoscopy,
      67, *68,* 69, *69*
   benign, 123–136
   malignant, 137–148
multicolored dermoscopy
   BCC patterns, 272, *272*
   malignant melanoma in situ, 274, *274*
   malignant nodular melanoma, *273,* 273–274
   SCC patterns, 272, *273*
   vascular red lacunae dermoscopic pattern, 261,
      261, 262, 262

F

Flat/elevated lesions
   milia/acne, 271, *271*
   sebaceous hyperplasia, 268, *269–270*
Flat lesions
   angiokeratoma, 264, *265, 266*
   blue-gray granularity, 17–18, *17–18,* 34
   clinically brown-black/dermoscopically brown
      benign, 203–212
      malignant, 212–214
   clinically brown-black/multicolored dermoscopy
      blue nevus, 232, *233*
      congenital nevus, 229, *229, 230, 232*
      dysplastic compound nevus, 238–241,
         239–241

early pigmented basal cell skin cancer,
      243–245, *243–245*
   junctional nevus dysplastic type, 242, *242, 243*
   LPLK, 227, *227, 228*
   malignant melanoma, 234–238, *234–238*
   melanocytic nevus, 229, *230, 231*
   traumatized nevus, 238, *239*
clinically dark brown/multicolored dermoscopy
   blue nevus, 232, *233*
   congenital nevus, 229, *229, 230, 232*
   dysplastic compound nevus, 238–241,
      239–241
   early pigmented basal cell skin cancer,
      243–245, *243–245*
   junctional nevus dysplastic type, 242,
      242, 243
   lichen planus-like keratosis (LPLK), 227,
      227, 228
   malignant melanoma, 234–238, *234–238*
   melanocytic nevus, 229, *230, 231*
   traumatized nevus, 238, *239*
clinically pale brown/dermoscopically brown
   benign, 150–159
   malignant, 159–170
clinically pale brown/multicolored dermoscopy
   benign, 172–184
   malignant, 184–188
clinically pink-clear/dermoscopically red
   benign, 59, 73–77
   malignant, 59, *61, 63,* 77–84
clinically pink-clear/multicolored dermoscopy,
      64–67, *64–67*
   benign, 105–112
   malignant, 112–121
vascular red lacunae dermoscopic pattern, 261,
      261, 262, 262
Focal pseudopods and radial streaming, 9–10, 19,
      20, 21, 161, *161, 162*

I

Ink-jet lentigo, 203, *204, 205*
Intradermal nevi (IN)
   clinically pink-clear/dermoscopically red/
      elevated, 86, *87, 88*
   clinically pink-clear/multicolored dermoscopy/
      elevated, 133–136, *133–136*
Irritated seborrheic keratosis. *See also* Lichen
      planus-like keratosis (LPLK)
   elevated lesions, 70, *71,* 199, *199–201*
   flat lesions, 59

J

Junctional nevi
   flat/clinically brown-black/dermoscopically
      brown
      dysplastic (atypical) nevus, 211, *212*
      symmetric reticular network pattern, 208,
         208–210

Junctional nevi (*Continued*)
  flat/clinically brown-black/multicolored
    dermoscopy, 229–232, *229–232*
  flat/clinically pale brown/dermoscopically
    brown, 154, *154*
  flat/clinically pale brown/multicolored
    dermoscopy, 172, *173–176*

L

Lacunae
  angiokeratoma, *264,* 265, *266*
  cherry angiomas, *261,* 261–262, *262*
Lentigo maligna, 150, 163, *164,* 165, *165–167, 169,*
    170, 203, *213,* 237, 238
Lichenoid keratosis, benign, 43–46, 75, *76,*
    177–181, 205–207, 226–228, *227, 228*
Lichen planus-like keratosis (LPLK)
  elevated/clinically pale brown/multicolored
    dermoscopy, 199, *199–201*
  elevated/clinically brown-black/multicolored
    dermoscopy, 251–255, *251–255*
  fingerprinting, *45,* 45–46, *46*
  flat/clinically brown-black/dermoscopically
    brown, 205–207, *205–207*
  flat/clinically pale brown/multicolored
    dermoscopy, 177–181, *177–181*
  flat/clinically pink-clear/multicolored dermoscopy
    crystalline scar-like pattern, 109, *110*
    inflammation, lesions, 109, *109*
    reticular pattern, 111, *111*
  flat lesions, 59
    clinically brown-black/multicolored
      dermoscopy, 226–228, *227, 228*
  moth-eaten borders and ridges, 44, *44*
  regression, 43
  vascular pattern, 4, *5*

M

Malignant lesions
  elevated/clinically brown-black/multicolored
    dermoscopy
    BCC, 257–259, *257–259*
    nodular melanoma, 256, *256*
  elevated/clinically pink-clear/dermoscopically red
    amelanotic melanoma, 94, *95*
    BCC, 98–103
    nonpigmented SCC, 95–98
  elevated/clinically pink-clear/multicolored
    dermoscopy, 137–148
    BCC, 142–148
    SCC, keratoacanthoma type, 137–142
  flat/clinically brown-black/dermoscopically
    brown, 212, *213 ,* 214, *214*
  flat/clinically brown-black/multicolored
    dermoscopy
    BCC, 242–245, *242–245*

dysplastic nevi, 238–242, *238–242*
  superficial spreading melanoma, 234–238,
    234–238
  flat/clinically pale brown/dermoscopically brown
    early pigmented BCC, 159, *160*
    early superficial spreading melanoma,
      161–163, *161–163*
    lentigo maligna, 163–167
    SCC, in situ, 168–170
  flat/clinically pale brown/multicolored dermoscopy
    BCC, 184, *185, 186, 188*
    malignant melanoma, 187, *187, 188*
    SCC, 184, *185*
  flat/clinically pink-clear/dermoscopically red
    BCC, 80–84
    SCC, 77–80
  flat/clinically pink-clear/multicolored dermoscopy
    BCC, 115–117
    early amelanotic melanoma, 118–121
    SCC, 112–114
Melanocytic patterns, malignant
  blue-gray granularity, 17–18
  blue-white veil, nodular melanomas, 18–20
  dysplastic nevi, 10, *10*
  focal pseudopods and radial streaming, 19–21
  globular disorganized, 13–14
  homogenous disorganized, 14–17
  indicative of melanoma, 11
  intraepidermal melanocytic proliferations, 10, *10*
  polymorphous and dotted vessels, 20–23
  reticular disorganized, 11–12
Melanoma
  malignant
    clinically elevated lesions//multicolored
      dermoscopy, *273,* 273–274, *274*
    elevated/brown-black/multicolored
      dermoscopy, 256, *256*
    flat/clinically pale brown/multicolored
      dermoscopy, 187, *187, 188*
    superficial spreading, *10,* 161–163, *161–163,*
      200, 212–214, 234–238, *234–238*
Milia/acne, 50–51, *51,* 268, 271, *271*

N

Nonmelanocytic patterns
  angiomas, 50
  benign lichenoid keratosis, 43–46
  clinically similar-appearing hyperpigmented
    lesions, 32, *33*
  dermatofibromas, 46–49
  LPLK, 43–46
  malignant
    BCC, 24, 25
    SCC, 23–24
  milia/acne, 50–51
  sebaceous hyperplasia, 50

seborrheic keratoses, 24–32
solar lentigines, 32–43
Nonpigmented seborrheic keratosis
    elevated/clinically pink-clear/multicolored
        dermoscopy, 123–125, *124–126*
    flat/clinically pink-clear/multicolored
        dermoscopy, 109–112

P

Pattern analysis
    benign melanocytic, 2–9
    description, 1
    malignant melanocytic, 9–23
    malignant nonmelanocytic, 23–24
    melanocytic/nonmelanocytic, 1
    noninvasive technology, 1
    nonmelanocytic (*see* Nonmelanocytic patterns)
    7-point checklist, 1
Peripheral erythema, 264, *266*
Polymorphous and dotted vessels
    amelanotic melanomas, 23, *23*
    malignant feature, 21, *21, 22*
    nonspecific faint pigmentation, 23
    vessel morphology, 20
Porokeratosis
    flat lesions, 59
    vascular dermoscopic pattern, 73, *74, 75*

R

Reticular pattern, 2–4, *2–4*
    disorganized, *3, 11,* 11–12, *12*

S

Sebaceous hyperplasia
    elevated/clinically pink-clear/multicolored
        dermoscopy, 129–132, *130–132*
    features, 50, *50*
    flat/elevated, clinically pink/skin-colored lesions,
        268, *269–270*
Seborrheic keratosis (SK)
    comedo-like openings, *27,* 27–28, *28, 34,* 220,
        220–224
    coral-like ridge pattern, *224*
    coral pattern
        fissures (sulci), 28, *28,* 30, *30*
        keratin-filled clefts, 30, *31*
        ridges (gyri), 28, *28, 29,* 30, *30*
    diffuse yellow pigmentation, 31
    elevated/clinically brown-black/multicolored
        dermoscopy, 251–255, *251–255*
    elevated/clinically pale brown/dermoscopically
        brown, 193, *193–195*
    epidermal features, 54, *54*

flat/clinically pale brown/dermoscopically
        brown, 155–157, *155–157*
focal thickening, 41, *41*
inflammation
    hairpin red vasculature, 93, *93*
    white halo, 92, *92*
milia-like cysts, 26, *26,* 220, *220–224*
nonpigmented, 54, *55*
sharp borders, 25, *25, 34,* 220, *220–224*
starry sky appearance, 220
white halo
    hairpin vessels, 31, *31, 32*
    looped vessels, 31, *31, 32*
Solar lentigines
    diffuse light brown structureless area, 35, *36, 37*
    fingerprinting pattern, 33, *34–36,* 40, 42, *43*
    flat/clinically pale brown/dermoscopically
        brown, 150–152, *150–153*
    moth-eaten borders, 37, *37, 38,* 40, *42–43*
    reticular pattern, 39, *39–40*
    sun exposure, 32, *34*
Spitz nevi, elevated lesions
    clinically pink-clear/dermoscopically red, 62
    clinically pink-clear/multicolored dermoscopy,
        70, *70*
Squamous cell cancer (SCC)
    characteristic patterns, 23–24, *24*
    clinically elevated lesions, multicolored
        dermoscopy, 272, *273*
    elevated/clinically pink-clear/multicolored
        dermoscopy
        keratoacanthoma type, 137, *138–141*
        nonpigmented squamous cells, 137, *137*
        peripheral keratinizing vessels, *139–141*
        white hyperreflective scale, 140, *142*
    flat lesions
        clinically pale brown/dermoscopically
            brown, 168, *168–170*
        clinically pale brown/multicolored dermos-
            copy, 184, *185*
        clinically pink-clear/multicolored dermos-
            copy, 65, 112–114, *113, 114*
        clinically pink-clear/dermoscopically red, 59, *62*
    nonpigmented, elevated/clinically pink-clear/
        dermoscopically red
        advanced lesions, 98, *98*
        glomeruloid/dotted vessels, 95, *96, 97*
    psoriasis and psoriasiform dermatitis, 78, *79, 80*

T

Telangiectasias, BCC, 24, 80, 82–84, 98, 100–103,
        100–103, 134, 146, *146*
Tumor/hyperkeratosis, *272–274*
Tyndall effect, 6, 14